Essential Paediatrics

CHURCHILL LIVINGSTONE INTERNATIONAL STUDENT EDITIONS

Essential Paediatrics

David Hull

BSc, MB, FRCP, DObst RCOG, DCH
Professor of Child Health, University of Nottingham

Derek I. Johnston

MA, MD, MRCP, DCH
Consultant Paediatrician, University Hospital, Nottingham

ILLUSTRATED BY GEOFFREY LYTH BA

CHURCHILL LIVINGSTONE
EDINBURGH LONDON MELBOURNE AND NEW YORK 1981

CHURCHILL LIVINGSTONE
Medical Division of Longman Group Limited

Distributed in the United States of America by
Churchill Livingstone Inc., 1560 Broadway, New York,
N.Y. 10036, and by associated companies, branches and
representatives throughout the world.

© Longman Group Limited 1981

First published 1981
  Reprinted 1981
  Reprinted 1982
  Reprinted 1984
  Reprinted 1985

ISBN 0 443 02202 X (cased)
ISBN 0-443-01953-3

British Library Cataloguing in Publication Data
Hull, David
  Essential paediatrics.
  1. Children — Diseases
  I. Title II. Johnston, Derek I
  618.9 2   RJ45   79-42809

Produced by Longman Group (FE) Ltd
Printed in Hong Kong

Preface

This book is intended primarily for medical students to help them master the essentials of paediatrics in the brief time provided for this purpose in their clinical course. It may also serve as a useful introduction to paediatrics for other health professionals.

Attention is mainly directed toward the common conditions. Genetics and heart disorders are considered in more detail than other areas because we believe it is important that they be understood thoroughly from the beginning. Many of the rare disorders are mentioned by name only just to note their existence. Occasionally they are discussed at more length because they are life-threatening or have genetic consequences or simply because they are of interest.

No book is an alternative to clinical experience acquired by talking to and examining children and discussing their problems with their parents. It is our hope that by providing a text which covers most aspects of paediatric practice, readers may feel more able to approach a sick child with confidence and that time spent in paediatric wards and clinics will be remembered with pleasure.

The authors are indebted to the contributors, listed on page vii, who offered expert advice regarding the accuracy, relevance and balance of the sections dealing with their respective specialties, in some cases virtually rewriting them. We also acknowledge our debt to medical artist Mr Geoffrey Lyth, whose contribution to the text is invaluable. Finally, we should like to thank Miss Kath Reed who typed tape recordings and handwritten drafts with unbelievable speed and accuracy.

Nottingham, 1981
D.H.
D.I.J.

Contributors

B. Roger Allen
MB, ChB, MRCP
Consultant Dermatologist, University Hospital, Nottingham.

Peter R. H. Barbor
MB, FRCP
Consultant Paediatrician, University Hospital, Nottingham.

Timothy L. Chambers
MB, BS, MRCP, DA, DObst RCOG, DCH
Consultant Paediatrician, Derby Children's Hospital.

Christopher L. Colton
MB FRCS
Consultant Orthopaedic Surgeon, University Hospital, Nottingham.

John S. Fitzsimmons
MB, FRCP(E), DCH
Consultant Paediatrician, City Hospital, Nottingham.

E. Joan Hiller
BSc, MB BS, FRCP, DObst RCOG
Consultant Paediatrician, City Hospital, Nottingham.

Margaret J. Mayell
MB, ChB, FRCS(Ed)
Consultant Paediatric Surgeon, City Hospital, Nottingham.

David H. Mellor
MD, FRCP, DCH
Consultant Paediatric Neurologist,
City and University Hospitals, Nottingham.

Anthony D. Milner
MD, FRCP, DCH
Reader in Child Health and Honorary Consultant Paediatrician, University of Nottingham.

Nicholas Rutter
BA, MB, BChir, MRCP
Senior Lecturer in Child Health and Honorary Consultant Paediatrician, University of Nottingham.

Contents

1
The Ill Child and his Doctor

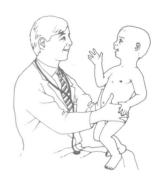

In paediatric practice it is not possible to make a full diagnosis or draw up an appropriate care programme without some knowledge of the child, his age, size, abilities and personality. Furthermore, a child is part of a family; to understand him one must know something of his family, particularly his parents, their life styles, their family life, their capacity to look after their children and in particular their relationships to our patient and attitudes towards his illness. Families live in communities and as the child grows older and becomes more independent he relates more directly to the community, in particular to his school and his peers. Thus, it is helpful to know the main features of that community and the child's and family's relationship to it. The mode of presentation, the symptoms and even the signs of disease may be influenced by the nature of the child, his family and their surroundings and experiences. Likewise, treatment will depend on the reserves and resources of the family and community.

THE INTERVIEW

First impressions are important. Even very young children are quick to sense an atmosphere and the reactions of their parents to it. As they grow older they become expert at masking their feelings. In uncertain situations they are more likely to demonstrate what they think by actions rather than words. They will look to and reach for those they trust. Children, not unlike adults, warm to those who like and admire them, and they are less suspicious than adults of ulterior motives. A relaxed, friendly beginning to the interview not only eases its passage, but is essential for its success.

It is a matter of sensitivity and judgement to know how to make the first introductions. In the U.K. shaking hands is probably right for most parents but not for most children. It is impolite not to know the child's name and what he would like to be called. All Susans do not like to be called 'Suzie'. The sex of the child is not always evident from appearances. Sometimes the dress and hair style may be very misleading and you may wonder why. Even under such circumstances, to call a boy 'she' is a mistake. His mother will not like it and neither will he if he is old enough to understand. Never refer to the baby as 'it'. Next ascertain the names and the relationship to the child of the adults who accompany him. Children belong to their parents, parents are responsible for their children so it is the parents point of view that, in the first instance, you want to know. Not infrequently parents differ in their interpretation of their child's symptoms and signs. Neither parent has a monopoly on objectivity. Sometimes unaccompanied mothers will say, referring to her husband, that 'he disagrees with me and says I fuss too much', or alternatively that 'he told me to bring the child along because he is not right'. Some grandparents are a tremendous support to their children when they start their own families but others tend to be interfering busybodies. The latter, if they are present at the interview, should be encouraged not to interrupt or enlarge upon the history given by the parents, though their attempts to do so may help in understanding the total situation.

The ability and willingness of children to describe their own symptoms varies widely. If in doubt always ask. It is instructive, for example, to find out why the child thinks he has been brought to see you. The answers are often revealing if not too helpful with the diagnosis. Another very important question, possibly best asked at the end of the interview, is what does the child and what do the parents think is the cause of the child's illness? In particular, what do they fear it might be?

In the main, children are not interested in adult talk so as the interview gets underway the majority of the younger ones will become restless and seek ways of entertaining themselves; but never make the mistake of thinking that they are not listening to what is being said. Toys for every age group should be scattered on the desk, shelves and floor. Play will not only occupy the youngster, it will also give valuable clues to his motor skills, mental abilities, interests and personality. So whilst taking the history watch the child. In particular, watch the way he moves, how he uses his eyes and ears and hands and feet. Does he follow up a challenge? Is he constructive? Is he relaxed? Watch the interplay between the child and his parents, and the child and yourself. It will not only help interpret the history but

The interview

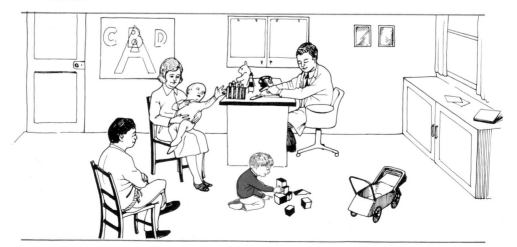

Suggested types of toys which should be at hand for children of varying ages

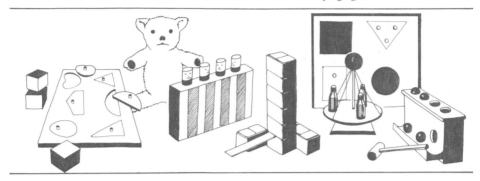

also give some indication of how best to examine the child later to get the most information. For example, if a four-year-old stays on his mother's knee and demands that the toys be brought to him, he is obviously feeling very threatened or is limited either by his illness or in his abilities. In these circumstances it is probably wisest to make the preliminary examination at least, whilst the child is on his mother's knee. Know something about the toys in the room; for example, at what stage can a child be expected to put a square block in a square hole, or to lift it out to find pictures underneath, or to name what he sees. If he does not do it you have not learnt much — it might be simply because of the situation — but if he does you may have learnt a great deal.

History
Every doctor develops his or her own way of collecting information. It is best to start by noting the main complaint or complaints. If there are a number, then a simple opening problem list helps. Then enlarge and define each problem and enquire about associated problems. An obsessional enquiry about all the bodily functions is not usually necessary, it wastes time and may interrupt the flow of the interview. However for most medical problems, and always for any child admitted to hospital, certain background information is essential.

Firstly, it is important to collect information about the child's own life. Was the pregnancy, labour and birth normal? What was the birth weight? How was he in the first days of life? It may be important to note whether he was breast or bottle fed and when he was weaned. Has he had the common childhood infections? Has he been immunised? Has he been treated in hospital and, if so, when and where and for what?

Secondly, an assessment should be made as to how the child is progressing. Full assessment of motor and language achievement and mental and social responses demands considerable skill and experience. However, for most purposes a simple enquiry about the principle stages of development is all that is required and should be within the competence of anyone presuming to advise parents about the care of their children. For the older child, ask about progress at school. It is not acceptable to make a note that the child is slow or retarded without indicating the basis for that conclusion. Indeed, labels of that nature are best avoided altogether. If a child is not speaking at three years of age, write that he has delayed speech, but do not guess at the likely cause, even if, for instance, his mother appears not to understand even your simplest questions.

The charts in this section highlight early development. Each step gives the approximate age range for the item listed. The infant is placed on the top line of the step if he achieves both items in each step, and on the bottom line if he achieves only one item. Three infants are illustrated in the first chart: The infant age 6 months achieved one item of Step 3 and is average; the infant age 14 months achieved both items of Step 6 and is advanced; the infant age 18 months achieved one item of Step 4 and is delayed. Further enquiries should be made about any child who scores below the line (modified from Barber *et al.*, 1976).

Eight steps in motor development

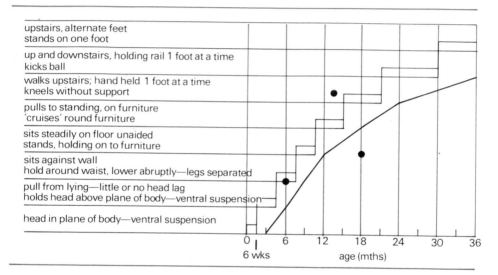

Eight steps in language development

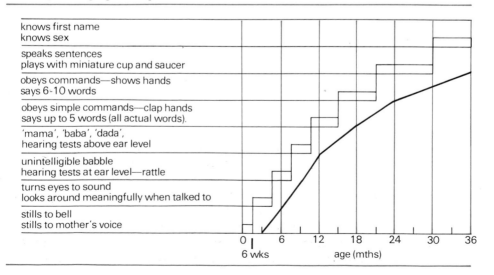

Eight steps in vision and fine motor development

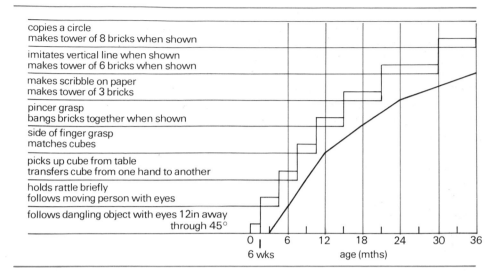

Eight steps in social development

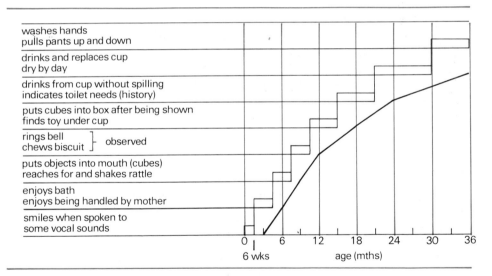

Always ask about the health of the rest of the family. This is important for a variety of reasons. The first, and perhaps the most obvious, is that the child might have an inherited disorder. Collect the information carefully and record it using accepted symbols and notation (see Ch. 2). Secondly, if environmental factors are important, then other members of the family may also be affected. This might include anything from respiratory infections to the inhalation of lead. Thirdly, the presence of chronic illness in other members of the family may be the reason why the parents are concerned about the child before you. It may be that the family's stress has helped precipitate the child's problems. The fourth, though not the most important, is probably the most interesting reason. There are often family complaints, headaches, stomach aches, weariness, which determine the family language of disease and colour the way the child and his parents interpret his symptoms and signs. This will be particularly so if there is a strong behavioural component to his problem.

Examination

Examining children can be fun, but it may involve games when you do not want to play, and occasionally it can be singularly frustrating. Children, even the smallest infants, will try and work out your intentions by looking into your eyes. People with kind eyes do not mean to hurt! The parents may be more nervous about what you might do than the child himself, so they need reassurance as well. Some parents attempt to comfort their child by telling him not to worry 'the doctor won't hurt you'. Up until that time it may not have entered his head that you might, so be prepared for the protests. Some mothers may say such things in an attempt to put you off any examination which might be uncomfortable or embarrassing. Always encourage the parents to help you with the examination by holding or distracting the child, unless, of course, the youngster is approaching puberty when his independence is to be respected.

Clinicians have different practices about clothes. Undressing disturbs babies and they do not like it. Older infants hold onto their clothes as a protection, so they may object to their removal. From three years onwards there is usually no problem until puberty. Then the youngster must be handled with all the care and sensitivity you would extend to royalty! So it can be very useful to make observations whilst the child is clothed and undisturbed. Palpation and auscultation can easily be performed through vest and pants. On the other hand, some babies and children will remain undisturbed and, indeed, may expect you to undress them, and you can learn a great deal by the handling involved. It is a form of palpation which the children understand and further palpation afterwards is usually acceptable. But if the child shows uncertainty ask the parents to undress him. Even the most defensive child is usually happy for you to observe him naked from a distance.

Although the collection of the information may be disorderly, its recording in the notes must not be. In most situations it is important to record aspects of the child's size. Weight and length or height must be measured accurately. In certain situations, skull circumference and very occasionally skin fold thicknesses may also be measured. The data is recorded in the notes and on the appropriate charts.

Note the child's general behaviour and awareness. You may wish to make your own evaluation of the child's capabilities and record them with the parents reports of his achievements.

Next, observe the child. Much of the information you seek may be obtained by careful observation. In general terms, is his appearance at all unusual? If so, try to define why, is it the shape of his head, the mould of his ears, the position of his eyes, his bodily proportions or the posture? Does he look like his parents? Has he got any of the recognised major or minor anomalies?

Then specifically assess his general size, proportions and nutritional state. Note the nature and distribution of any skin lesions or rashes. Then examine the system or systems that are the source of the complaint.

Examination

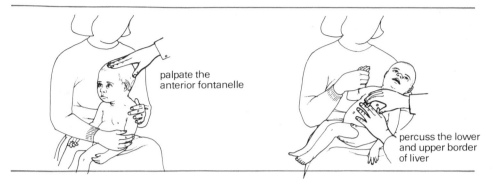

palpate the
anterior fontanelle

percuss the lower
and upper border
of liver

Respiratory disorders are often most easily observed. Avoid percussion or auscultation until you have noted the respiratory rate and the movement of the diaphragm and chest wall with quiet breathing and the effect of an stronger respiratory effort performed on request in an older child, or with a cry in a baby. Determine whether or not the lung is over-inflated by percussion of the upper edge of the liver.

Interpretation of breath sounds and additional noises can be difficult in the very young. Fine crackling noises on inspiration (crepitations) may be heard on careful auscultation in apparently normal babies. If they are persistent and bilateral in a distressed toddler they usually indicate bronchiolitis or, very rarely, left heart failure. Coarse intermittent noises during both inspiration and expiration (rales) usually signify liquid debris in the larger airways. They may be transmitted from the back of the throat. Harsh and more persistent noises superadded on the breath sounds (rhonchi), indicating a more persistent obstruction, are less fequently heard in children. Continuous noises, hardening and extending the breath sounds (bronchial breathing) may be heard in babies over most of the upper back, and usually are transmitted sounds from the main airway. When the airway is partially obstructed the noise becomes harsher and more vibrant and is called a stridor. This term covers a wide range of sounds, some fine and high pitched, some low and coarse. The character depends on the site, the nature of the obstruction and the narrowness of the aperture. Wheezing is heard when the mid airways are narrowed; always check if it is bilateral.

Examination of the cardiovascular system begins by recording the rate, rhythm, strength and character of the peripheral pulses. Palpate and percuss the anterior chest wall to determine the heart size, the site and nature of the apex beat and to detect the presence, if any, of a thrill. Then listen to the first heart sound, then the second, then the sounds in between and then the murmurs between the heart sounds. For each murmur you will wish to know its timing, character, loudness, site and distribution. Check if it is transmitted into the neck.

Always observe the abdomen before you palpate. Look for swellings and movements. Ask if anywhere is tender, and if you can, watch the child's face and not his abdomen whilst you palpate. After general palpation in the four quadrants, systematically determine the position and size of the liver, spleen, kidneys and bladder. If an organ is enlarged, note its position, size, surface and texture, the

Examination

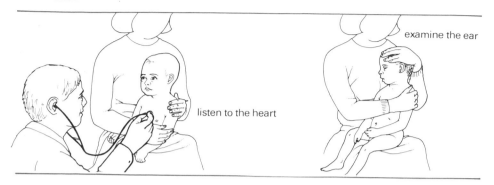

listen to the heart

examine the ear

character of the edge if it has one, and whether or not it is tender. When examining the back of the chest, look at the spine, particularly the lower end.

Again, examination of the locomotor and nervous systems is more by observation than manipulation. In babies and infants always palpate the anterior fontanelle or head 'soft spot'. It usually closes in the middle of the second year. Note if it is pulsating: it usually does. You can record the heart rate from it. The fontanelle may be full or flat. Ask yourself the following questions: Can the child see? Can he hear? Does he move his eyes and head well and in all directions? Does he move all limbs, is the movement normal and full? Is the contour and position of each limb normal? Is the power good? When you handle the infant, note the tone on passive movement of the limb. Is there any limitation in the movement at any joint? Are the joints unduly lax and hyperextendable? Again, watch the child's face whilst you move his limbs. Eliciting the reflex responses rarely adds useful information in children but it is as well to keep up the habit for the odd occasion when it does. In the infant the percussing finger can be used as the hammer.

Finally, examine with the light. If necessary, check the eyes and then the ear drums and finally the throat. Never force yourself upon the child. Never force his mouth open against his will: be patient. Ask yourself, is the information you wish to gather as important as all that? Why use a nasty dry stick to depress the tongue when a smooth tea-spoon handle will do just as well, and spoons are meant to go into mouths anyway.

Before you finish, should you bother to record the blood pressure? If disease of the kidney or heart is suspected, the answer is yes.

This completes the general examination. During it you may have included specific observations or examinations, for example, to see if the testes are in the scrotum, femoral pulses are present, the hips in joint, the characteristic of unusual lumps, the presence of the signs of puberty, etcetera.

Once the clinical enquiry is complete the next step is to re-examine the initial list of problems, some may be easily dealt with by appropriate advice, on the other hand new problems may have arisen. Draw up a new list and indicate what steps by way of further enquiry, investigation or treatment you propose to follow, and discuss these with the parents and to the extent that he may understand it, with your patient.

THE PROBLEMS

Every week a practising paediatrician sees a condition, anomaly, or a sign that he has never seen before and in such a situation his actions depend on his basic scientific knowledge. Every month he will treat a condition which is known but rare, then he relies on colleagues who have reported their observations in the medical literature. However, the substance of a doctor's practice is with diseases he has seen before, and his management of these problems will be influenced as much by his own previous experience and by his knowledge of his own patients and their community, as it is by therapies recommended in text books. What are these common problems? Obviously, this will vary from place to place and from community to community. The following is a description of the experience in one town in the centre of England in 1978.

The child may be seen by his family doctor, by a medical officer at a child health clinic or by a hospital doctor in the local district hospital. Each family doctor has about 2500 people in his practice. This means that with a birth rate running at 12.0 births per 1000 population, there will be 30 births in the practice each year and 450 child patients spread between 0 and 15 years of age. Between 15 and 20 per cent of the family doctor's work is with children. Disorders of the respiratory system are by far the commonest, followed by skin conditions, infectious diseases, gastrointestinal disorders, problems with eyes, ears and teeth. Social and administrative problems form the bulk of the remainder. Only 10 per cent of children's disorders are judged to be serious and in need of specific therapy, though it is likely that medicine will be prescribed in over half the cases.

Many family doctors work in group practices in health centres. Working with them in the primary care team are health visitors. In some centres one doctor in the group, with the health visitors, holds regular child health clinics in order to examine routinely every child and provide a preventive health service. In others a special clinical medical officer attends the clinic. Healthy babies are examined routinely at six weeks of age and then at regular intervals afterwards. The predominant problems in the early months are related to feeding, nutrition, bowels and general growth and development. Hearing is assessed at 6 to 9 months of age. The infants are examined for vision abnormalities and the development of squints. The clinics also have responsibilities for the immunisation programme

Paediatric experience in general practice

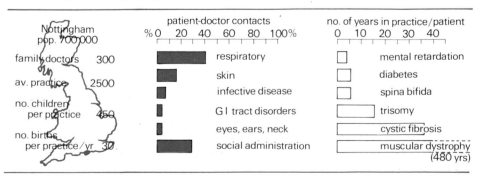

and health education. After the age of five years surveillance is continued by the school health services.

The preventive role of the child health clinic

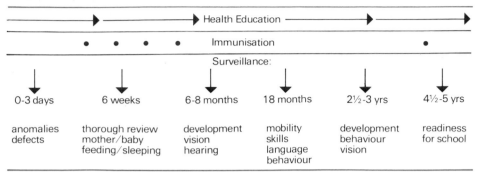

0-3 days	6 weeks	6-8 months	18 months	2½-3 yrs	4½-5 yrs
anomalies defects	thorough review mother/baby feeding/sleeping	development vision hearing	mobility skills language behaviour	development behaviour vision	readiness for school

Children who fall ill suddenly are usually brought directly to the hospital emergency and accident department. Over half of the children admitted to hospital are brought by their parents directly to hospital. Here the conditions commonly seen are home and road accidents, accidental poisoning, acute respiratory illness, fevers, convulsions and acute bowel upsets.

Patients referred to the Paediatric consultancy service usually have less acute conditions. The commoner problems include recurrent respiratory infections, asthma, failure to thrive, small size, suspected developmental delay, convulsions or suspected convulsions, nocturnal enuresis and constipation. There are special clinics for children with chronic illnesses, for example for children with diabetes, leukaemia, epilepsy, short stature, cystic fibrosis and renal disorders. Children with physical and mental handicaps are assessed in a special developmental assessment unit by a team which includes physiotherapists, occupational therapists, psychologists, teachers, audiometricians as well as doctors from various disciplines.

Paediatric experience in hospital. For a population of 750 000, special out-patient clinics are needed for a variety of chronic illnesses

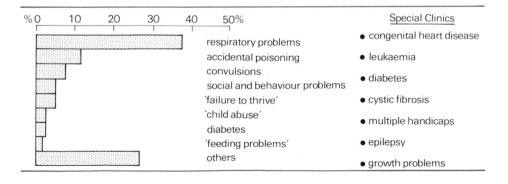

About half the people of Nottingham live within the old city boundary. Within that boundary are the deprived inner city areas. The children living in these areas are at greater risk to most health hazards from conception

	Deprived areas	Average
admitted to Neonatal Unit/100 births	27.8	12.2
admitted to Hospital in 1st Year of life/100 births	55	27
on Child Abuse Register/1000 children	4.5	1.5
infant deaths 0-1 yr/1000 children	40	15.8

deprived areas

Deprivation Nottingham City

The distribution of health problems differs across the town. Certain inner city areas, deprived by most material and social standards, have a higher incidence of most medical problems and the children who live there are, in general, less physically, mentally and socially able. At a disadvantage from birth, these children 'born to fail', are less able to form the secure relationships and thus are themselves less likely to establish a strong family environment for the own children. Breaking this circle of events is one of the major tasks of community paediatric care. It is a challenge that the health service staff share with social workers and teachers.

Mortality

Happily, infant and child mortality rates continue to fall. The rates are highest for the very young. In over 40 per cent of neonatal deaths, the infant has a congenital abnormality incompatible with independent life, and over 40 per cent are very immature and even with artificial respiratory and nutritional support do not survive the first few days after birth. Improvements in general health, antenatal care, and appropriate genetic counselling may accelerate the fall in the perinatal mortality rate.

Mortality rates in England and Wales, and the causes of neonatal deaths in Nottingham 1976-1977

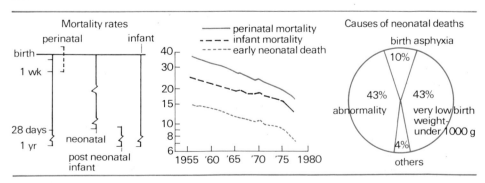

Post-neonatal infants deaths according to age at death, place of death, birth weight and social class in Nottingham, 1975-1977 (Madeley, 1977)

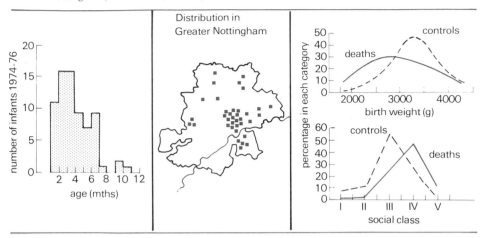

Older infants rarely die in hospital. The majority of children dying between four weeks and one year, post-neonatal infant deaths, die suddenly at home. The 'sudden infant death syndrome' or 'cot death' has received considerable attention recently. There is undoubtedly a small group of infants who die suddenly and nothing abnormal is found at post mortem. Some consider that death might be due to a confusion in respiratory control precipitated by a respiratory infection or unexpected regurgitation. However, many of the infants who die unexpectedly do have evidence of known disease, or non-specific signs of illness at autopsy. The incidence is higher in families living in poor housing, when the parents are inexperienced or of limited ability, or when there is domestic stress. Early infant death occurs more often in babies born prematurely or experiencing problems in the newborn period. These characteristics can be identified at birth and if the

Major causes of death in childhood

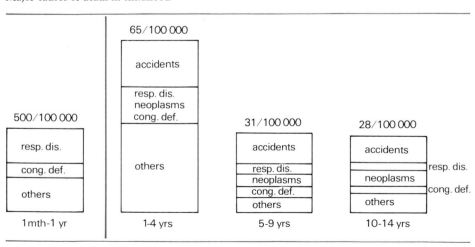

families are given extra advice and support during the early months the number of post-neonatal infant deaths might be reduced.

An unexpected death of a child over the age of one year is rare. Many are due to accidents; others are due to previously diagnosed malignancies. The remainder include children with inherited diseases, for example, cystic fibrosis, muscular dystrophies, and progressive encephalopathies. Acute infections, which used to be a major cause of death, are usually controllable; but occasionally the onset can be so sudden and death follows so quickly that therapeutic measures cannot be introduced in time, for example in meningitis with septicaemia or an intravascular coagulopathy, severe gastroenteritis, acute epiglottitis and fulminating respiratory infections.

BIBLIOGRAPHY

Barber J H, Bootham R, Stanfield J P 1976 A new visual chart for pre-school developmental screening. Health Bulletin 34: 80

The county deprived area study 1975 Nottinghamshire County Council

Fit for the future. The report of the Committee on Child Health Services. Chairman Court S D M. 1976 H.M.S.O. London. Cmnd. 6684

Hicks D 1976 Primary health care — a review. H.M.S.O., London

Madeley R J 1977 Social factors associated with post neonatal death in Nottingham 1974-76. Archives of Disease in Childhood 52: 809

2

Genes

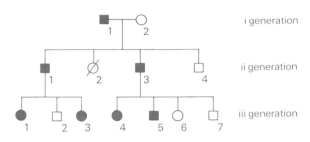

i generation

ii generation

iii generation

Pedigree: congenital cataracts

The differences between people result from the interaction between our genetic inheritance, or genotype, and the environment in which we develop and live. Most of us are fortunate and the eventual product of this interaction, our phenotype, is normal. Others, as a result of faulty gene action with or without a hostile environment, may be subject to various types of disease. This effect may be obvious at birth as a congenital abnormality or it may become evident only later in life as a consequence of growth or environmental factors. Since about 1 in 40 pregnancies results in the birth of a child with a serious congenital abnormality and about 30 per cent of children admitted to paediatric wards have a significant inherited disease, some knowledge of genetics is essential for those working with children. In many patients, it may be difficult to decide the importance of genetic or environmental factors and it is important, therefore, in all patients, to take a detailed family history. In those patients suffering from a disorder thought to be the result of abnormal gene action a comprehensive family pedigree is essential. The pedigree may be of considerable help with the diagnosis and without them affected families cannot be offered sensible advice for the future.

Diseases in man thought to be genetic in origin may be divided into those

Pedigree notation

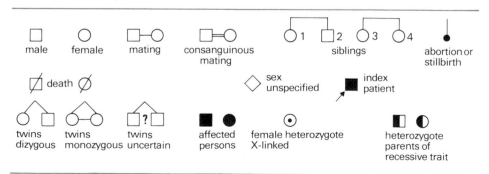

resulting from the action of single major genes, those due to chromosomal abnormalities and those in which there is a genetic component acting in conjunction with environmental factors.

SINGLE GENE INHERITANCE

The mode of single gene inheritance may be autosomal or sex-linked, dominant or recessive.

Autosomal dominant inheritance

Over 700 diseases are known to result from this mode of inheritance. Although individually rare and responsible for less than 1 per cent of total human illness, they may nevertheless present very striking clinical features.

In this form of inheritance the abnormal gene responsible for the disease is carried on one of a pair of autosomes, and the heterozygote manifests the condition. In most instances the specific chromosome involved is not known but both sexes are affected. As each parent contributes only one of the two genes to the gamete, each offspring has a 1 in 2 chance of inheriting the abnormal gene and hence manifesting the disease. The risk remains the same for each successive pregnancy, irrespective of the outcome of the preceding one. This all sounds very obvious, but when parents have had two affected children they do feel that the next should be normal or at least the risk should be better than 50:50. Unfortunately, it is not.

As in many other forms of disease, irrespective of the cause, the severity of the condition may vary considerably from one individual to another. This variation is referred to as expressivity and points to the importance of examining patients thoroughly before declaring them free of the disease. Some of those affected may have only minor manifestations but, by passing on the responsible gene, may have a child with much more serious problems. This is very well illustrated by a family with tuberose sclerosis. The features of this disease are mental retardation, a characteristic facial rash and epilepsy. In the family illustrated below, the mother has epilepsy and the facial rash but she was able to attend a secondary modern school where she managed, albeit with some difficulty. Early in life her daughter developed a particular form of epilepsy called infantile spasms, and she was left

Dominant inheritance

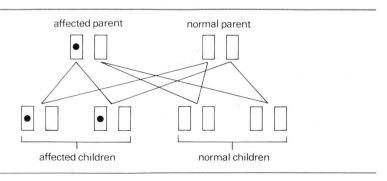

affected parent   normal parent

affected children   normal children

severely mentally retarded. She has not yet, but may later, develop the characteristic facial rash. When these parents were informed of the genetic implications of the condition, they decided not to have further children.

This particular form of mental retardation, as with other types of dominantly inherited disease, may occur in the offspring of normal parents. When this happens the abnormal gene is not found in either parent but arises as a mutation in the gametes, either in the ova or sperm. The risk of another mutation in future pregnancies is very low but the affected child will have the same risk of passing on the abnormal gene as any other affected person. In achondroplasia, a skeletal abnormality producing dwarfism, as many as 80 per cent have normal parents, and are the result of a new mutations. Paternal age at the time of conception appears to be a significant factor in the mutation rate in achondroplasia as in many other inherited disorders and the older the father the greater the risk. It occasionally happens that a gene disorder present in one generation fails to appear in the next but reappears in subsequent generations. In these circumstances the gene is said to lack penetrance. Such a skip-generation is not a common occurrence and apparent cases of it may well only illustrate our inability to detect minor expressions of the abnormal gene.

The concept of dominance and recessiveness is useful but it is as well to remember that genes cannot work in isolation and their actions may be modified by many factors.

Dominantly inherited conditions, example: tuberose sclerosis

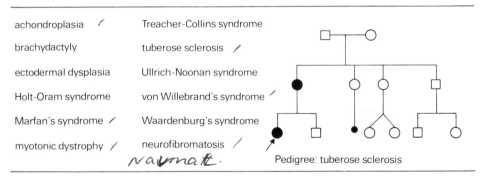

achondroplasia	Treacher-Collins syndrome
brachydactyly	tuberose sclerosis
ectodermal dysplasia	Ullrich-Noonan syndrome
Holt-Oram syndrome	von Willebrand's syndrome
Marfan's syndrome	Waardenburg's syndrome
myotonic dystrophy	neurofibromatosis

Naumatt.

Pedigree: tuberose sclerosis

Autosomal recessive inheritance

There are approximately 500 diseases known to be transmitted by the autosomal recessive mode. Whereas autosomal dominant diseases tend to produce gross structural defects and clinically obvious abnormalities, recessively inherited disorders commonly result in biochemical disturbances. Although in some the defect may be of a single enzyme, the clinical effects may be widespread and very serious. In phenylketonuria, for example, the end result of such a deficiency may be severe mental retardation, whilst in congenital adrenal hyperplasia it may cause a life-threatening electrolyte disturbance.

In recessive inheritance neither parent shows any signs of the disease but the risk of their offspring being affected is 1 in 4. There is a 1 in 2 chance of a child being a carrier like the parent and only a 1 in 4 chance that their offspring will be

PKU – auto. rec.
absent Phe ala – OH lase
pheala Hs tyroine
↳ PPA (urine).

Recessive inheritance

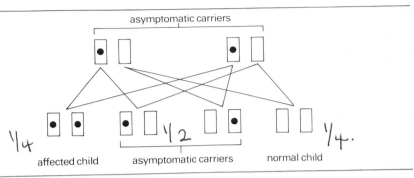

```
asymptomatic carriers
```

¼   affected child   asymptomatic carriers   ½   normal child   ¼.

normal both phenotypically and genotypically. Those with the disease do not usually have affected children and the asymptomatic carriers will only have become aware of their carrier status with the birth of an affected child.

Many of us carry abnormal genes but fortunately our spouse, although also carrying some abnormal genes, usually carries different ones. However the possibility of the spouse carrying the same abnormal gene is considerably increased in first cousin marriages. First cousins share one eighth of their total genetic complement, their genome, with each other and thus the opportunity for similar recessive genes to come together and hence produce disease is increased. As the biochemical deficiency resulting may well cause mental retardation it is not surprising that there is concern about first cousin marriages.

As with dominantly inherited disease, the action of the gene is not an all or none phenomenon and in recessive disease the heterozygote may well manifest some biochemical evidence of the condition. This is illustrated by Tay-Sach's disease. This disorder is seen most frequently in the Ashkenazi Jewish population on the North-Eastern American seaboard. It causes mental retardation, blindness and a variety of neurological abnormalities, all the result of the deficiency of the enzyme hexosaminidase-A. Minor deficiencies of this enzyme can be detected in heterozygotes, but they remain clinically unaffected. As individual carriers can be detected it is possible to screen large populations at special risk. Such a screening

Recessively inherited conditions, example: cystic fibrosis

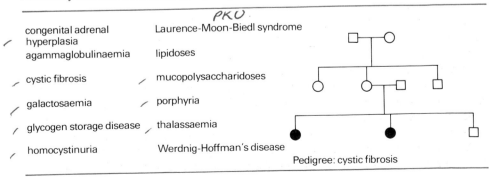

PKU

congenital adrenal hyperplasia	Laurence-Moon-Biedl syndrome
agammaglobulinaemia	lipidoses
cystic fibrosis	mucopolysaccharidoses
galactosaemia	porphyria
glycogen storage disease	thalassaemia
homocystinuria	Werdnig-Hoffman's disease

Pedigree: cystic fibrosis

MP GIRG

programme has had considerable success in American Ashkenazi Jews in selected areas.

The gene loci responsible for most recessive disease have not been assigned to specific chromosomes. One possible exception however is the gene responsible for a particular type of congenital adrenal hyperplasia, the variety associated with 21-hydroxylase deficiency. It has recently been demonstrated that this gene lies close to the gene loci for the important histocompatibility antigens comprising the HLA system. These gene loci are known to be on chromosome No. 6 and although this association does not help in the management of the disease, it may offer an opportunity for prenatal diagnosis in the future.

Sex-linked disorders

There are 100 or so sex-linked diseases described to date. They include several common and serious childhood problems. So far, no serious disability has been reported due to genes carried on the Y chromosome and sex-linked normally means X-linked. In addition, although dominantly inherited sex-linked disorders do occur, for example a variety of vitamin D resistant rickets is transmitted in this fashion, they are rare and the common sex-linked diseases are recessively inherited. Because the gene for colour blindness is carried on the X chromosome, mapping of the gene loci on this chromosome is further advanced than on most others.

Sex-linked recessive inheritance

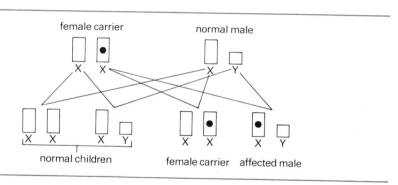

In these disorders the abnormal gene is carried on the X chromosome. In the female, the presence of the normal allele on her other X chromosome protects from the disease but she is a carrier. In the male, however, the abnormal gene on his X chromosome is not balanced by a normal allele and he manifests the disease. Any son born to a carrier female will have a 1 in 2 chance of having the condition. Equally any daughter has a 1 in 2 chance of being a carrier, like mother. Because it is the X chromosome which carries the abnormal gene an affected male can never transfer the disease to his sons but all his daughters will be carriers.

The illustrated pedigree is of a family in which several children are affected by Duchenne's muscular dystrophy. In generation II, a male child (II 3) developed evidence of the disease by the age of four years and subsequently died from the

Sex-linked inherited conditions, example: muscular dystrophy

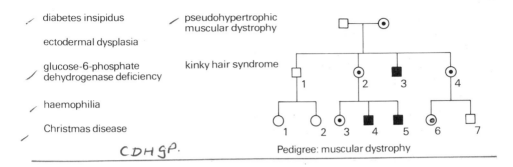

diabetes insipidus

ectodermal dysplasia

glucose-6-phosphate dehydrogenase deficiency

haemophilia

Christmas disease

CDH gP.

pseudohypertrophic muscular dystrophy

kinky hair syndrome

Pedigree: muscular dystrophy

condition at the age of 16 years. Unfortunately, unaware of the genetic implications of her brother's disease, his sister already having one daughter, had another child, a boy, and before his disease became obvious she had a second affected son. Both developed clinical evidence of the disease before starting school and both will probably die before the age of 20. Her sister was more fortunate and despite the fact that she was subsequently shown to be a carrier, she already had a son who was unaffected and a daughter who in turn was shown to be a carrier.

Genetic counselling. Such a situation would hopefully be avoided today. When genetic disease of whatever type occurs in a family it is the responsibility of the family doctor or the doctor consulted to ensure that the relevant members of the family receive genetic counselling. The counsellor's task in the family described above would be to present the parents of the affected boys with an explanation of why the disease has occurred and its mode of inheritance. In this, as in other situations, it is important that this information is imparted in a sympathetic and unhurried manner and in a way which is understood. If, as a result of the explanation, the parents decide not to have further children they could then be directed to the appropriate agency for family planning advice. However, if they were very anxious to have another child, a number of possibilities need to be discussed; for example, they might want to consider adoption. Unfortunately, in many parts of the world this is not an easy option as the number of children for adoption is insufficient to meet the demand. Parents without a handicapped child and without illness in the family are more favoured by adoption societies. As an alternative it is possible to offer fetal sex determination. If the fetus is proven to be male, the parents might decide to have the pregnancy terminated with the hope that the next fertilised ovum would produce a girl. Such an approach is not common in the U.K. although it is popular in other parts of the world. It has the disadvantage that each male infant lost has a 50/50 chance of being normal. A much more positive approach is likely to be available with improvements in the technique of fetoscopy and fetal blood sampling. By this procedure it is possible to obtain a sufficient quantity of fetal blood to estimate the concentration of the enzyme, creatinine phosphokinase. It has recently been confirmed that this is elevated in some affected male infants very early in development. Where a mother can be shown to carry a male with the disease she can be offered termination. Obviously this selective reproduction will not suit everyone. However it does permit some couples to have a family with the reassurance that they will not produce children suffering from this tragic disease.

It is equally important in such families to identify those females carrying the abnormal gene before they have an affected child. In Duchenne's muscular dystrophy it seems likely that there is a basic abnormality of the membranes of many structures other than those surrounding muscle fibres. As a result of this membrane disorder, the muscle enzymes, particularly CPK, leak into the blood stream and in frank muscle disease the CPK level may be very high. In female carriers the level may also be increased but to a much lesser extent and in practice it is found that the level shows considerable variation. It seems that this variation is due to the fact that one X chromosome in the female is normally inactive and may or may not be the one containing the abnormal gene. The inactivation of one of the sex chromosomes does not occur immediately at fertilization but some little time later, thus the female has essentially two cell lines; one containing the chromosome with the abnormal gene and one with the normal gene. The proportion varies and this variation permits some female carriers to be identified; the more cells there are with the abnormal gene the more likely it is to find a raised CPK level. Hopefully, it may be possible in the future to detect elevation of other substances as a result of the increased membrane permeability and to make the identification of carriers easier. Recently, increased levels of myoglobin have been described in the serum of parients with the disease and in a number of carriers.

Referrals to Nottingham Genetic Counselling Service 1973 to 1978

	Condition	No. of cases	%
Single gene abnormalities	Dominant	88	12.7
	Recessive	70	10.2
	X-linked	40	5.8
Chromosomal abnormalities	Autosomal	73	10.5
	Sex	10	1.5
Multifactorial conditions		164	23.8
Miscellaneous		244	35.5
e.g., mental retardation			
congenital abnormalities			
epilepsy			
recurrent miscarriage			
Total		689	100

The principles of genetic counselling discussed here apply equally to other genetic disease and they are an important aspect of the medical management. Currently only a small percentage of parents who would benefit from genetic counselling are receiving it.

CHROMOSOMAL ABNORMALITIES

Whereas genes, a specific sequence of nucleotide bases, cannot be visualised, it is possible to detect alterations in both the number and the structure of chromo-

Normal male karyotype; female XX in box

somes by direct examination of cells during cell division. Peripheral blood lymphocytes are the cells usually studied. Mitotic division is stimulated by agents such as phytohaemaglutinin and then the chromosomes are fixed, stained, identified and arranged in matching pairs, the karyotype.

Chromosomes consist of two halves, the chromatids, joined at a point called the centromere. With special stains the chromosomes can be shown to have heterochromic bands alternating with lighter non-staining areas. For very accurate identification these light and dark areas are assigned special numbers so that it is possible to detect loss or deletion of even a small portion of a chromosome. Chromosomes contain many hundreds of genes and loss of any of these may have serious consequences. For reasons which are less clear, additional genetic material in the form of an extra chromosome may have just as serious an effect.

There are 46 chromosomes in the nucleus of each body cell, of these 22 are matching pairs with matching genes and are called autosomes. The remaining pair, the sex chromosomes, are alike in the female and labelled XX but in the male there is only one X and a smaller chromosome, Y. In the gamete, ovum or sperm, there are only 23 chrosomes, half the somatic cell number, and this ensures that at fertilisation the normal human chromosomal complement is reconstituted.

Somatic cells grow by the process of mitosis, each daughter cell having the same chromosomal complement as the parent cell. This is made possible by each chromosome splitting longitudinally into two. Gametes are the result of a different process called meiosis in which, as a result of two nuclear divisions, the total number of chromosomes is halved. By this means the germ cells contain only one of each pair of chromosomes and hence only one of each equivalent pairs of genes. This reduction division is an essential factor in the inheritance of diseases resulting from abnormalities of genes. Meiosis also affords the opportunity for exchange of genetic material between homozygous chromosomes and hence forms the basis of the wide variation of human characteristics.

Diseases associated with chromosomal abnormalities may result from changes in the number of either the autosomes or sex chromosomes, aneuploidy; or from alterations in chromosomal structure, for example loss or deletion of a portion of a chromosome; or interchange of chromosomal material from one chromosome to another, translocation.

Trisomy 21. Female karyotype

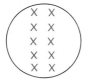

Down's syndrome, trisomy 21

The illustrated karyotype is from a child with Down's syndrome, one of the common causes of mental retardation. There is an extra chromosome in the No. 21 group or Group G. This is referred to as trisomy 21. Theoretically it is possible to have trisomy of any of the autosomes but for some, as yet unknown reason, trisomy 21 is by far the commonest. In normal circumstances, during meiosis there is equal distribution of single chromosomes to each daughter cell. In trisomies where there is an extra chromosome, normal separation fails to occur, one pair of chromosomes remain together and the result is one gamete with two homologous chromosomes and another gamete devoid of these chromosomes. At fertilisation the union of a normal gamete carrying one chromosome and the abnormal gamete containing two of the same chromosome produces trisomy for that particular chromosome. This unequal distribution of chromosomes is referred to as non-disjunction.

The incidence of Down's syndrome as with some other trisomic anomalies increases with maternal age. It is possible that as the female ages, her ovaries are increasingly subject to environmental hazards. However, mothers of any age can have infants with Down's syndrome and, as few women over the age of 40 years have babies, the majority of affected infants are born to younger women and non-disjunction is the usual cause. However, not all infants with trisomy 21 are a consequence of non-disjunction. About 6 per cent are associated with chromo-

Non-disjunction

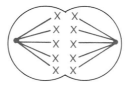
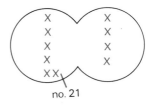

no. 21

somal re-arrangements, so-called translocations, and approximately 2 per cent with mosaicism.

In mosaicism some of the body cells have a normal complement of chromosomes, 46, others have 47 chromosomes, the extra one being an additional No. 21. This abnormality may be a result of mitotic non-disjunction after formation of the zygote. Babies with Down's syndrome due to mosaicism usually do not differ from those with the full trisomy 21 abnormality, but some may be less obviously unusual either in their physical appearance or intellectual ability. Presumably the greater the proportion of trisomic cells the greater the degree of abnormality. It could be that this proportion alters during growth with the relative contribution of abnormal cell line gradually decreasing. A better understanding of the mechanisms involved might prove to be of practical value in the management of some of these children.

Clinical features. The diagnosis of Down's syndrome is usually suspected soon after birth. In the majority a confident diagnosis can be made on clinical criteria alone but occasionally the diagnosis may not be suspected for weeks, or in some cases, months after birth. Chromosome studies are important to help in the

Trisomy 21. Clinical features

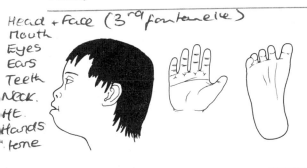

Head + Face (3rd fontanelle)
Mouth
Eyes
Ears
Teeth
Neck.
Ht.
Hands
· feme

1. Mental retardation

2. Hypotonia

3. Cranio-facial abnormalities
    a. flat occiput
    b. oval face-mongoloid
    c. epicanthic folds
    d. Brushfield spots

4. Increased incidence of
    congenital heart defects

5. Abnormal dermatoglyphics

diagnosis when there is doubt, and to identify the rarer chromosomal anomalies even when the diagnosis is certain. As in other chromosomal anomalies, abnormalities of the dermal ridge patterns may occur and in association with other features may suggest the need for chromosomal analysis in some dysmorphic infants. Once the diagnosis is firm it is important to discuss the implications thoroughly with both parents. Medical opinion varies as to whether this is best done in the first few days after birth or sometime later when parental attachment is stronger. Making the diagnosis is usually the easiest aspect of the problem; helping the parents to accept the child and make the most of his disabilities may be more difficult.

A number of societies are very helpful. They provide a forum for parents to discuss their problem with others who have had similar experience. The parents will ask many questions, in particular why did it happen to their child, and will it happen again? If mother is under 36 the risk of a further child being affected is not high and certainly not greater than 1/100. However, despite this low risk, many

Incidence of trisomy 21 according to maternal age

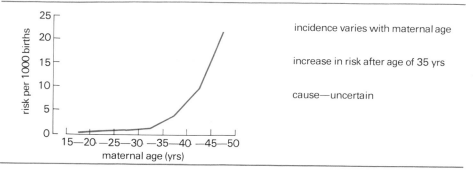

incidence varies with maternal age

increase in risk after age of 35 yrs

cause—uncertain

couples are sufficiently concerned to request diagnostic amniocentesis in future pregnancies. This is usually performed between the 14th and 16th week of pregnancy and involves taking a sample of amniotic fluid containing fetal cells, which are cultured *in vitro* and the chromosomal complement analysed. The procedure is technically easy; but the delay between the performance of the amniocentesis and the completion of the cytology examination is very upsetting for some parents. Happily in the majority the findings are normal and the parents can be reassured. In those families where the child has a translocation however, the risks of recurrence are very much greater.

The other trisomies

Trisomy of some of the other chromosomes have been described but they are rare. In most cases the patients suffer from a combination of physical abnormalities and mental retardation. Despite their rarity, new syndromes resulting from chromosomal abnormalities are regularly described, and it is important to examine the karyotype of any baby with an unexplained cluster of congenital abnormalities, particularly any infant who has an odd facial appearance and developmental delay.

Trisomy 18. Edward's syndrome

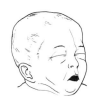

1. Mental retardation

2. Cranio-facial anomalies
   a. micrognathia
   b. prominent occiput
   c. low-set, faun-like ears

3. Abnormalities of limbs

4. Cardiac and other abnormalities

5. Abnormal dermatoglyphics

Sex chromosome anomalies

Survival without one of a matching pair of autosomes does not appear to occur.

Turner's syndrome (XO). Clinical features

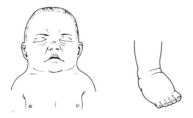

Short stature

Cranio-facial abnormalities
  a. webbing of neck
  b. down-turned mouth
  c. micrognathia
  d. downward slanting palprebral fissures

Abnormalities of limbs and trunk
  a. lymphoedema
  b. cubitus valgus
  c. widely-separated nipples

Ovarian dysgenesis with infertility

Increased incidence of heart defects

However it is possible to lose one X chromosome and survive. This is referred to as monosomy and is usually written XO.

Turner's syndrome. The diagnosis can be confirmed by chromosomal analysis but additional information may be obtained by examining the buccal mucosal cells for the presence of the Barr body. This chromatin mass, almost certainly an inactivated X chromosome, is seen in a higher percentage of cells in the female than in the male, females are normally reported as chromatin positive and males as chromatin negative. In Turner's syndrome, with only one X chromosome, girls are chromatin negative. When there is an extra X chromosome, for example in an XXX female, there are two Barr bodies to be seen in the buccal cells. The XO constitution is common in abortuses but due to a high fetal loss rate the incidence of Turner's syndrome is only about 0.3/1000 live births.

Klinefelter's syndrome. Although the Y chromosome is small, it does carry the coded information for maleness and even though there is an extra X chromosome in this syndrome the patients are male in appearance. It occurs in 1 in every 400 to 600 births and often passes undetected. The men are usually tall

Klinefelter's syndrome (XXY). Clinical features

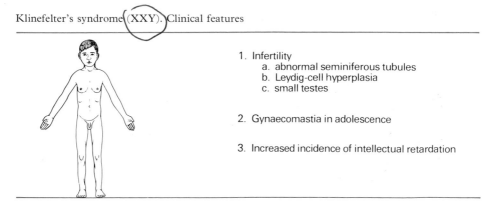

1. Infertility
  a. abnormal seminiferous tubules
  b. Leydig-cell hyperplasia
  c. small testes

2. Gynaecomastia in adolescence

3. Increased incidence of intellectual retardation

and thin, and have infertility and hypogonadism.
They contrast with those males with an XYY chromosomal constitution.

Individuals with an extra Y chromosome are thought to be more common in prison communities and to have an increased tendency to psychiatric illness.

Structural changes in chromosomes

Sometimes a portion of one chromosome is transposed or translocated onto another chromosome. If, during this process of translocation no important genetic information is lost, then there may be no obvious clinical effects of the re-arrangement and the translocation is said to be balanced. However, the possessor of this abnormality, particularly if it is the mother, is <u>very prone to produce offspring with an unbalanced translocation</u> with resultant serious congenital abnormalities. This type of structural rearrangement between chromosomes is responsible for about 6 per cent of all children with Down's syndrome and

Pedigree illustrating translocation

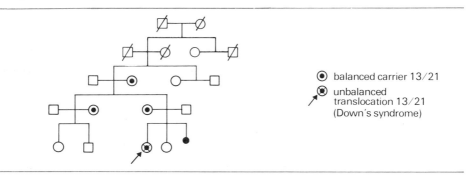

◉ balanced carrier 13/21
⊗ unbalanced
   translocation 13/21
   (Down's syndrome)

commonly involves chromosomes in Groups D and G. It is possible for it to arise *de novo* in the infant but more commonly it results from a parental balanced translocation. If the latter is the case the risk of Down's syndrome in further children is high, <u>around 1 in 8 if the mother</u> carries the translocation and <u>1 in 20 if the father is the carrier</u>. It is important to study all the siblings and the chromosomal make-up of the relatives of the carrier parent, if the risk of their producing abnormal infants is to be recognised and reduced.

Translocations may be found in other conditions, for example in about <u>10 per</u>

Down's syndrome 13/21 translocation karyotype

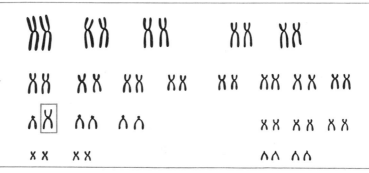

Cri-du-chat (deletion short arm, Chromosome No. 5)

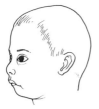

1. Mental retardation

2. Cranio-facial abnormalities
    a. microcephaly
    b. moon-faced
    c. hypertelorism
    d. epicanthic folds
    c. alert expression

3. Abnormal cry in infancy

4. Spasticity

cent of women who have frequent miscarriages or failed pregnancies. Should such a person have a successful pregnancy there is a real risk that her child will have an unbalanced translocation and be abnormal.

It has been suggested that chromosomal abnormalities account for around one per cent of all disease in childhood. This figure is undoubtedly an under-estimate. In a recent report 7 per cent of infants dead at birth or dying in the first year of life were found to have a chromosomal anomaly. A chromosomal anomaly is found in about 25 to 30 per cent of early abortions.

POLYGENIC OR MULTIFACTORIAL INHERITANCE

The inherited diseases discussed so far have resulted from either a fault in a single gene or an alteration in chromosomal structure or number. There are, however, many commoner disorders in which there is a genetic component where the inheritance pattern cannot be explained simply in terms of dominant or recessive traits or chromosomal rearrangement. In these it appears that it is the cumulative action of a number of genes, a polygenic effect, which is important and it is this factor which is responsible for the familial tendency or predisposition to various diseases. However, as the expression of the disease depends on environmental factors as well as genetic ones, the aetiology of this group of conditions is more correctly described as multifactorial. Many human traits, for example height and

Polygenic inheritance

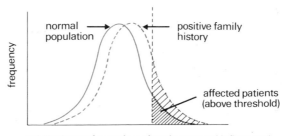

liability (sum of genetic and environmental influences)

intelligence, are inherited in this way and these characteristics in a given population follow a Gaussian or normal distribution. The liability of any individual to develop a disease of multifactorial aetiology also has a normal distribution, and the condition occurs when a certain threshold level is exceeded.

When one member of a family is affected then relatives sharing some of the responsible genes are at an increased risk and as expected this risk is higher for a first degree relative, that is sons and daughters, than for second degree relatives, cousins and nephews.

Examples of polygenic inheritance, example: spina bifida

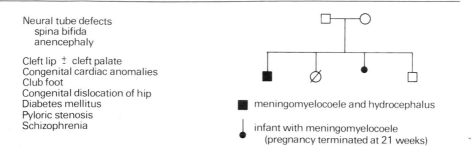

Neural tube defects
  spina bifida
  anencephaly

Cleft lip ± cleft palate
Congenital cardiac anomalies
Club foot
Congenital dislocation of hip
Diabetes mellitus
Pyloric stenosis
Schizophrenia

■ meningomyelocoele and hydrocephalus

infant with meningomyelocoele
(pregnancy terminated at 21 weeks)

The neural tube defects are the most common serious congenital abnormalities in the United Kingdom and their distribution within the community fits a multifactorial aetiology. The risk of any mother having a baby with this condition is about 1 in 200. Following the birth of an affected child the risk for subsequent infants is about 1 in 20. Should she be unlucky enough to have a second affected child then the risk for subsequent pregnancies rises to approximately 1 in 8. With three affected children the risk rises even higher, probably 1 in 4. Families with such tragic histories were encountered before it was possible to diagnose the condition early in pregnancy. The chances of both identical twins being affected is less than 10 per cent.

The geographical distribution of this abnormality emphasises its multifactorial origin. In Belfast the incidence is 7:1000 and in South Wales even higher, whereas in East Anglia and South East England the incidence is only about 2:1000. The increased tendency of those of Irish stock to have affected children persists even in those Irish who move to live in other parts of the world. This suggests a genetic contribution. The births of children with neural tube abnormalities have a definite seasonal incidence; they are more common in lower social classes; and they are more likely to affect the first and fourth children in a family. These various elements could be considered to reflect environmental factors.

Epidemiological studies in the future should identify further environmental factors in multifactorial conditions. Recently, studies in Liverpool suggested that a preceding abortion or failed pregnancy might act as the stimulus for the production of some form of antibody which could damage the developing neural tube in a subsequent pregnancy. Despite the failure to identify a specific causative factor in neural tube abnormalities, pre-natal diagnosis of the condition has been possible for some time. It had been shown that in anencephaly or open meningomyelocele a normal fetal blood constituent, alpha-fetoprotein, is increased in the amniotic fluid. This increase can be detected sufficiently early for termination of the pregnancy to be offered to the parents. Initially, amniocentesis and estimation of the alpha-fetoprotein was only considered in those couples who already had an affected child. However, when it was confirmed that a rise in the maternal serum alpha-fetoprotein was also present in many cases of neural tube defect it became possible to offer a routine screening procedure for all mothers irrespective of their previous history. Despite the problems inherent in such a widescale population screening procedure it is already producing a significant decrease in the number of children born with this abnormality in our community.

The pedigree of a family in which the first child was born with severe meningomyelocele and hydrocephalus is illustrated. Although treated surgically he remains retarded and severely crippled at the age of 16 years. A second infant died at the age of three months from meningitis. Not surprisingly, the parents at this stage were very concerned about the outcome of any children born to them. In her third pregnancy the mother had a routine serum alpha-fetoprotein screen. This was reported as raised and a repeat examination confirmed that it was abnormal. She and her husband were given an explanation of the possible significance of this finding and it was recommended that she should have amniocentesis. This confirmed a high level and the parents requested termination. A stillborn infant of 21 weeks gestation was delivered and on examination

Amniocentesis

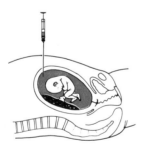

Indications for Amniocentesis:

1. neural tube defects

2. chromosomal anomalies

3. sex-linked disease

4. biochemical abnormalities

was found to have a large meningomyelocele. Some months later the parents decided on a further pregnancy. On this occasion both the serum and liquor alpha-fetoproteins were normal and mother was eventually delivered of a healthy girl with no evidence of a congenital disorder.

BIBLIOGRAPHY

Emery A E H 1979 Elements of medical genetics, 5th edn. Churchill Livingstone, Edinburgh
McKusick V A 1969 Human genetics. Prentice-Hall, New Jersey
McKusick V A 1978 Mendelian inheritance in man, 6th edn. The Johns Hopkins University Press, Baltimore
Salmon M A, Lenderbaum R H 1978 Developmental defects and syndrome. H. M. & M. Publishers,
Smith D W 1970 Recognisable patterns of human malfunction Saunders, Philadelphia

3
Fetus

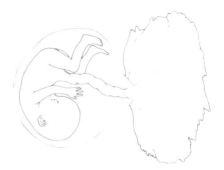

Since the fetus lies hidden, unobserved within the uterus, he can fall ill, lose parts, even die, without the mother being aware of what is happening. In the main, he is protected against diseases which attack the mother, and his favoured status allows him to thrive and grow even though the mother's reserves are under pressure. Paradoxically there are some situations, fortunately rare, when the fetus is seriously harmed by agents which either have little effect on the mother, for example the virus of german measles, or which might even benefit her, for example various drugs. Towards the end of pregnancy fetal demands for oxygen and nutrients reach a point where they may challenge the capacity of the utero-placental unit to supply them. At this stage, any disturbance of that supply line might interfere with fetal growth or damage sometimes permanently the delicate rapidly growing tissues, particularly in the brain.

EXAMINATION OF THE FETUS

In the past, the assessment of fetal growth depended on a knowledge of the date of the last menstrual period and the estimation of fetal size by palpation, but recently developed ultrasound techniques have provided more accurate means of measuring growth.

However, evaluation of fetal health is more difficult. Some indication of fetal well-being is gained by measuring maternal blood levels of placental lactogen, a protein synthesised by the placenta, or the maternal 24-hour urinary output of oestrogens which reflect the rate of steroid synthesis by the feto-placental unit. Normal values of these biochemical measurements are available for the different stages of gestation. Repeated measurements which show falling levels indicate that the fetus is under increasing difficulty.

If it is suspected that the fetus is structurally or biochemically abnormal, then more invasive procedures which involve entering the uterus might be justified. Withdrawing fluid through a needle inserted into the amniotic space (amniocentesis) involves a slight risk of fetal injury or premature birth. It does, however,

Measurements of fetal head growth and two indices of placento-fetal well being. The examples are serial measurements in individual situations where the fetus was in difficulties

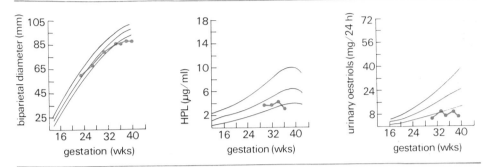

allow analysis of fetal cells for a wide range of inherited biochemical disorders and chromosomal abnormalities. In later pregnancy an index of the maturity of the fetal lungs, and thus the capacity of the infant to survive if delivered prematurely, can be gained from measuring the ratio of lecithin to sphingomyelin in the amniotic fluid. In rhesus incompatibility, when the infant is suspected of being severely affected, the concentration of bilirubin in amniotic fluid can be a guide to management.

Fetoscopy requires the introduction of an instrument with a larger bore, but it does permit the fetus to be viewed, in part at least, so that it is possible to identify a placental vessel and collect some fetal blood samples. The latter procedure enables conditions to be diagnosed which currently escape detection by analysis of amniotic fluid. This technique has allowed programmes for the antenatal detection of thalassaemia to be successfully established.

Once labour starts some indication of the ability of the fetus to tolerate it can be gained by analysis of the fetal heart rate, particularly in relation to the uterine contractions, and pH measured on capillary blood samples from the presenting part may indicate the degree of asphyxia that the fetus is experiencing.

FETAL INFECTIONS

The list of organisms that have been proven to cross the placenta and affect the

Fetal infections

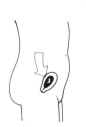
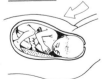

Transplacental:

Treponema pallidum (syphilis)

rubella virus
cytomegalovirus
plasmodia (malaria)
Toxoplasma gondii

Birth canal:

Neisseria gonorrhoea
Listeria monocytogenes
Herpes virus hominis

Candida albucans
enteropathogenic
—Escherichia coli

fetus is relatively short. It is possible that a much larger number might on rare occasions cause fetal disease or death, but gathering evidence for this relationship is difficult.

Rubella

A small percentage of women have their first attack of german measles during early pregnancy, and they may or may not have a suggestive rash. The risks to the fetus are considerable, particularly if a viraemia occurs in the first trimester; a large percentage of pregnancies abort or the surviving fetus is seriously damaged. The viraemia may persist throughout pregnancy and the infant may continue to excrete virus for many years afterwards. During this time the disease process continues. It is because of these terrible consequence of this otherwise trivial infection, that rubella immunisation is offered to all teenage girls. Older women may be immunised but should not become pregnant for at least three months.

Rubella. Clinical features in mothers; the HI antibodies in the affected and non-affected infants after birth; and the percentage of children at different age groups with antibody

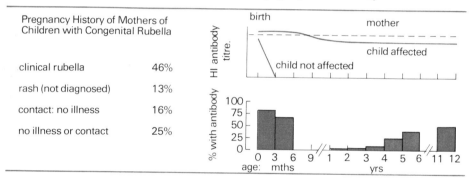

Clinical features. A surviving fetus may be left with congenital heart defects, defects of the ears with deafness, and eye disorders, particularly cataracts. A small percentage present at birth with purpura, thrombocytopenia, hepatosplenomegaly and have X-ray evidence of bony lesions. Many have an associated encephalopathy and are subsequently mentally retarded.

If a pregnant woman has contact with suspected rubella it is essential to

Congenital rubella. Clinical features

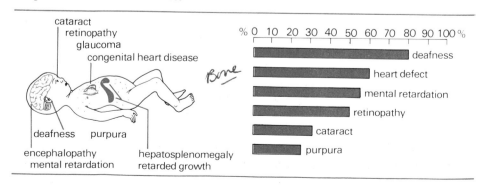

determine whether she is vulnerable to primary infection or whether she has protection from previous exposure. If the diagnosis is suspected, blood is taken and tested for serum haemagglutinin inhibition antibodies (HI) for rubella. If antibodies are high within the incubation period, the patient can be considered to be protected by a previous infection. If they are low, a further sample should be taken 7 to 10 days and if possible 17 to 21 days after first exposure. A rise in titre confirms primary infection and the risk of fetal damage and many consider this grounds for a therapeutic abortion. Diagnosis in the newborn is confirmed by the presence of a specific rubella IgM antibody.

Cytomegalovirus disease (CMV)

In common with rubella virus, CMV produces a mild disease in adults. It is also widespread in the community, 50 per cent of pregnant English women have antibodies to CMV. It has been estimated that between 1 and 6 per cent of pregnant women contract CMV infections and that the fetus is affected in around 50 per cent. Infection in early pregnancy may cause abortion or a spectrum of malformations including growth failure, microcephaly, cerebral calcifications, cataracts, cardiac lesions and deafness. CMV may be a significant cause of mental handicap, epilepsy and nerve deafness, problems which become manifest in later life when the relationship with intrauterine infection is less likely to be appreciated. CMV infection in late pregnancy may produce a systemic illness comprising purpura, hepatosplenomegaly, pneumonia and encephalitis.

Due to the absence of clinical illness in the adult, the infection in the mother often passes undetected. Even routine screening of the newborn for raised CMV specific IgM levels can be misleading. However, the presence of virus in the urine of the newborn with raised cytomegalovirus specific IgM antibody confirms the diagnosis. At present there is no reliable vaccine available for the protection against CMV infections.

Toxoplasmosis

Toxoplasma gondii, a protozoon parasite, is found around the world and affects animals as well as man. Again, the maternal infection may not produce any clinical symptoms. Only a small percentage of women contract the infection in the first part of pregnancy but when they do so the organism may invade the placenta and spread to the fetus.

Toxoplasmosis has widespread effects on the developing brain, causing hydrocephalus or microcephaly with cerebral calcification and a chorioretinitis. There is usually resultant mental handicap with other neurological abnormalities.

A diagnosis is made on the basis of rising antibody titres. In the newborn, the toxoplasma specific IgM fluorescent antibody test will be positive in those infants who have been infected, but the absence of antibodies does not rule out the possibility of a congenital infection. Infants thought to have the disease should be followed up both clinically and serologically.

Others

Syphilis used to be the most commonly recognised organism that attacked the fetus but happily it is now very rare in the United Kingdom. The same is true for congenital tuberculosis. Malaria commonly affects the placenta and may interfere with the fetal growth. Mothers with malaria have babies of relatively low birth weight. Occasionally the parasites cross to the fetus and cause fetal disease.

INFECTIONS ACQUIRED DURING PASSAGE THROUGH THE BIRTH CANAL

A sterile infant passing through the birth canal is at risk of contracting a wide range of infections, particularly from pathogenic organisms in the maternal bowel. If the membranes have ruptured prematurely, the infant may be infected two to three days prior to birth by organisms entering the uterus via the birth canal. There has been recent concern that, even without rupture of the membranes, infection can pass up the birth canal to produce an infection of the placenta and the fetus.

Gonococcal ophthalmia
Infection due to *Neisseria gonorrhoea* acquired during the birth can lead to a purulent conjunctivitis, which if not treated promptly, results in corneal ulceration and perforation. Frequent irrigation with antibiotic eye drops are recommended together with a course of systemic penicillin or, if the organism is insensitive to penicillin, a broad spectrum antibiotic.

Congenital pneumonia
So-called congenital pneumonia is in most instances not due to a bacterial infection. However, occasionally listeria or group B streptococcal organisms in the birth canal can be drawn into the respiratory tract and produce a bacterial pneumonia in the first few days of life. The possibility needs to be recognised and vigorous antibiotic therapy given.

Herpes virus hominis infections
Herpes virus Type 2 infection is a sexually transmitted disease. The cervicitis is frequently asymptomatic but it creates a major risk for the fetus. Ascending infection may result in abortion or, in later pregnancy, premature birth. There is a high (40 per cent) risk of direct infection during the infant's passage through the birth canal. Neonatal herpes infection is frequently fatal and some obstetricians regard herpetic cervicitis an indication for elective Caesarean section.

DRUGS ACROSS THE PLACENTA

There is no doubt that some drugs cause embryopathy. There is some suspicion that many others may under some circumstances have harmful effects, but it is very difficult to establish beyond doubt that they have made a contribution to the production of an abnormality in one particular child. Difficulty establishing the association is due in part to the fact that the drug may only occasionally have this harmful effect, and in part to the fact that the end pathology may not be specific.

Thalidomide
It was the damaging effect of this drug which highlighted the need for caution

when introducing new agents for treating women during pregnancy. The drug damaged a large percentage of the fetuses of women who received it in early pregnancy. Characteristically it affected the skeletal system, causing unusual defects of the arms and legs, phocomelia. The limbs may be absent, shortened, or hypoplastic. Less frequently there may be abnormalities of the intestinal tract, of the heart or kidneys, or there may be a harelip and eye defects.

Other drugs causing embryopathies

Cytotoxic agents may kill the fetus, indeed aminopterin was used to terminate pregnancies, but if the pregnancy continues the fetus may survive with many deformities. Progesterone preparations will masculinise the female fetus. Alcohol has recently been linked to facial abnormalities, growth retardation and mental handicap. Such abnormalities are not an unusual occurrence in babies of women who are chronic alcoholics. Anti-convulsant drugs have been suspected of being responsible for an increased incidence in facial clefts and congenital heart disease. Certainly there is sufficient evidence to recommend that they are not given during pregnancy unless there are sound clinical indications.

Drugs given to fetus which affect neonatal behaviour

Drugs administered to the mother during the time prior to delivery may affect the baby's behaviour immediately after birth. Obviously sedatives and anaesthetics which cross the placenta will make the baby sleepy and inactive. This is the reason why many babies after Caesarean section used to require resuscitation. Mothers who are on long-term anticonvulsant therapy may have babies with withdrawal symptoms. The babies on the second and third day become hyperactive and difficult to feed and some have 'jittery' episodes. It is important to reassure mother of the nature of these episodes as she may fear that her baby is going to have fits like herself. Mothers who are drug addicts have babies who are undersized but their maturation may be advanced so that they have a lower incidence of respiratory distress syndrome. However, the babies may show severe withdrawal symptoms and require careful management over the first few weeks of life. Any drugs that the obstetrician uses to accelerate labour, may interfere with the fetus and the development of the baby after birth. For example, it has been suspected

Drugs affecting the embryo and fetus

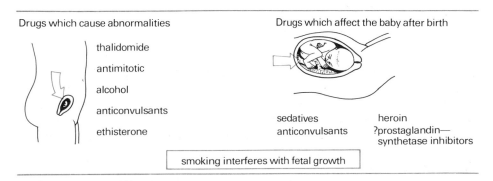

Drugs which cause abnormalities	Drugs which affect the baby after birth	
thalidomide		
antimitotic		
alcohol		
anticonvulsants	sedatives	heroin
ethisterone	anticonvulsants	?prostaglandin—synthetase inhibitors

smoking interferes with fetal growth

that the prostaglandin and antiprostaglandin agents may interfere with the balance between patency and closure of the ductus arteriosus. Oxytocin administered to control labour causes a small increase in bilirubin levels in the infant after birth.

MATERNAL IMMUNOGLOBULINS

The immune defence mechanisms develop early in fetal life, but in the absence of stimulation, specific antibodies are not produced. The human fetus gains some specific protection by the transfer of maternal IgG across the placenta. In general the maternal immunoglobulins confer benefit but they can produce disease. The commonest example is the transfer of maternal antibodies against the fetal blood cells as in rhesus and ABO incompatibility. Less commonly, mothers suffering from the so-called autoimmune diseases may transfer damaging antibodies to the fetus. Thus, mothers with platelet antibodies, who may or may not themselves have clinical features of idiopathic thrombocytopenia, may have babies who develop purpura in the first two to three days of life due to the transfer of platelet antibodies across the placenta. Similarly, mothers with systemic lupus erythematosis may have infants who have either systemic disease, which is usually lethal, or transient lupus rashes on the face. Likewise, babies of mothers with myasthenia gravis may have transient but severe hypotonia, and infants of mothers with ulcerative colitis may have transient melaena. Finally, mothers with circulating thyroid antibodies, irrespective of whether they are themselves thyrotoxic or even in a hypothyroid state during pregnancy may have infants who develop all the signs of thyrotoxicosis after birth including exophthalmos. There may be little indication that the baby is affected until they develop heart failure in the second week or so of life. It is as well to keep an eye on all infants at risk.

Transient disorders in the newborn caused by maternal immunoglobulin

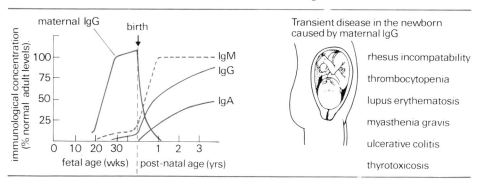

maternal IgG   birth

immunological concentration (% normal adult levels).

100
75
50
25

0 10 20 30   1   2   3
fetal age (wks) post-natal age (yrs)

IgM
IgG
IgA

Transient disease in the newborn caused by maternal IgG

rhesus incompatability

thrombocytopenia

lupus erythematosis

myasthenia gravis

ulcerative colitis

thyrotoxicosis

BIBLIOGRAPHY

Campbell S 1976 Fetal growth. In: Beard R W, Nathanielsz P W (Eds.) Fetal physiology and medicine. Saunders, Philadelphia

Davies P A 1974 Maternal and fetal infection. Clinics in Obstetrics and Gynaecology 1: 17-34

Dudgeon J A 1976 Infective causes of human malformations. British Medical Bulletin 32: 77-83

Hanshaw J B, Dudgeon J A 1978 Viral diseases of the fetus and newborn. Saunders, Philadelphia

Hull M G R, Chard T 1976 Hormonal aspects of feto-placental function. In: Beard R W, Nathanielsz P W (Eds.) Fetal physiology and medicine. Saunders, Philadelphia

Marshall W C 1977 The child with congenital rubella. Journal of Maternal and Child Health 2: 94-102

Smithells R W 1978 Drugs, infections and congenital abnormalities. Archives of Disease in Childhood 53: 93-96

4
Newborn

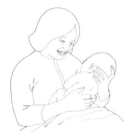

In our concern to provide every mother and her child with a safe birth we may overlook the importance of their first meeting face to face. They have a deep basic need to 'recognise' and respond to each other. Fascinating research in recent years has demonstrated how very aware and responsive the human newborn is to his new environment. If the mother is ill or the delivery is difficult or the newborn infant is sick or weak it is even more important for the caring staff to encourage the establishment and the strengthening of the bond between mother and child. Failure to do so may lead subsequently to poor feeding patterns, failure to thrive, and the longer term consequences of maternal neglect. When mother and infant have failed to establish a mutually satisfying relationship there is an increased risk of child abuse and post-neonatal infant death.

ROUTINE EXAMINATION OF THE NEWBORN

'Is my baby all right?' is often the first question that mothers ask after delivery and it is so difficult to answer if he is not! As soon as the baby is born a quick but careful scrutiny of the face, eyes, mouth, chest, abdomen and limbs should exclude major blemishes; a lusty cry and the development of a suffuse pink blush over the face and body denotes satisfactory immediate adjustment to independent existence. Together they are sufficient to answer the mother's pressing question. If you are not sure of the sex of the infant do not make a guess. Explain to the parents that occasionally it can be difficult to tell immediately and that tests may be necessary. If there is difficulty establishing adequate breathing, then the appropriate steps in resuscitation should be taken. If the baby is small, immature or injured, he must be given extra support and protection. If the mother has had hydramnios then a firm tube must be passed into the stomach to exclude oesophageal atresia, a congenital abnormality which is usually associated with a tracheo-oesophageal fistula.

Over the next 48 hours all infants should be examined thoroughly and at leisure, preferably in the mother's presence, ideally with both parents, and only after the

Incidence of the commoner malformations in England and Wales. (These figures are only approximate; see Carter 1976)

Malformation	%
Anencephaly	0.20
Spina bifida	0.25
Cleft lip and cleft palate	0.10
Club foot	0.07
Congenital hip dislocation	0.10
Congenital heart malformations	0.60
Down's syndrome	.14–.18
Pyloric stenosis	0.30

details of the medical history of the family, the pregnancy and labour are known. This first medical examination is a screening procedure, and its aim is to discover disorders which are open to early management. The baby should be naked in a warm room. The examination should be systematic; first assess overall size, proportions and maturity, then look for structural abnormalities, starting with the head and eyes and then the ears, mouth, chest, abdomen and limbs, hands and feet. Note any accessory tags, digits and dimples. Many abnormalities follow failure of complete union in the midline, so a quick check along the midline is worthwhile, and this should include a close look at the palate and anus. Respiratory disorders are more easily seen than heard. Palpating the peripheral pulses may suggest, if full, a ductus arteriosus, or, if weak, a major defect causing poor systemic cardiac output. The presence or absence of femoral pulsations must always be noted. Abnormal heart sounds and murmurs are more difficult to interpret; if there is doubt, it is better to find an opportunity to re-examine the baby later. If the murmur persists but the baby is otherwise well, then the parents are told of the finding and a follow-up examination is arranged. Two other conditions are specifically sought; congenital dislocation of the hips, and in boys, the presence of testes in the scrotum.

The third stage of this examination is to assess the baby's behaviour and responsiveness. The mother and the midwife will usually be quick to tell you about the baby's feeding, behaviour, crying and sleeping patterns. An unduly floppy or sleepy baby, an irritable or restless baby, or a poor 'suckler' all call for more careful evaluation, particularly in relation to the establishment or otherwise of satisfactory breast feeding.

Minor anomalies
Parents should be reassured about the following minor anomalies:

Capillary or macular haemangioma (stork bites, salmon patch) around the eyes and at the nape of the neck are seen in 30 to 50 per cent of babies. Those around the eyes usually disappear in the first year. Those at the nape may persist.

Blue-black pigmented areas (Mongolian spots) at the base of the back and on the buttocks are unimportant and are common in infants of dark skinned parents but can also occur in Caucasian infants. They usually fade over the first year or so.

Urticaria of the newborn (erythema toxicum) is a fluctuating, widespread, erythematous maculopapular rash which is usually most marked on the trunk and is most evident on the second day. It disappears spontaneously, requiring no treatment.

Heat rash (miliaria) is seen in mature infants nursed in warm humid atmospheres. Both red, macular patches and superficial, clear vesicles may be seen, most evident on the forehead and around the neck. The lesions clear in a cool environment.

Breast enlargement. Both girl and boy infants may develop breast enlargement and even secrete small amounts of milk (witches milk). Girls may discharge a mucous plug from the vagina and there may be a little vaginal bleeding.

White pimples (milia) on the nose and cheeks are very common and are found in about 40 per cent of infants. They are tiny epidermal cysts. Similar larger lesions may be seen in the mouth (Epstein's pearls). They rupture spontaneously and disappear. Cysts attached to the mucosa in the mouth and even 'teeth' may be present at birth.

Accessory skin tags on the face, anterior to the ears (accessory auricles) or loosely attached, vestigial, extra digits can usually be dealt with easily but this should preferably be done by the surgical team.

Sacral dimples should be explored gently to exclude underlying sinuses.

Minor anomalies

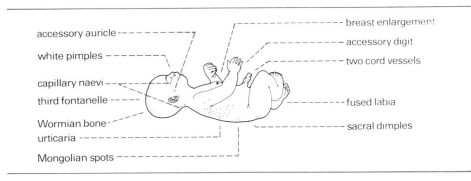

Some anomalies, although relatively unimportant in themselves, may be associated with more important abnormalities. The fontanelles (head 'soft spots') are occasionally very wide and not infrequently extra bones float in the space, Wormian bones. If skin defects overlie the posterior fontanelle the possibility of chromosomal abnormalities should be considered. A third fontanelle is occasionally found between the anterior and posterior fontanelles and is common in trisomy 21. Oddly shaped ears and two cord vessels may be associated with renal abnormalities. Normal kidneys are best palpated immediately after birth before the bowel fills with gas.

Congenital postural deformities
The posture of the infant after birth often reflects his position *in utero*. However,

Intrauterine postures

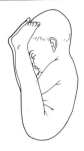 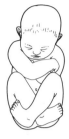 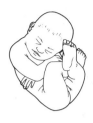

with more freedom, the infant soon chooses to curl into a compact shape with arms and legs flexed. If there is less than an average amount of amniotic fluid to cushion the fetus, then towards the end of gestation the infant may be so tightly packed within the uterus that deformations of the musculoskeletal system develop. These congenital postural deformities may mould the head into odd shapes (dolichocephaly, plagiocephaly) suppress or distort the chin, resulting in its being unduly small (micrognathia), or cause mandibular assymetry or neck muscle contractures and torticollis. The shoulders may be dislocated, the chest wall compressed, the hands and feet distorted (club hand, club foot). These effects are usually multiple and are seen in their extreme form when the kidneys are absent in renal agenesis, and very little amniotic fluid is present (oligohydramnios). The presenting part is often the most deformed. One special example of postural deformity associated with intrauterine position is dislocation of the hip, which is more common in breech presentation.

Disorders detected by the Massachusetts Metabolic Disorders Screening Program (Levy, 1976).

Disorder	Newborns screened	Number with disorder	Frequency
Phenylketonuria (PKU)	1 095 519	78	1: 14 000
Atypical PKU	1 095 519	64	1: 17 000
Galactosaemia	690 000	7	1:100 000
Maple syrup urine disease (MSUD)	956 162	3	1:300 000
MSUD (intermediate)	956 162	2	1:450 000
Homocystinuria	563 773	3	1:190 000
Argininosuccinic acidaemia	414 329	6	1: 70 000
Cystinuria	414 329	27	1: 15 000
Cystathioninuria (B6 responsive)	414 329	4	1:100 000
Cystathioninuria (B6 resistant)	414 329	1	—
Vit. D. resistant rickets	414 329	1	—
Fanconi syndrome	414 329	1	—
Propionic acidaemia	414 329	1	—
Benign disorders			
Histidinaemia	414 329	22	1: 20 000
Iminoglycinuria	414 329	?40	?1:10 000
Hartnup 'disease'	414 329	23	1: 18 000
Hyperprolinaemia	414 329	2	1:200 000
Hyperlysinaemia	414 329	1	—

Biochemical screening

The number of inherited biochemical disorders or variations which can be recognised by relatively simple and cheap biochemical tests increases yearly. It is the simplicity and cheapness of the test which makes it feasible to test the blood of every newborn infant. The tests are primarily intended to screen for phenylketonuria, but other conditions including galactosaemia, maple syrup urine disease and homocystinuria may be identified. Many countries are now testing the blood in an attempt to recognise early hypothyroidism. Amino acid and galactose disorders may be detected by a blood test performed when milk feeding has been established, usually on the fourth or fifth day of life.

BIRTH INJURIES

The short journey down the birth canal is not without hazards for the infant but fortunately the risks are becoming less as the techniques for recognising fetal distress improve. Infants who are judged to be too big for the birth canal or who fail to advance during labour and become distressed are now delivered by Caesarean section, making heroic obstetric manipulations to achieve vaginal birth rarely necessary. The risk of birth trauma is greater in breech deliveries, in premature births, in precipitate deliveries and when the baby is unexpectedly large.

Some of the damage caused by the birth is unsightly but quickly resolves. Inevitably, the presenting part becomes oedematous and bruised. This caput succedaneum is commonly found on the back of the head and happily it clears spontaneously in a few days. However, the swelling looks uncomfortable when it involves the breech and scrotum and very unpleasant in a face presentation. The face also looks bloated, blue and bruised when the cord is pulled tightly around the neck and there may also be retinal and conjunctival haemorrhages. As the fetal head is pushed down the birth canal it rotates and the apex of the parietal bones may catch the ischeal spines and be dented like a ping pong ball or the outer shelf may be cracked and crepitus may be felt, or the periosteum may separate and a cephalhaematoma form beneath the periosteum producing a lump the size of a small hen's egg. Again, these injuries are of little import although the cephalhaematoma may take many months before it finally disappears. Very rarely a bleed may occur under the aponeurosis (sub-aponeurotic haemorrhage) when the bleeding is not confined to a single cranial bone like a cephalhaematoma but spreads rapidly over the head and down towards the eyes. A significant fraction of the blood volume may be lost into this haematoma.

Severe compression with extreme moulding of the skull can tear the tentorium cerebri and its accompanying vein. The resulting haemorrhage is likely to cause permanent damage or death. The baby may be born in a state of shock and may not respond to resuscitative procedures.

Manipulation of the spine and arms, which is most likely to be required for breech deliveries, may damage the cervical spinal cord with residual palsies in arms and legs, or lead to stretching and damage of the upper part of the brachial plexus causing weakness or paralysis of abduction at the shoulder, flexion at the elbow and extension and supination of the wrist (Erb's palsy). The arm is dropped

Birth injuries

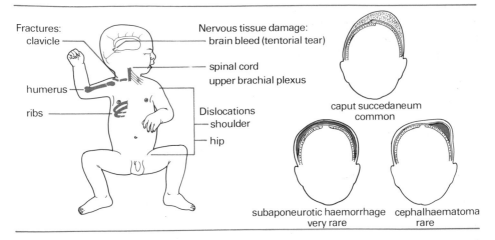

Fractures:
    clavicle
    humerus
    ribs

Nervous tissue damage:
    brain bleed (tentorial tear)
    spinal cord
    upper brachial plexus

Dislocations
    shoulder
    hip

caput succedaneum
common

subaponeurotic haemorrhage   cephalhaematoma
very rare   rare

into the position a waiter adopts in the expectation of a tip. The weakness may resolve spontaneously in a few weeks, or the paralysis may remain.

Rough handling may lead not only to fracture of the skull but also of the clavicle, humerus or ribs. These 'non-accidental injuries' may pass undetected in the newborn period and be unknown to parents and medical attendants alike.

Forceps blades may compress the facial nerve as it leaves the parotid gland. Usually the resultant facial palsy is transient, occasionally the pressure causes overlying fat necrosis with permanent scarring and a residual palsy.

BIRTH ASPHYXIA

The fetus, floating in the amniotic fluid, 'breathes', 'feeds' and 'excretes' through the placenta. The fetal lungs are filled with fluid secreted by the alveolar cells to a volume close to the functional residual capacity found after birth. Following delivery, the placenta is discarded and 'dies' whilst the independent infant activates his own system for obtaining oxygen and nutrients and discarding waste.

The most urgent requirement is to breathe. To do this the lung liquid must be displaced by air. During a vaginal birth the thorax is squeezed in the birth canal and the lung liquid can sometimes be seen pouring out of the baby's nose when his head is just emerging from the birth canal. Once the infant gasps, air is drawn into the lung and lung liquid disappears to the periphery of the respiratory tree. From there it is cleared by the pulmonary circulation and lymphatics. Failure to complete this process satisfactorily is one important factor leading to transient tachypnoea.

As the infant passes down the birth canal his head is squeezed and then released and exposed to the cooling air. His limbs are pushed, pulled and finally allowed to drop into positions they have never occupied before. His umbilical cord is intermittently obstructed, stretched and finally clamped. His arterial concentration of oxygen falls and that of carbon dioxide rises. Many of these stimuli are known to provoke a gasp.

The onset of breathing and circulatory adjustments after birth

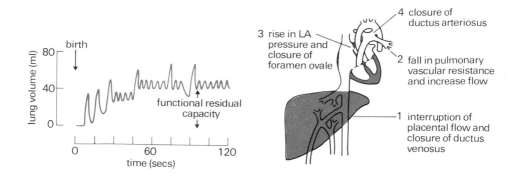

On average, newborn infants gasp after six seconds and the majority have done so by twenty seconds. With these efforts the lungs rapidly fill with air and a residual lung volume is formed. Once this is achieved, tidal breathing begins. It occurs on average after thirty seconds and the majority of infants are breathing regularly by ninety seconds.

As the lungs expand and fill with gas, the pulmonary vascular resistance falls, the pulmonary blood flow increases and the pressure in the left atrium rises closing the foramen ovale. As a consequence of these changes, oxygenated blood passes through the ductus arteriosus; oxygen has a direct effect on the muscle of the ductus causing contraction and physiological closure, anatomical closure proceeds more slowly over the following weeks. Occasionally, in cyanosed infants, the ductus may remain open or the physiologically closed ductus may reopen, and so add to the infant's problems sometimes to the point of precipitating heart failure.

Infants may be asphyxiated *in utero* for a variety of reasons. If the disorder is not reversed they will be asphyxiated at birth and they must be resuscitated immediately. Many of the babies who appear all but dead at birth but who

Causes of intrauterine asphyxia

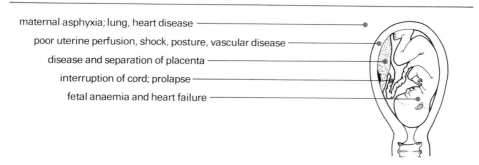

respond promptly to active resuscitation may make a full recovery. More commonly, infants are reasonably oxygenated at birth but due to previous asphyxia or sedative drugs given to the mother they fail to begin adequate ventilation, and then become asphyxiated and require resuscitation. Many factors are associated with birth asphyxia including the general wellbeing of the mother and the maturity and nutrition of the infant.

With increasing asphyxia the infant becomes blue or white, hypotonic, unresponding, and the heart rate begins to fall. These features, colour, tone, motor reactions, respiratory response and heart rate were arranged into a scoring system by an American anaesthetist, Dr Virginia Apgar. The main features to watch are the infant's attempts to breathe and the rate and strength of the pulse. Those who fail to breathe and become asphyxiated should be actively resuscitated when the heart rate begins to fall.

Resuscitation

The newly born baby is gently dried and wrapped in a warm towel. The time of birth is noted. The upper airway is cleared by gentle suction of excess fluid and any inhaled vernix, blood or meconium. If during this procedure the infant fails to make any respiratory effort then a gasp may be provoked by blowing cold oxygen on the nose. If this is not effective then the other bizarre methods used in the past, for example pinching, slapping, injecting respiratory stimulants, putting champagne or pepper on the nasal mucosa, are not likely to work.

The next step is to expand and ventilate the lungs. Often inflation of the lungs itself will initiate a gasp with spontaneous breathing. If it does not, the lung should be ventilated at a rate between 30 and 50 inflations per minute with pressures below 30 cm H_2O. The majority of infants will quickly become pink and begin breathing within two to five minutes.

The most effective method of inflating the lungs is via an endotracheal tube. To insert the tube, the infant's head must be carefully positioned in slight extension, the small finger of the hand holding the endoscope pushes the larynx into view. If either the skill or the equipment is not available for intubation then the infant can be resuscitated nearly as well with a face mask which fits snugly over his mouth and nose, and a bag which delivers small volumes of gas. It is essential to hold the lower jaw forward to ensure a clear airway; over-inflation of the stomach should be

Steps in resuscitation

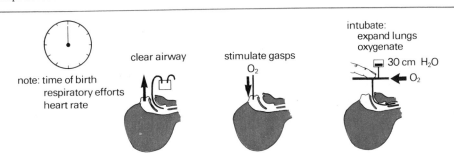

note: time of birth
respiratory efforts
heart rate

clear airway

stimulate gasps
O_2

intubate:
expand lungs
oxygenate
30 cm H_2O
O_2

avoided by passing a nasogastric tube and putting gentle hand pressure on the upper abdomen.

If the infant fails to become pink with good expansion of the lung then he is probably in a state of shock. Cardiac massage using two finger pressure on the lower half of the sternum at a rate of 140 taps per minute is occasionally necessary. Correction of respiratory acidosis by alkali injections into the umbilical vein can be helpful but it is important that the alkali is washed through with saline to avoid liver damage.

If the lungs do not expand then either there is a rare abnormality of the airways or lungs, of the endotracheal tube is not in the trachea. Clumsy insertion of the tube can damage the upper airways; energetic and faulty inflation may damage the lungs. Occasionally, the difficult decision of whether to resuscitate or not has to be made. If the baby is physically normal and can be resuscitated then recent reports suggest that he will probably survive intact, although he may have a stormy few days rather like an older child after a head injury. If the baby is physically abnormal then one must ask oneself firstly, could this child survive even if resuscitation is successful, and secondly, has the infant's brain developed adequately? If the answer to either is no, then resuscitation is not justifiable. If there is uncertainty, call a colleague, remembering that in general parents would wish us to respond to their offspring as we would wish others to respond to our own.

Effects of asphyxia

Birth asphyxia may have both immediate and long term effects. Acute total asphyxia seen, for example with cord prolapse, may by haemorrhage and oedema damage and interfere with brain function causing profound hypotonia followed by irritability and fitting; there may be an abnormal cry and poor sucking patterns. The breathing pattern may be so disturbed as to suggest a primary respiratory problem. Loss of homeostatic control may lead to hypoglycaemia, hypocalcaemia and hypothermia. But asphyxia may damage many other organs as well: in the

Reasons for failure to resuscitate and the immediate effects of severe birth asphyxia

Brain damage:
  haemorrhage

Upper airway obstruction:
  laryngeal spasm
  laryngeal stenosis

Lung pathology:
  pneumothorax
  hypoplasia
  effusion
  diaphragmatic hernia

Small chest cage:

Shock due to ruptured viscera

Brain:
  fits, irritability
  abnormal tone
  hypo and hyperventilation
  hypoglycaemia

Lungs:
  aspiration, RDS
  haemorrhage

Kidneys:
  vein thrombosis
  tubular necrosis

Bowels:
  ileus, perforation

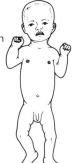

lungs it causes oedema; in the myocardium changes resembling an infarct; in the bowel it causes an ileus or ischaemic perforations; in the kidneys it may result in renal vein thrombosis or tubular necrosis; and in the liver disorders of metabolism and haemostasis may be caused. In premature infants, birth asphyxia increases the risk of idiopathic respiratory distress syndrome and lethal intraventricular haemorrhages.

The immediate post natal effects of chronic intermittent prenatal asphyxia are more difficult to assess for invariably asphyxia is not the only noxious factor affecting the infant.

Cerebral oedema and haemorrhage may lead to necrosis with permanent brain damage and resultant cerebral palsy and mental handicap. That less severe degrees of asphyxia can lead to less severe evidence of brain damage, for example, fits, hyperactivity and learning problems is generally accepted but the extent to which it is responsible for these disorders in the community is difficult to assess.

We are still left with the problem of trying to determine which infants asphyxiated before or during the birth are likely to be permanently affected. Some infants make remarkable recoveries so that parents should be encouraged to be reasonably optimistic. It has been estimated that only 1 in 10 of infants showing evidence of brain asphyxia in the week or so after birth are subsequently found to have evidence of brain damage.

SIZE AT BIRTH

Fetal growth, and thus the size at birth, is determined by both genetic and environmental factors. Many disturbances affecting the mother, the utero-placental unit or the fetus may alter fetal growth patterns. Most adverse influences retard or distort growth but occasionally growth is accelerated. Diabetes in the mother is the commonest clinical disorder leading to an over-sized baby.

The infant of a diabetic mother is large and obese. Not many years ago many of them were stillborn. Now with improved antenatal care the majority survive but they are still at a slightly greater risk of having a congenital

Weight at birth and fetal weight curves

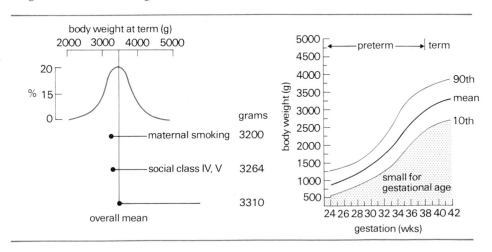

Clinical features of the oversized infant of a diabetic mother, and an undersized, under-nourished infant

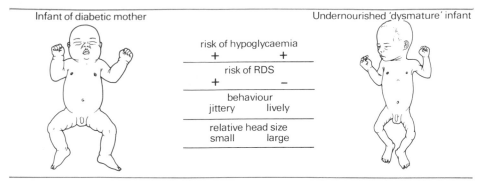

Infant of diabetic mother		Undernourished 'dysmature' infant
	risk of hypoglycaemia	
+		+
	risk of RDS	
+		−
	behaviour	
jittery		lively
	relative head size	
small		large

abnormality; their broad shoulders may give problems during the birth (shoulder dystocia) and after birth they are more likely to develop hypoglycaemia, respiratory distress and to become jaundiced. Their hyperexcitability, jitteriness and immaturity may initially cause feeding difficulties. With meticulous control of the diabetic state during the whole of pregnancy, many if not all these problems can be avoided. The exciting question is whether or not good control in early pregnancy will reduce the incidence of congenital abnormalities.

Undersized infants

'Small for dates', 'light for dates', dystrophic, and dysmature are some of the many terms used to describe undersized but mature infants. As a group they are not easily defined. If they are identified by their weight, for example those in the lowest 10 per cent of the normal distribution, and this is the common practice, then by definition the group will include normal small children as well as those subject to growth restraint.

There are three main clinical categories. The first comprises infants with chromosomal or severe structural abnormalities. The average body weights of children with Down's syndrome or tracheo-oesophageal fistula are all well below the average. In this group also are those infants who have suffered intrauterine infections. Secondly, there is a group typified by the perfect miniature, small infants who have the proportions of a mature baby. These infants may well have been small throughout gestation and are likely to become small adults. The third group comprises the undernourished infants. Characteristically they have big hands and feet, little subcutaneous fat, they look long and ungainly and it is not difficult to imagine that they have relatively large brains and small livers. In these infants the growth rate probably fell off towards term.

It would be helpful if undersized babies could be slotted easily into these three main categories but in practice this is not possible. In their body proportions the majority fall somewhere between the two last extremes.

It is important to recognise those infants who are born undernourished irrespective of their birthweight, for they are particularly susceptible to damaging hypoglycaemia. Usually they look anxious, lively and hungry; their crinkly skin reflects their mild dehydration and limited fat reserves. If there is any doubt four-hourly estimations of blood glucose concentration should be made and early generous feeding commenced. Should the blood glucose concentration fall below 1.2 μmol/l, intravenous glucose therapy should be given.

Light-for-dates babies have a lower mortality rate than babies of similar weight born prematurely but their eventual outlook may not be so good. The 'balanced' small infants may remain small and their abilities are more likely to fall below the average. The situation is complex for such babies are more frequently born to parents of low socio-economic status.

Premature infants

Human pregnancy lasts about 40 weeks. Premature birth is usually taken to mean birth before the 37th week of gestation. If the uterus is structurally abnormal, the fetus awkwardly implanted, if more than one fetus is present, or if excess fluid collects around the fetus (hydramnios) then premature delivery is more likely to occur. But in many instances the cause of the early delivery is not known. It is more common in teenagers, in first pregnancies, in the unhappy, the unfortunate and the sick, and too often it occurs before the mother has had any antenatal care.

The survival rates of premature infants has improved over the years. Some highly specialised units are achieving excellent results. It is now expected that babies over 32 weeks gestation who weigh over 1.5 kg without major pre-natal pathology should survive and survive intact. However, pre-term birth brings with it a number of problems.

Nutrition. As the ability of the weak, pre-term infant to suckle is limited, they often require to be fed some weeks after birth using a nasogastric tube. Breast milk and various artificial milks have been given with success but there is still uncertainty as to the most appropriate nutrient mixture for a prematurely born infant. The immature bowel adjusts surprisingly well, although by adult standards the stools contain a relatively high fat content.

Thermal stability. Premature babies have high surface area to body weight ratio and little subcutaneous fat, and over the first few days they lose water rapidly through their skin (transepidermal water loss). These physical characteristics make it difficult for them to maintain thermal stability. As cold exposure jeopardises their survival, great attention must be paid to keeping them warm. To provide a controlled ambient temperature it is current practice to nurse premature infants in incubators or under radiant heaters, but reducing heat losses by oiling the skin and insulating the infant with clothing and light blankets makes more sense.

Respiratory difficulties. Because of their immaturity many, but not all, prematurely born infants have difficulty opening their lungs and forming and maintaining a functional residual capacity. Failure to do so leads to a mixture of primary and secondary atelectasis, the idiopathic respiratory distress syndrome. Their respiratory drive varies, this is apparent in their periodic breathing pattern, and becomes troublesome when it leads to long apnoeic spells. Asphyxial episodes during birth or apnoeic attacks afterwards may cause ischaemic necrosis in the germinal cell layer lining the lateral ventricles of the brain. When these necrotic areas break down, local haematomas form which often progress to intraventricular haemorrhages which may result in death or permanent brain damage. Idiopathic respiratory distress syndrome and intraventricular haemorrhages are two pathologies peculiar to premature birth.

Liver immaturity. Physiological jaundice is often more marked and more prolonged in immature infants but with careful nursing and early establishment of feeding, exchange transfusions should rarely be necessary. It is thought that the pre-term brain is more at risk from damage due to high bilirubin levels.

Infections. Because of their delicate surfaces and limited immunological competence, premature babies are more susceptible to infections. Because of their weak defence systems, they do not show the symptoms and signs that are seen in older infants. Their clinical state changes rapidly from bacteraemia, to septicaemia, to death. Associated meningitis can easily pass undetected. Therefore in any infant suspected of having an infection, it is necessary to culture both blood and cerebrospinal fluid and to commence therapy with broad spectrum antibiotics before the results come back.

Other hazards. Premature babies are often born unexpectedly and are therefore more likely to experience asphyxia during birth and their delicate tissues are more likely to be damaged. They are susceptible to hypoglycaemia, metabolic acidosis, peripheral oedema, and irritability and fits due to birth injury and asphyxia.

The delicate pre-term infant is also more easily damaged by nursing and medical procedures. In particular, inhalation of gas mixtures with high concentrations of oxygen, if they lead to high arterial concentrations, may stimulate abnormal vascularisation in the eye (retrolental fibroplasia) with subsequent blindness. Thus, if high oxygen-gas mixtures are given to preterm infants, it is mandatory to monitor arterial blood concentrations.

Once they have adjusted to extrauterine life and feeding has been established,

Survival rates in prematurely-born infants

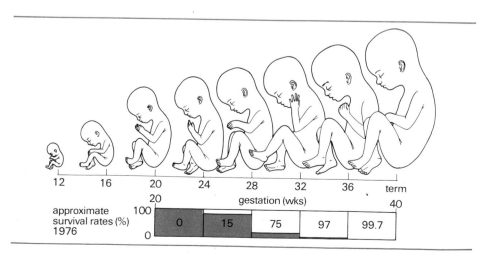

gestation (wks)	12	16	20	24	28	32	36	term
			20					40

approximate survival rates (%) 1976	0	15	75	97	99.7

premature babies can grow at a rate similar to that which they would have achieved *in utero*. This high growth rate can lead to anaemia and vitamin deficiency so it is common practice to give supplements of both iron and vitamins from the fourth week.

The outlook of prematurely born infants, particularly those with only moderate problems adjusting to extrauterine life, is good. The majority reach their expected size and ability level.

Infants of very low birth weight. Until recently infants born before 28 weeks' gestation were thought not to be viable. It was exceedingly rare for infants weighing less than 1 kg to survive. Now, with intensive care, including if necessary artificial ventilation and intravenous nutrition, more and more of these infants of very low birth weight are surviving. Experts have been optimistic about their subsequent development but it is still too early to be confident about their prognosis.

Inevitably, however, intensive neonatal care interferes with the normal establishment of the parent-child relationship and this, with adverse social factors, contributes to the increased risk of cot death and child abuse in babies born before their time.

RESPIRATORY PROBLEMS IN THE NEWBORN

There are a number of clinical syndromes presenting with respiratory difficulties in the first weeks of life. It is convenient to describe them as separate entities but in practice the situation is usually complex with a variety of factors contributing to any individual infant's respiratory problem.

Lung disorders due to aspiration

An infant may aspirate foreign material before, during and after birth.

Intrauterine pneumonia. Occasionally babies are born with lung consolidation due to material aspirated from the amniotic fluid. This 'congenital pneumonia' is associated with prolonged rupture of the fetal membranes, amnionitis and fetal asphyxia. The aspirated material may or may not contain organisms. It is rare to find an inflammatory response in the infants lungs. If organisms are present they are usually *E. coli*, paracolon bacillus, *Staphylococcus aureus*, and *albus*, and the other bacteria which might be expected on the mother's perineum. The babies develop respiratory distress after birth and this may last a few days. A chest X-ray will show patchy shadowing. Inevitably the infants will be given broad spectrum antibiotics but it is probable that the infants would manage as well without them. This condition must be distinguished from fetal lung infection due to transplacental transmission of *Listeria monocytogenes*. This condition is preceded by a febrile illness in the mother and the placenta may show listerial abscesses.

Meconium aspiration. Asphyxia during birth will provoke mature infants to make vigorous efforts to breathe in. If there is meconium in the amniotic fluid, or if the baby's head is in the birth canal surrounded by vernix, meconium and blood,

Lung disorders in the newborn

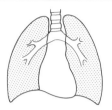
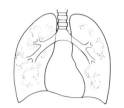
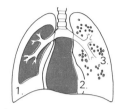

air bronchogram:
idiopathic respiratory
distress syndrome

patch collapse with overinflation.
meconium aspirate

1. pneumothorax
2. pneumomediastinum
3. interstitial emphysema

then these tenacious materials may be drawn into the upper airway. Prompt clearing of the airways by gentle suction at birth may be life-saving. Once the debris is drawn into the respiratory tree, patches of lung collapse and over-inflation develops. The infants may have severe respiratory difficulties for some days and complications like pneumothorax and pneumomediastinum are common and may be fatal. Gentle supportive therapy with minimal interference probably achieves the best results. Supportive ventilation may aggravate the lung disorders.

Transient tachypnoea of the newborn. Rapid breathing for some hours after birth is relatively common and usually resolves spontaneously. It may in part be due to failure to clear lung liquid, particularly during the birth.

Milk aspiration. It is quite a challenge to the newborn infant to separate in the pharynx the air breathed in through the nose and milk sucked in through the mouth. They often get it wrong and swallow air; and they occasionally get it wrong and inhale milk. Obviously the latter is the more dangerous and every effort must be made to anticipate and avoid it. The risks are higher in certain groups of infants:

1. Those with depressed central control, for example after birth asphyxia or heavy sedation, and in infants with central nervous system abnormalities;
2. Breathless infants with lung or cardiac lesions;
3. Infants with structural anomalies of the nose, mouth and oesophagus, for example cleft palate, choanal atresia, oesophageal atresia and in infants with oesophageal incoordination.
4. The immature who, although they may be able to make sucking and swallowing movements, are unable to sustain their effort to take in sufficient nutrient.

An infant is particularly at risk of aspiration after an apnoeic attack. Management of these babies requires considerable nursing skill and judgement. The introduction of plastic feeding tubes was a major advance.

Disorders due to lung immaturity

Idiopathic respiratory distress syndrome. The more immature the infant the greater is the risk of respiratory distress and the lower the survival rate. In the adult, alveolar spaces are clustered around the terminal bronchioli; in the infant at term a single, simple sac is found at the end of each bronchiole. Lining the sac are two types of alveolar cells, A and B. Cell type B secretes a lipoprotein, surfactant, which plays a critical role in determining the physicochemical characteristics of the gas-liquid interface in the air sacs. In some prematurely born infants these cells seem unable to release or produce enough surfactant and the air sacs collapse. The pulmonary capillaries ooze liquid and red cells into the interstitial space causing oedema and haemorrhage. The protein leaked into the alveolar sacs forms 'hyaline' membranes which can be clearly seen on light microscopy. This finding led to the disorder being called hyaline membrane disease, but in early severe forms, membranes may not have had sufficient time to form.

The ability of the B cells to release surfactant can be assessed before birth by measuring the ratio of lecithin and sphingomyelin in the amniotic fluid. Certain stimuli, maternal ill health, intermittent asphyxia, uterine contractions and drugs may induce the cells to begin secreting earlier in gestation. Asphyxia may have the opposite effect and possibly increases the need for surfactant. Within a few days of birth, whatever the gestation, the cells appear to function adequately.

As the affected infants have difficulty forming and maintaining a functional residual capacity, they are recognised clinically by their struggle to draw in air and to hold it. Each diaphragmatic tug pulls in the lower rib cage and soft tissues of the neck. An expiratory grunt accompanies each effort. The signs appear at birth or soon after, with apparent increasing severity. If the infant survives then improvement is usually seen after the second or third day and the lungs appear to recover fully. It might be deduced from the pathogenesis that the disorder will vary in severity and this is true; at one extreme it produces an unimportant transient disturbance in the respiratory pattern, at the other it leads to increasing cyanosis, acidosis and death in the first few hours of life. In these infants, a chest X-ray will show a diffuse ground glass appearance with an air bronchogram. At necropsy, the lungs look like liver.

The management of idiopathic respiratory distress syndrome requires considerable medical and nursing skill and involves continuous monitoring of many features of the baby (HR, RR, PaO_2) and of his environment (T^0, FiO_2) as guides for respiratory support, nutrition programmes, and intravenous therapy. Inept enthusiastic interference does more harm than good; the alternative to expert intensive care is to allow the infant to nestle in a warm, humid, oxygen-enriched (but not more than 40 per cent) environment to take his own chance.

Wilson-Mikity syndrome. One consequence of patchy collapse of lung segments is over inflation of other areas leading to patchy emphysema. This complication may become an increasing embarrassment over the first few weeks of life in immature infants.

Pulmonary haemorrhage may complicate asphyxia and atelectasis or occasionally appear to be a primary problem. It also occurs during recovery from hypothermia.

Apnoeic attacks are a common problem in sick and premature newborn infants. The respiration of infants at risk must be continually monitored. Physical stimuli are usually sufficient to provoke a gasp and the recommencement of breathing. Occasionally intubation and supportive ventilation may be required. Respiratory stimulants like theophylline may help.

Three non-lung diseases may present with respiratory symptoms. Cerebral anoxia can produce bizarre respiratory patterns mimicking dyspnoea though more commonly cerebral asphyxia leads to hypoventilation. If lung expansion matches respiratory effort this possibility should be considered. Metabolic acidosis, frequently an outcome of disorders of aminoacid metabolism presents with hyperventilation, deep and effective breaths. Congenital heart disease is perhaps the most difficult to exclude. Auscultation may not help or be positively misleading; assessment of peripheral perfusion, an electrocardiograph and chest X-ray are often more helpful.

JAUNDICE IN THE NEWBORN

Many healthy normal newborn infants develop jaundice after birth. *In utero*, bilirubin crosses the placenta and is excreted by the mother. After birth, the infant must activate his own excretory systems but there is some delay and blood bilirubin concentrations rise. This 'physiological' jaundice appears over the first 48 hours and begins disappearing towards the end of the first week; the bilirubin is largely unconjugated and the baby remains generally well. There is considerable variation from one infant to another. The condition may be more severe and prolonged in immature infants, if hypoxia and hypoglycaemia further limit bilirubin conjugation, and if the infant is constipated then there may be increased enteric reabsorption of bilirubin.

Kernicterus

Unconjugated bilirubin is lipid soluble and travels in the circulation largely bound to albumin. It is the small fraction of free bilirubin which escapes from the vascular compartment and enters the cellular lipid fractions of the brain cells, which may cause transient or permanent damage, kernicterus. When this happens the infant behaves abnormally, feeds badly and may fit and develop opisthotonus

The average and range of bilirubin concentrations in infants during the newborn period, and bile pigment metabolism

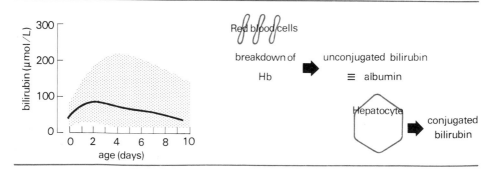

when the back is arched and the head thrown back. If the infant recovers there is usually residual brain damage, often with severe choreoathetosis and mental handicap.

In full term infants serum bilirubin concentrations above 340 μmol/l are considered dangerous. The risks are greater when albumin levels are low or when there is competition for albumin binding by, for example free fatty acids and drugs like sulphonamides and aspirins. Various diseases can aggravate this situation causing unconjugated bilirubin to rise to dangerous levels.

Haemolytic disease of the newborn

Jaundice appearing in the first 24 hours of life is usually due to excess haemolysis of the newborn red cells by antibody from the mother. This will only happen if the maternal and fetal blood are incompatible. The haemolytic jaundice which causes most clinical problems is due to Rh incompatibility. ABO and rarer blood groups may produce a similar but usually milder clinical picture. The problems occur after the mother has been sensitized by either a mismatched blood transfusion, or from fetal blood entering her circulation during a miscarriage or, more commonly, at the end of a previous pregnancy during labour and delivery. She reacts to the fetal blood by producing antibodies. The concentration of the antibodies are measured serially during pregnancy in affected mothers. It is these globulin antibodies which cross the placenta in increasing concentrations, during the pregnancy which attack and haemolyse the red cells in the fetal circulation.

Clinical features. When the condition is mild, the fetus and newborn tolerate the small increase in haemolysis rate, although after birth the baby may become moderately jaundiced and have mild anaemia. With higher rates of haemolysis, the bilirubin levels in the fetus may still stay low because the unconjugated bilirubin passes back across the placenta and the fetus can tolerate moderate anaemia, but after birth the bilirubin concentrations rise rapidly and dangerous bilirubin levels may be reached within 24 hours. In the severe forms with high rates of haemolysis the fetus is unable to maintain his haemoglobin and becomes

Mild, moderate and severe rhesus incompatibility

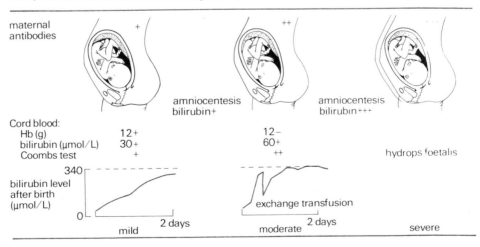

severely anaemic, and this with an associated general disturbance in fetal metabolism leads to severe oedema (hydrops fetalis) a condition which is usually fatal.

Management. The aim of obstetric management is to deliver the baby before the anaemia becomes critical. A measure of the state of the fetus can be gained by serial analysis of amniotic fluid taken by amniocentesis for bilirubin products. Very rarely if the fetus is severely affected and too immature to be delivered, fetal blood transfusions have been given to correct the infant anaemia.

When any baby suspected of Rh incompatibility is born, cord blood is collected and analysed for haemoglobin, bilirubin and antibody concentrations. If the cord blood tests suggest that the infant is affected, bilirubin concentrations are measured serially every four to six hours. If there is a risk that they will rise to dangerous levels an exchange transfusion is performed. During this procedure blood is alternatively withdrawn and transfused in 10 to 20 ml units, via a catheter in the umbilical vein, until 60 to 70 per cent of the infant's red blood cells have been replaced. Good hydration and phototherapy are helpful in reducing the need to perform exchange transfusions.

Rhesus incompatibility is now far less common following the discovery that administration of Anti-D antibodies to the mother immediately after birth destroys any red cells which might have leaked into the maternal circulation and so reduces the risks of the mother producing antibodies.

Causes of early and late neonatal jaundice.

Early neonatal	Prolonged neonatal
Haemolytic disease of newborn	Liver disease
Bruising and petechia, haemorrhages due to asphyxia and birth trauma	Infection
	Infants of diabetic mother
Glucose G6PD deficiency	Hypothyroidism
Inherited red cell anomalies	Galactosaemia
E. coli septicaemia.	Breast milk jaundice
	Biliary atresia

GASTROINTESTINAL PROBLEMS

Oesophageal atresia

Oesophageal atresia (incidence 1:2500) is usually associated with a tracheo-oesophageal fistula. In every infant born to a mother with hydramnios, it should be excluded by passing a firm, large-bore (12 G) tube through the mouth into the stomach. After birth, the affected infant is unable to swallow his own saliva and bubbles fluid from the mouth, another sign requiring investigation. It is always a sad event when the diagnosis is made only after the child has choked over his first feed. It is the condition of the lungs as well as the extent of the abnormality which dictates the success of surgical correction.

The diagnosis is confirmed radiologically by passing a firm, radio-opaque tube into the upper pouch and taking a lateral film of the chest, and an antero-posterior film of the chest and abdomen. Air in the stomach confirms the presence of a fistula. Associated anomalies may include ano-rectal agenesis and cardiac defects, particularly Fallot's tetralogy.

Oesophageal atresia with diaphragmatic hernia

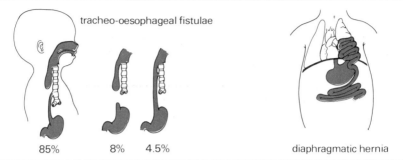

tracheo-oesophageal fistulae

85%   8%   4.5%

diaphragmatic hernia

Congenital diaphragmatic hernia

Congential diaphragmatic hermia (incidence 1:2200) is due to a defect of the hemidiaphragm, usually the left. Where the diaphragmatic defect is the only anomaly, the baby may appear well at birth, but observation will show a deep chest and a scaphoid abdomen. Respiratory distress develops as the child swallows air, which passes into the small bowel within the chest cavity. The resulting mediastinal shift leads to compression of the previously unaffected lung. The diagnosis is confirmed by X-rays of chest and abdomen. Once respiratory distress is present surgery is urgent. A nasogastric tube should be passed to empty the stomach and small bowel. Endotracheal intubation and ventilation may be necessary pre-operatively.

Babies with diaphragmatic hernias may also have bilateral pulmonary hypoplasia when even initial resuscitation may be impossible, or a major heart defect.

All cases of diaphragmatic hernia are associated with abnormalities of gut rotation.

Small bowel obstruction

In the newborn period 'functional ileus' is the most common form of small bowel obstruction and settles with conservative measures. The most common form of organic obstruction of the small bowel is meconium ileus. Other causes of small

Duodenal atresia and small bowel atresia

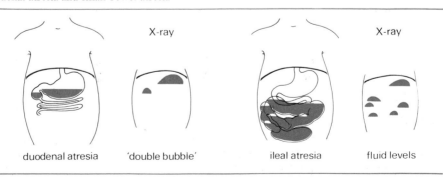

X-ray   X-ray

duodenal atresia   'double bubble'   ileal atresia   fluid levels

bowel obstruction in the neonatal period include atresia, stenosis and diaphragms of the duodenum, jejunum or ileum, midgut volvulus 'volvulus neonatorum', Ladd's band associated with failure of caecal descent, enterogenous cyst and milk curd obstruction. Meconium ileus and atretic lesions will present very early with distension and vomiting within hours of birth. The other lesions may not produce symptoms for some days or even a week or two after birth.

Vomiting of green rather than yellow bile-stained material is suggestive of organic obstruction. Meconium may or may not have been passed in the early hours of life. The area of distension will depend on the level of the obstruction; in duodenal obstruction it is confined to the upper abdomen, in ileal obstruction it is generalised. Erect X-rays of the abdomen should be taken, and may be diagnostic, for example, the double-bubble of duodenal atresia, the ground glass appearance of some cases of meconium ileus, and the calcification of an ileal atresia with prenatal perforation. In other cases fluid levels may be present but these do not necessarily indicate mechanical obstruction. They will be present in functional ileus, and in a baby with ileus secondary to septicaemia.

Large bowel obstruction

In the neonate there are only two causes of large bowel obstruction, Hirschsprung's disease and ano-rectal agenesis. The former is the more common, and it is suggested by delay in the passage of meconium beyond 24 hours. The baby may appear otherwise well for a few days but is liable to become suddenly and acutely distended, with peripheral circulatory collapse, a feature of a 'Hirschsprung's enterocolitis'.

Ano-rectal agenesis is an all embracing name for a very large number of anatomical anomalies. Basically there are two types of ano-rectal agenesis, high and low, depending on whether the bowel ends above or below the pelvic floor. All low anomalies are easily corrected at birth by a perineal procedure. High anomalies require a temporary colostomy; in boys there is always a fistula into bladder or urethra; in girls there may be a fistula into the vagina.

Most babies with ano-rectal agenesis have no visible anus at birth: it is extremely rare for the anal canal to be present but not communicating with the upper bowel (rectal atresia).

Rectal agenesis

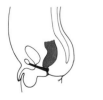 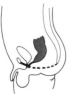 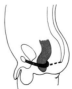 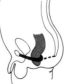

| normal | 'High' agenesis with or without fistula into urogenital tract | 'Low' agenesis—covered or anterior ectopic anus, both usually with stenosis |

Exomphalos and gastroschisis

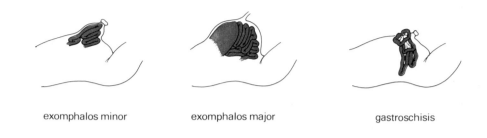

exomphalos minor   exomphalos major   gastroschisis

Exomphalos

Exomphalos is a persistence of the herniation of the gut into the extra-embryonic part of the umbilical cord which is normally present between the sixth and four-teenth weeks of intrauterine life. Occasionally complete return of the gut into the abdominal cavity does not occur, the bowel which remains outside will be obvious at birth. In its mild form one or two loops of bowel are seen in the base of the cord, exomphalos minor; at its most severe a huge swelling occurs in the centre of the abdomen containing most of the abdominal contents (exomphalos major). The gut is covered by membrane. In gastroschisis there is a defect in the abdominal wall to the right of a normal umbilical cord. Gut prolapses through the defect and has no covering.

NEONATAL INFECTIONS

Sticky eye

Sticky eye is a common problem. Usually there is no underlying infection. However, conjunctivitis can occur sometimes due to a staphylococcus or occasionally a streptococcus but it may also be caused by organisms acquired from the mother's birth canal, in particular *Neisseria gonorrhoeae* and *Chlamydia trachomatis*. Both are sexually transmitted diseases. The latter is also responsible for the eye disease, trachoma, If conjunctival inflammation and pus is present then swabs should be taken for Gram and Giemsa staining and appropriate culture.

If no organisms are found, then conjunctival washes with normal saline is usually all that is required. For presumptive gonococcal infections local penicillin eye drops every two hours for the first 24 hours and then for three times a day for the next three days should be given with systemic penicillin. If the organisms prove to be penicillin insensitive then chlortetracycline eye ointment with erythromycin systemically should be given. *Chlamydia trachomatis* infections also respond to the latter.

Sticky cord

The umbilical cord dries and usually drops off after a few days. The residual sticky stump may become infected and if this happens requires immediate attention. Local antiseptic powders usually suffice, but the infant should be observed for signs of a more general infections.

Septic spots

Small septic blisters in the skin creases are not unusual and are commonly due to staphylococcal infections. Again local treatment is usually all that is required.

Septicaemia and meningitis

Newborn babies can die from infections before anyone is aware that they are ill. Thus, if an infant goes 'off his feed', handles badly, has an unexpected body temperature either up or down, or develops unusual respiratory patterns, fits or apnoeic spells, he should be thoroughly examined and a blood sample should be taken for culture and cerebro-spinal fluid should be taken for examination and culture. If in doubt broad spectrum antibiotics to cover *E. coli*, staphylococcal, Group B streptococcal and pseudomonas infections should be given whilst awaiting the results of the investigations. Neonatal meningitis has a high mortality and high morbidity rate.

Causes of convulsions in newborn infants

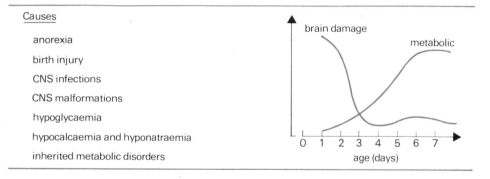

Causes

anorexia

birth injury

CNS infections

CNS malformations

hypoglycaemia

hypocalcaemia and hyponatraemia

inherited metabolic disorders

NEONATAL CONVULSIONS

Many disorders may cause fits in the newborn period. The treatment is directed at the cause.

BIBLIOGRAPHY

Behrman R E 1977 (Ed) Neonatal-perinatal medicine. Mosby, St Louis
Brazelton T B 1972 Infants and mothers. Hutchinson, London
British Births 1970. Volume 1 (1975) The first week of life. Heinemann, London
Carter C O Genetics of Common Single Malformations. British Medical Bulletin 32: 21-26
Cockburn F and Drillien C M 1974 Neonatal Medicine. Blackwell, Oxford
Dunn P M 1976 Congenital Postural Deformation. British Medical Bulletin 32: 71-76
Klaus M H, Kennell J H 1976 Maternal-infant bonding. Mosby, St. Louis
Leck I 1976 Descriptive epidermiology of common malformations. British Medical Bulletin 32: 45-52
Levy H L 1976 Screening: perinatal aspects. In: Kelly S, Hook E B, Janerick D J, Porter I H (eds) Birth defects: risks and consequences. Academic Press, London
Schaffer A J, Avery M E 1977 Diseases of the newborn. Saunders, Philadelphia
Solomon L M, Esterly N B 1973 Neonatal dermatology. Saunders, Philadelphia
Strange L B 1977 Neonatal respiration physiology and clinical studies. Blackwell, Oxford

5
Nutrition

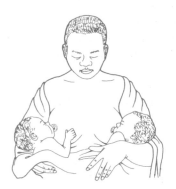

The nutrients supplied to the young in early development are uniquely and sensitively adjusted to their requirements. During intrauterine life a mixture of water, salts, proteins, carbohydrates and fats, which are drawn from the maternal blood stream and processed by the placenta, enters the fetal circulation and determines the substrates that are available for growth and energy metabolism. After birth, the breast produces a specialised total food in an acceptable and digestable form. Breast milk production is a characteristic of mammals. The mixture of nutrients in their milk varies widely from one species to another and this is to be expected for the rates of growth of the young at birth and their motor activities are very different. In view of this it is perhaps surprising that the young of one species can be reared effectively on the milk of another. But this is so, for some decades now it has been a common practice to rear human infants on cow's milk. So successful has it been in Western Societies that the advantages of human breast milk are being questioned! Breast feeding benefits both mother and child in many ways and therefore mothers should be given every encouragement to breast feed their infants, however for those who are unable to do so it is important to reassure them that there are other ways of rearing their infant successfully.

Major constituents of various mammalian milks

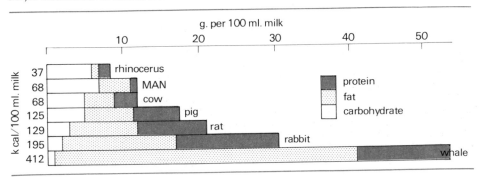

Hormones involved in lactation

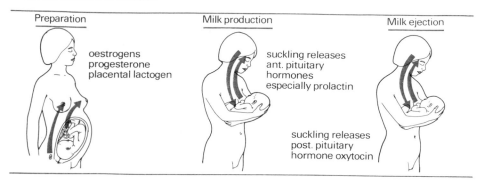

BREAST FEEDING

During pregnancy many endocrine agents prepare the breast for lactation. These include lactogen (human chorionic somatomammotropin), which is secreted by the placenta, and prolactin which is released by the pituitary gland and is important not only in initiating milk secretion but also in maintaining milk production after birth. Suckling is a powerful stimulus both to prolactin release from the anterior pituitary gland and to the secretion of oxytocin from the posterior pituitary gland. Oxytocin stimulates the ejection or 'let down' of milk by acting on the myoepithelial cells which surround the alveoli and ductules.

Even from this brief outline, it is obvious that breast feeding is a complex process which might break down at a number of stages. For example, the breast and nipple may be ill-formed, although appropriate care during pregnancy can do much to encourage adequate development. Milk production may not be initiated and maintained at a rate fast enough to suit a hungry baby or may flow too quickly for an ill or sleepy infant. If the full breast is not emptied then it may become engorged and inflamed, and the resulting pressure and pain will inhibit further milk production. Gentle manual expression of milk will avoid this complication. Finally, the unhappy, nervous, drowsy or sick mother may not be able to 'let down' her milk as she would wish or a lethargic, sick, newborn baby may not stimulate her to do so.

Breast anatomy and milk production

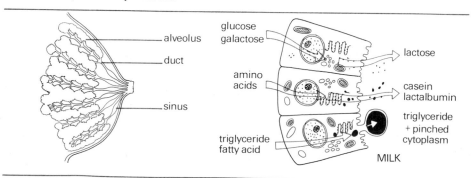

Breast feeding does not seem to be a basic instinct; many mothers who have not seen others breast feeding need considerable guidance initially. A simple explanation of how the breast works is often very helpful and avoids unnecessary anxiety. Should it be desirable to discontinue breast feeding, this can be achieved most simply by firm breast support and analgesia.

As a food, milk has some remarkable characteristics. Most of the carbohydrate is in the form of a disaccharide, lactose, which requires a specific disaccharidase for its digestion. The fats are present mainly as triglyceride in globules surrounded by lipoproteins which are probably remnants of the walls of the alveolar cells. The individual fatty acids reflect the mother's diet and her fat stores. If mothers are on low fat diets then the alveolar cells themselves make saturated fatty acid with chain lengths of 12 to 16 carbons. The protein content of human milk is surprisingly low but a large percentage is in the form of the more easily digestible whey, rather than indigestible curds. Whey contains in addition to lactalbumin, proteins which influence the infant's bowel bacterial flora, namely lactoferrin, lysozyme and IgA. Breast milk also contains vitamins, minerals, enzymes, especially lipase, and cells. The latter are predominantly macrophages and act either to keep the lacteals free from infection or to assist in the defence of the intestinal tract.

The relative amounts of the constituents vary. The first milk produced after birth, colostrum, is rich in protein and cells but the volume is small. When feeding is established, the mature milk constituents vary diurnally and from day to day. The milk at the end of a feed, hind milk, has a higher fat content than fore milk. The content of milk is also modified by the maternal diet and well-being, and by the mother's general level of nutrition.

Points in favour of breast feeding

If a mother wishes and is able to breast feed then she should be supported in this and given every encouragement to do so. Human milk is an excellent nutrient mixture which also gives the baby some protection against infection. Its protein content is less likely to induce allergic reactions and the infant may be less at risk from unexplained sudden death. The process of breast feeding usually gives satisfaction and pleasure to mother and child and this in itself will be of lasting benefit to both.

Technically, breast feeding is easier than bottle feeding in as much as the mother is not required to make up the mixture according to instruction, and sterilising bottles is not a problem.

In western societies breast feeding may be economic, but elsewhere it certainly is.

Some mothers are anxious that breast feeding or, alternatively, not breast feeding may alter the contour of the breast but there is little evidence one way or the other. Under non-lactating conditions the shape of the breast is largely determined by fat cells rather than the mammary gland. However, pregnancies and age are certainly two major factors leading to change.

Approximately 9 out of 10 women who are feeding their babies do not ovulate; but nevertheless breast feeding should not be regarded as a method of contraception.

Breast milk

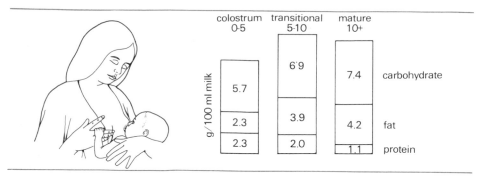

	colostrum 0-5	transitional 5-10	mature 10+	
		6.9	7.4	carbohydrate
g/100 ml milk	5.7			
	2.3	3.9	4.2	fat
	2.3	2.0	1.1	protein

Cancer of the breast is less common in women who have borne children and breast fed them.

When breast feeding is difficult

Mothers give a variety of reasons when asked why they have chosen not to breast feed. Some women just do not like the thought of breast feeding and, given an alternative, they take it. Others are embarrassed or uncertain and fear that they will fail or develop sore nipples and swollen, painful breasts. Some mothers obviously believe that bottle feeding is an easier and more certain way of ensuring their baby grows well and sleeps regularly. Others feel that bottle feeding offers greater freedom by, for instance, making it possible for them to return to work and to take the contraceptive pill. They might, perhaps, feel differently if they were better informed and more carefully prepared during the antenatal period; for example, once lactation is established, the contraceptive pill can be taken without its influencing breast feeding.

For some mothers, breast feeding is just not possible or may be contraindicated. For example, successful breast feeding is difficult with twins and virtually impossible with triplets; and in a premature birth, neither breasts nor baby are prepared for feeding. It is possible with manual techniques to establish breast feeding for these infants who initially are unable to suckle satisfactorily, but it requires a great deal of resolve on the mother's part.

If the mother has been chronically ill, severely undernourished, subject to severe asthmatic episodes or has limited renal function, breast feeding may be an unacceptable drain on her reserves. Similarly, mothers with diabetes may find that the metabolic challenge of producing milk upsets their diabetic state. Active tuberculosis in the mother is a contraindication to breast feeding until the infant has been immunised.

Most drugs taken by the mother enter the milk. For practical purposes it can be estimated that one-tenth of the dose given to the mother enters the milk so that the possibility that a drug given to a breast-feeding mother may affect her baby must always be kept in mind.

Some babies with abnormalities of the mouth, particularly cleft palate, are unable to suckle satisfactorily and breast feeding is virtually impossible. Tongue tie, unless it is in a very extreme form with forking of the tongue, should not interfere with the baby's ability to suckle.

Babies with inherited disorders of digestion or metabolism may not be able to tolerate the nutrients in human or other natural milks and special formulae have to be prepared. The inherited mono- and disaccharide intolerances, galactosaemia and phenylketonuria fall into this group.

ARTIFICIAL FEEDING

Artificial feeding in babies who suck well is usually by the bottle, but a spoon, cup, or plastic feeding tube may be used. The currently fashionable bottle sits on its base and has a wide neck surmounted by a rubber teat or nipple. Between feeds it must be washed with cold and then warm water and sterilised. The hole in the teat must be large enough to allow the baby to take his feeds in under fifteen minutes but not so large that the feed flows so quickly as to cause the baby to splutter and choke. If a baby is unable to suck or swallow, or too weak or breathless to complete the feed, then he can be fed via a fine plastic nasogastric tube. This procedure properly performed is simple, safe and well tolerated by the infants. It has probably saved more lives than any other innovation in neonatal care. In certain situations the end of the tube may be advanced into the duodenum or jejunum.

The feed is usually cow's milk modified in some way. Many babies have been reared successfully on ordinary pasteurised or sterilised cow's milk, reconstituted evaporated liquid, or dried powdered cow's milk, but there have been problems. Some have been due to the way cow's milk differs from human milk. Cow's milk contains more protein, in particular more curd protein or casein, and these thick curds being less easy to digest have caused bowel obstruction. Cow's milk contains more fat and phosphorus. In the early weeks of life, particularly from 5 to 15 days of age, this may lead to hypocalcaemia with subsequent fitting. Cow's milk has a relatively high sodium content and this, with the tendency of mothers to make strong or concentrated feeds from powdered or condensed milks leads to hypernatraemia, which may cause fits and brain damage, complications which are more likely during superimposed episodes of infection, particularly gastro-enteritis. Some infants are allergic to cow's milk protein; they may react to feeding with perioral rashes and oedema or by vomiting or passing frequent loose stools which usually contain blood.

Comparison of human, cow's and 'humanised' milk

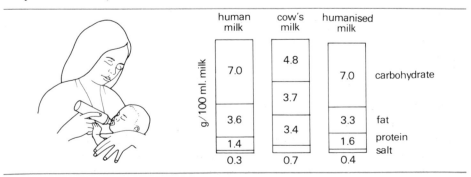

Makers of infant feeds now prepare a variety of modified cow's milk formulae, which have been 'humanised' in that the mixture more closely resembles that found in average mature human milk. This has posed considerable problems for manufacturers, for milk is a complex colloid mixture and, as such, it is very sensitive to any attempts to change it. In addition, manufacturers can only modify and supplement cow's milk to resemble human milk as far as their knowledge of the constituents of human milk permits. Pyridoxine was added to formulae only after its deficiency had led to fits in artificially fed babies. They cannot of course add the 'living elements', cells and enzymes, and at the moment we do not know how important these are.

Nutritional requirements

If a breast-fed child is content and growing, one need not trouble to consider the volume and nutrient value of each feed. There are, however, many reasons why an adequately breast-fed child may not be content or may not be growing satisfactorily. The nutrient intake of artificially fed infants is as much determined by the giver as the receiver and is more easily assessed. It is this facility which tempts some mothers whose infants are not thriving on the breast to change to bottle feeding, for then she and her health advisers can at least see the feed going in! Thus, it is essential in both breast and artificially fed infants to be able to assess their nutrient intake and their nutritional status.

Nutrient intake in breast-fed babies may be assessed by weighing the baby before and after feeds, that is by carrying out a test feed. In artificially-fed babies it is advisable to watch the mother make up and give at least one feed before calculating a daily intake from the history of feed volume and frequency. Nutritional status is usually assessed from the infant's weight, a visual evaluation of the quality of the skin and by the amount and distribution of subcutaneous fat. More information can be gained by measuring length or height and skin fold thicknesses. Appetite and metabolic efficiency vary from infant to infant, much as they do in adults. The average intake of healthy infants can be used as a guide, but

Daily milk intake of healthy, thriving, free-feeding babies. Just for interest, breast milk consumption is expressed per baby, artificial feeding is given per kg body weight

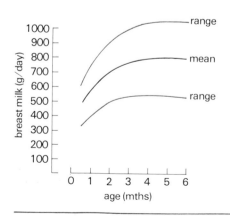
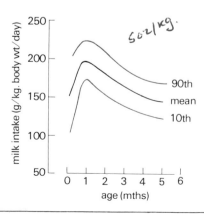

it must be remembered that the range is wide and each infant's needs must be assessed individually.

FEEDING PROBLEMS

New mothers often wish to be reassured that their babies are feeding normally. If there are problems, they may seek advice from more experienced members of the family or from shop keepers who sell milk foods, or midwives, community nurses and health visitors and it is to be expected that they will be given differing opinions. Occasionally, the problem is of such magnitude that medical advice is sought. The doctor must be aware of, or take advice about, the general abilities, approach and attitudes of the parents, the mother's feeding technique and the infant's nutrient intake, before considering the possibility of more serious underlying conditions.

Vomiting

Most babies swallow air with their milk. Gentle patting or massage of their backs helps them bring back the 'wind'. Most babies bring up a little milk as well; this is called posseting and is unimportant.

Occasionally, infants regurgitate large amounts of milk, either immediately after a feed or between feeds. It is rare for this to be sufficiently severe to affect the infant's nutrition but it does distress his mother; and, apart from other considerations, it makes all her clothes and furnishings smell and it fills her washing basket. Various strategies may be tried. By not allowing the baby to cry or become too upset before a feed and using good feeding techniques excess air swallowing can be avoided. Using agents which thicken the feed in the stomach also reduces the baby's ability to bring them back. Propping the baby up after a feed may also help.

Some babies enjoy bringing their feeds back, 'ruminating' like a cow. This habit may be difficult to break but it will become less of a problem as the infant's diet, abilities and interests change.

There is no clear distinction between regurgitation and vomiting. An underlying cause must be sought if a baby suddenly starts to be sick, if the vomit contains blood or bile, if the vomiting persists to the point of dehydration or malnutrition, or is associated with other signs and symptoms. Vomiting may be the first indication of a general infection; it may be the only clue to an infected throat is common in pyelonephritis and is usual in meningitis and gastroenteritis. Certain disorders of the oesophagus and stomach must also be considered.

Hiatus hernia of infancy is always sliding in type; 70 per cent are without a peritoneal sac. The congenital anomaly seems to be of the oesophageal hiatus itself which is lax, and the diaphragmatic grip is weaker than normal. The cardia of the stomach may remain competent even within the chest. Vomiting is usual from birth and eventually bleeding may occur due to ulceration of the oesophagus following persistent reflux. If untreated, this will give rise to a stricture. The clinical diagnosis is confirmed radiologically by a barium swallow.

Most infants improve if they are nursed upright in a hiatus hernia 'box' or chair,

Hiatus hernia

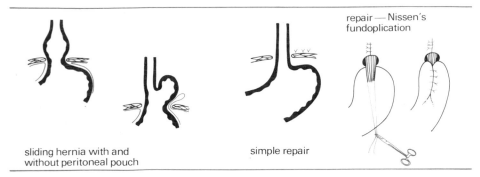

repair — Nissen's
fundoplication

sliding hernia with and
without peritoneal pouch

simple repair

and if the feeds are thickened and alkalis given. Usually the hernia resolves spontaneously by the time the child is getting onto his feet. However, if oesophagitis is present or vomiting persists after one year of age, surgery is likely to be necessary. Hiatus hernia seems more common in children with mental handicap.

Oesophageal incoordination leads to dribbling, choking and aspiration of milk as well as regurgitation and vomiting. It may be due to a wide variety of conditions all of which are rare, or sometimes it may be an isolated problem. It can be recognised by cine radiography.

Pyloric stenosis is due to hypertrophy and hyperplasia of the pyloric muscle mainly the circular fibres. It usually develops in the first four to six weeks of life. The condition is inherited by the multifactorial mode and is commonest in first-born, male children. Characteristically, the vomiting is projectile and may be so persistent that the baby becomes undernourished or even dehydrated. Being hungry, the baby is eager to feed again soon after he has vomited. On examination, stomach wall peristalsis may be visible and a rubbery tumour is felt by gentle deep finger palpation in the area half way between the mid-point of anterior margin of the right rib cage and the umbilicus. The diagnosis is entirely clinical and X-rays are not indicated. Treatment is surgical after the infant's fluid deficit has been corrected.

Pyloric stenosis

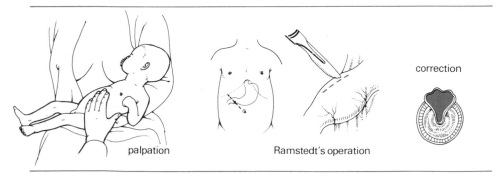

palpation

Ramstedt's operation

correction

Failure to thrive

Mothers are naturally anxious if their infants do not appear to be growing fast enough. In most western societies now, babies are measured at regular intervals and if they fail to grow satisfactorily compared with the average for that community, further enquiry is made.

Failure to thrive can be the first indication of a serious underlying problem, such as chronic renal failure and congenital heart disease, but this is rare. More often than not, it reflects difficulties in the home, limitations in the parents, unhappiness in the relationship between mother and child or uncertain feeding methods. Many women feel 'down' after pregnancy and their unhappiness and nervousness may be communicated to their babies who in turn become irritable and restless so that a vicious spiral is begun which ultimately leaves both mother and child exhausted. Bringing one or both of them into hospital to permit both to have a good night's sleep may go a long way to easing the problem.

If a baby is undersized, and it has been established that he was of normal birth weight, that he is receiving an adequate diet in a settled home and that he has no obvious serious underlying disorder then investigation should be made for the various causes of malabsorption.

Crying and 'three month colic'

Babies cry when they are hungry. They also cry for other reasons, such as cold or discomfort and as they get older they cry when they are cross or frustrated. With experience their mothers are usually able to distinguish a cry for food and a cry in pain, but it can be difficult. Not many parents can stand a baby crying intermittently throughout the night and the temptation is to feed him, not so much for his nutrition as to keep him quiet. He may react to this by vomiting. Some babies, particularly at feeding time, but at other times as well, may have inconsolable outbursts of crying, sometimes to the point of screaming for no obvious reason. During the attacks they may draw their knees up and go red in the face. It is difficult to believe that they are not having colic. It is possible that some infants have inflamed Peyer's patches and resulting painful bowel contractions. Drug therapy is seldom justified for they do not appear to come to any harm. Bowel relaxants like dicyclomine may help. This so-called 'three month colic' may last well beyond three months of age.

Diarrhoea, constipation and nappy rashes

There is no doubt that what an infant eats influences the frequency and nature of his stool and the effect the stool has on the skin of the buttocks. It is normal for a baby to have a loose yellow bowel motion with every feed, and it is equally acceptable that he has a bowel action every other day passing a firm large brown stool. But it is not acceptable that he passes frequent stools which are green and watery, or large stools which are pale and oily, or very occasional stools which are hard enough to tear the anal mucosa causing pain and bleeding. All require investigation. They may respond to simple dietary adjustments. Stool gazing is a dying art, for the information it yields is disappointingly small, but occasionally it can be instructive.

NUTRITIONAL DEFICIENCIES

Vitamin and mineral deficiencies

When unexpected symptoms or signs appear in infants and children on odd diets or with major feeding problems, the possibility of a vitamin or mineral deficiency should be considered. Clinical syndromes due to deficiency of most vitamins and many trace elements have been reported.

Scurvy is due to vitamin C deficiency. Cow's milk contains little vitamin C and most of this may disappear if the milk is stored or heated. Before artificial milks were fortified with extra vitamin C to a level similar to that in human milk, artificially-fed babies were at risk of developing scurvy. In this disorder connective tissues and structural membranes break down, small vessels bleed and wounds are slow to heal. The infants present with bruises, painful periosteal bleeds or persistent superficial haemorrhages.

Rickets is due to vitamin D deficiency. The body obtains the vitamin by the action of ultraviolet light on the ergosterols in the deeper layers of the skin or from certain foods, including fish, eggs, butter and margarine. Lack of sunshine, a pigmented skin or a poor diet leaves a child at risk. It is important that lactating mothers have adequate vitamin D so that her milk will contain sufficient for her rapidly growing infant.

Vitamin D aids the absorption of calcium from the bowel and the formation and calcification of bone. Deficiency leads to softening and deformity, particularly of the long bones. In early life rickets may be suspected if the skull bones are soft, craniotabes; in the 3 to 6 month old child the enlargement of the ends of ribs produces a rachitic 'rosary'. In a child 12 to 18 months of age just beginning to walk, the ends of the long bones may be bowed either in or out by the strain. This is a tragedy if it occurs because the deformity is easily and cheaply avoided by vitamin D supplementation of the diet.

Vitamin D deficiency. Rickets

craniotabes
delayed closure
of fontanelle

rickety rosary
chest deformity

swelling of metaphyses

genu—varum
valgum

Dental caries is due to progressive decay of teeth by organic acids produced locally by bacteria that ferment dietary carbohydrate, particularly sucrose. Fluoride reduces the incidence and severity of caries, by converting the enamel mineral, hydroxyapatite to fluorapatite which is more acid resistant, by promoting

Dental caries

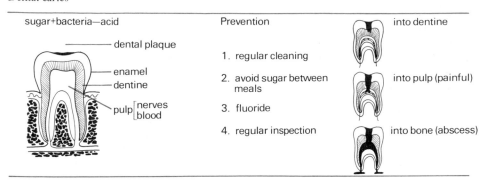

sugar+bacteria—acid

— dental plaque

— enamel
— dentine

pulp [nerves, blood]

Prevention

1. regular cleaning

2. avoid sugar between meals

3. fluoride

4. regular inspection

into dentine

into pulp (painful)

into bone (abscess)

remineralisation, and by antibacterial effects which reduce acid production. Thus, tooth decay may be considered to be a nutritional disorder, in part due to a deficiency of fluoride and in part due to excess of simple sugars. The risks of dental caries may be reduced by avoiding food between meals, particularly sticky sweets or sweet drinks in nursing bottles or pacifiers; by regularly cleaning the teeth; and by an adequate intake of fluoride either in the water, toothpaste or if necessary by tablet.

MALNUTRITION

Protein-energy deficiency syndromes
Many children in some parts of the world simply do not get enough to eat. Following a political or natural disaster, the news media have been quick to make us more aware of the severe forms of childhood malnutrition which are prevalent during famine.

A WHO Expert Committee divided the protein-energy deficiency syndromes into marasmus, where failure to grow is associated with emaciation and a fair appetite; kwashiorkor, where malnutrition is associated with oedema and loss of appetite; and 'unspecified' where growth retardation and undernutrition are evident without frank emaciation or oedema. These terms describe the various ways by which starvation can affect the growing child.

With starvation of whatever degree comes misery and an increased risk of infections. Both add to domestic problems and increase the risk of death or permanent damage.

Marasmus in western societies may be seen in infants born severely undernourished, or after severe chronic illnesses, particularly affecting the bowel. In poorer communities, nutritional marasmus commonly occurs due to failure of lactation in people who just cannot afford artificial milks. Thus it is more common in low-birth-weight infants, twins and in infants after infection, particularly gastroenteritis.

The infant's survival depends on the mother's ability to maintain lactation, even if the infant is unable to suckle for a few days. If food can be found, the prognosis of these infants is good. During a famine children of all ages may

Malnutrition

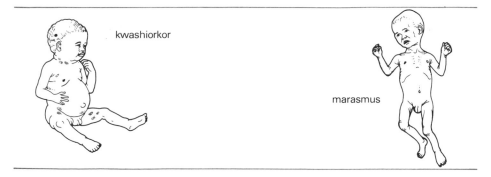

become marasmic and the recovery of older children may take longer. The risk of death due to superadded infection during the recovery phase is also higher.

Kwashiorkor is a colourful word that gives the impression of a specific disease entity but it is but one end of a spectrum. Most commonly, it occurs in children 18 to 24 months old at the time of weaning. The marasmic child receives a little of a balanced diet; in the child with kwashiorkor the energy intake may be just about adequate but the protein content is insufficient for growth. As a consequence there is muscle wasting but preservation of some subcutaneous fat.

The infant is oedematous, listless and irritable. There may be a 'flaky paint' dermatitis of a depigmented skin and the hair is sparse and friable. The liver may be large due to fatty infiltration and the serum albumin concentration may be reduced.

The complications include hypothermia, hypoglycaemia, drowsiness, severe diarrhoea, cardiac failure and all these are compounded by superimposed infections.

An inadequate supply of food is not primarily a medical problem. However the health service can help in the following ways:

1. By encouraging and supporting the lactating mother; there is no reason why breast feeding should not be continued for 18 or 24 months.
2. By advising parents about weaning.
3. By recommending those local foods which will meet the protein needs of the growing child.
4. By the early recognition of children in difficulties so that limited food resources can be optimally deployed.
5. By the treatment of associated infections and vitamin deficiency states.

OBESITY

Obesity is a common health problem when food is in abundance. Fat parents tend to have fat children for there is a genetic component in the aetiology. Fat children tend to but do not invariably become fat adults. Fat people die on average at a younger age than thin people. In particular, fat adults are more likely to develop diabetes and hypertension; they weather chronic chest disease, heart failure and

Skin fold thickness

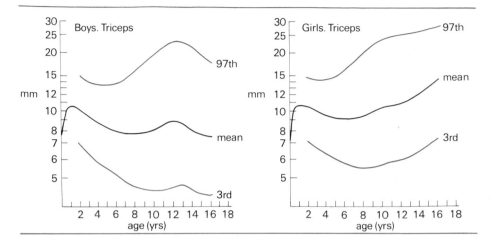

abdominal operations badly; and they have more problems with varicose veins, piles and skin crease ailments.

Obesity can be assessed reasonably well just by looking at the child and by plotting body weight on a centile chart. The height:weight ratio and skin fold thicknesses can be measured if more accurate analysis is required.

Prevention. As obesity is so difficult to treat it is best to avoid it. There is some evidence that bottle-fed babies are more likely to become overweight than breast-fed infants. This may be because the baby is less able to resist pressures to finish the bottle. Obesity may develop in the months after weaning when clearing the plate or emptying the cup becomes a virtue. Early weaning encourages this development. There is little virtue in commencing weaning before four or five months of age. One big meal a day appears to be more fattening than many small ones amounting to similar caloric value. Thus, the best prophylaxis for infants at risk of obesity because of fat parents is for them to be breast fed and weaned late; overfeeding should be avoided, particularly during the weaning period and the habit of taking regular exercise and eating small frequent meals should be established.

Who is for dieting

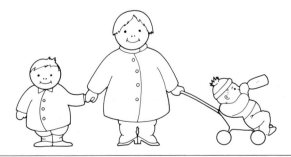

Treatment. Obese children may be referred for medical advice for a variety of reasons. The child may be concerned because of his appearance or the clothes he is required to wear or because he is teased. His parents may be concerned for the same reasons but also because they fear it may affect his health in other ways. His teachers may be concerned because of his lack of physical fitness. If the child really wants to be thinner and his parents are prepared to put themselves out to help him then there is some hope that a diet and exercise regimen will work. However, occasionally over-eating is an outward sign of inner confusion and unhappiness. This needs to be recognised and discussed. But in the majority of cases a detailed enquiry brings little to light except bad parental dietary attitudes and practices. One mother still gave her child aged seven years a breast feed at night; another considered that a bumper gorge was a high treat; a third used food to settle a particularly active and demanding baby.

BIBLIOGRAPHY

McClaren D S, Burman D 1976 Textbook of paediatric nutrition. Churchill Livingstone, Edinburgh.
Foman S J 1976 Nutritional disorders of children. D. H. & W. Publication No. (HSA) 76-5612
Gunther M 1970 Infant feeding. Methuen, London
Jelliffe D B, Jelliffe P E F 1979 Human milk in the modern world. Oxford University Press, Oxford
McKeith R, Wood C 1977 Infant feeding and feeding difficulties. Churchill Livingstone, Edinburgh
Paul A M, Southgate D A T 1978 The composition of foods. H.M.S.O., London

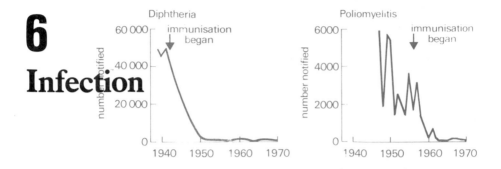

6
Infection

Infections spread readily among children. Acute respiratory infections, gastroenteritis and the main subject of this Chapter, the infectious 'fevers' account for a very large part of childhood illness, although scourges of the past, such as diphtheria and poliomyelitis, have now virtually disappeared. Infections are most likely to occur when the child first mixes with others, at a nursery, a playgroup or at primary school, and he may bring them home to his younger siblings. Often the infectious fever is diagnosed by the mother and the child is not very ill and can usually be looked after at home. If hospital admission is required it is often for social rather than medical reasons, however occasionally complications arise which are potentially damaging or life threatening.

MEASLES

Measles is a common and very infectious viral disease. The incubation period of about ten days is followed by a prodromal illness with fever, coryza, conjunctivitis and cough. Generalised lymphadenopathy may be found, and tiny white spots on a bright red background, Koplik's spots, are present on the buccal mucosa of the

Measles

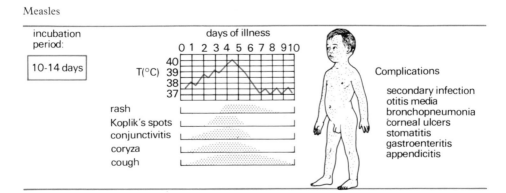

cheeks. After three or four days a florid maculopapular rash appears, and spreads downwards from the head and neck to cover the whole body. The earlier lesions are more numerous and become confluent and blotchy. The rash begins to fade by the third day and the child's general condition improves steadily.

Respiratory complications, particularly bronchopneumonia and otitis media are common. Encephalitis occurs in about one in 1000 affected children and is manifested by headache, drowsiness and vomiting. Convulsions and coma begin 7 to 10 days after the onset of the illness. The course of encephalitis is unpredictable but about 15 per cent of cases die, and 25 per cent suffer brain damage resulting in mental retardation, fits, deafness, or behaviour disorders. Measles may be associated with a disturbance of immune mechanisms, especially lymphopenia. Defective immune response may also be the basis of the rare late complication, subacute sclerosing panencephalitis, which occurs 4 to 10 years after an attack of measles and is characterised by slow, progressive neurological deterioration. There are very high levels of measles antibody in the blood and cerebrospinal fluid, and measles virus antigen has been demonstrated in brain tissue.

In developing countries, measles carries a high morbidity and mortality. It tends to occur in younger children than in the U.K. (median age 17 months in Nigeria, 52 months in England and Wales). Reported mortality rates range from 5.5 per cent in East Africa to between 20 and 40 per cent in a selected hospital series in West Africa. In the malnourished child, a severe form of measles may occur with a confluent rash that darkens to deep red or purple, and then desquamates. This is followed by depigmentation of the skin which lasts for several weeks and may be associated with pyodermia. A sore mouth is common during the acute illness and may lead to cancrum oris; invariably breast feeding is disturbed. Diarrhoea is common and may persist for a long time, further aggravating any underlying malnutrition. Measles mortality rate is directly related to socio-economic conditions, and there is a strong correlation with the distribution of kwashiorkor. In young, susceptible children measles itself causes loss of weight. In a village in Nigeria almost 1 in 4 of children lost more than 10 per cent of their weight following an attack of measles, and the average time to regain the previous weight was seven weeks (Morley, 1973). It is, therefore, important to maintain the child's hydration and nutrition during the illness and afterwards. Measles immunisation is now being used widely in developing countries with the result that there is a fall in rates of mortality and a reduction of malnutrition. In these countries it should be given at 9 to 10 months of age.

RUBELLA

Rubella or German measles, is usually a mild illness, and may pass unrecognised. The incubation period is 14 to 21 days and there may be little or no fever or malaise before the appearance of the pink macular rash which lasts for about three days. Generalised lymphadenopathy, especially involving the suboccipital nodes may be present. A rising haemagglutinin inhibition antibody titre confirms the diagnosis. This test is seldom necessary in children but is essential when the possibility arises of rubella in early pregnancy. Complications of rubella, such a thrombocytopenia and encephalitis, do occur but they are rare. Arthritis may occur in adolescents.

German measles

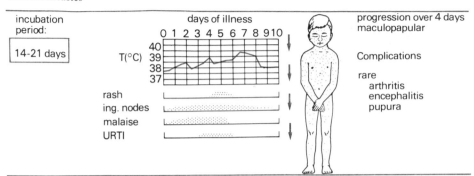

incubation period:	days of illness	progression over 4 days maculopapular

14-21 days

T(°C) 40 39 38 37
0 1 2 3 4 5 6 7 8 9 10

rash
ing. nodes
malaise
URTI

Complications

rare
arthritis
encephalitis
pupura

The importance of this disease lies in its devastating effect on the developing fetus if the mother contracts the infection during the first three months of pregnancy (see Ch. 3). A generalised viraemia may lead to fetal death and spontaneous abortion, or may affect the growth and development of the fetus resulting in a severely handicapped child with multiple congenital defects, classically including cataracts, deafness and congenital heart disease. It is in an attempt to prevent this disaster that immunisation against rubella has been introduced using an attenuated virus. Some countries, including the U.K., offer it to girls before leaving school; others (e.g. the U.S.A.) offer it to all school children. In the U.K. at present only 64 per cent of girls are actually receiving it.

ROSEOLA INFANTUM (EXANTHEM SUBITUM)

The patient is usually under two years of age. He develops a high fever, often without appearing particularly ill, though convulsions may occur. Examination reveals only a mild pharyngitis and lymphadenopathy. After three or four days the temperature drops suddenly to normal, and a macular rash appears which lasts for a few hours or a day or two. The child then makes an uneventful and rapid recovery.

SCARLET FEVER

Group A haemolytic streptococci are responsible for a variety of problems in children, especially tonsillitis. Sequelae such as rheumatic fever and acute glomerulonephritis are important, but have become rare in western societies. Scarlet fever results from infection with a strain of the organism which produces an erythrogenic toxin. After an incubation period of two to four days, the child develops tonsillitis, fever, headache and malaise. The rash develops within 12 hours of the onset and rapidly becomes generalised. It consists of a fine punctate erythema which blanches on pressure. The face is spared, but the cheeks are flushed so that the child is indeed 'scarlet', apart from the area around the mouth. The tongue has a thick white coating through which the inflamed papillae project, the 'white strawberry tongue'. By day four or five the tongue peels, leaving a 'red strawberry' appearance. The skin rash fades after a few days, or sooner if

Scarlet fever

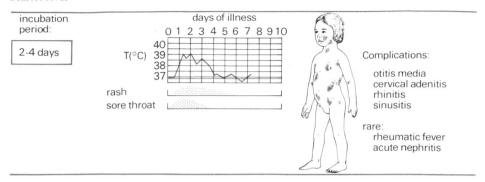

incubation period:

2-4 days

days of illness

0 1 2 3 4 5 6 7 8 9 10

T(°C)

rash

sore throat

Complications:

otitis media
cervical adenitis
rhinitis
sinusitis

rare:
rheumatic fever
acute nephritis

penicillin is given, followed by desquamation, especially on the hands and feet. This may persist for some time and is useful in making a retrospective diagnosis. Scarlet fever may also follow infection of wounds or burns. Treatment with penicillin leads to a rapid recovery, but a ten day course is necessary to eradicate the streptococci.

CHICKENPOX (VARICELLA)

Chickenpox is a common and highly infectious disease but is usually mild in children. The same virus produces herpes zoster. The incubation period is 14 to 16 days. There may be no symptoms apart from the rash and a low grade fever. Chickenpox spots appear in crops, progressing rapidly from macule to papule to vesicle. The vesicle soon dries and crusts and the scabs separate without scarring. Lesions may also occur on mucous membranes, especially in the mouth where they quickly rupture to produce shallow ulcers. Now that smallpox has been virtually eradicated from the world, problems of differential diagnosis are rare. The character and distribution of the rash are different, but expert virological help is necessary where modified forms of smallpox exist.

Complications of chickenpox are uncommon in healthy children. Encephalitis is rare but when it does occur there is often cerebellar involvement. The child presents with ataxia three to eight days after the onset of the rash. At least 80 per

Chicken pox

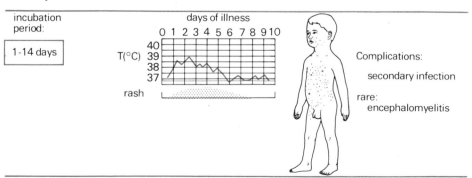

incubation period:

1-14 days

days of illness

0 1 2 3 4 5 6 7 8 9 10

T(°C)

rash

Complications:

secondary infection

rare:
encephalomyelitis

cent of affected children make a complete recovery. Pneumonia is a rare complication in children, but it may be part of the very rare severe form of the illness when the rash is haemorrhagic. This is more likely to occur in children with immune deficiency, in particular children treated for leukaemia.

HERPES SIMPLEX INFECTIONS

Infection with this virus is extremely common and usually asymptomatic, less than 10 per cent of children with primary infections becoming clinically ill.

Newborn infants may be infected during delivery by maternal genital herpes infection (Type 2) or, less commonly, by the usual Type 1 virus in the postnatal period. Infection may result in a severe, disseminated disease characterised by lethargy, vesicular rash, hepatosplenomegaly, bleeding and neurological symptoms. Mortality is about 70 per cent and there is a high morbidity rate among the survivors. The risk of this severe illness is about 40 per cent if the mother has active genital herpes at the time of delivery, and an elective Caesarean section should be considered.

Herpes virus Type 1 is spread by infected saliva and transmission therefore requires close personal contact. Primary infection may affect the mouth, skin or eyes. Acute gingivostomatitis is most common, particularly in preschool children from poor socio-economic circumstances. It is characterised by high fever, swelling and bleeding of the gums and extensive ulceration of the buccal mucosa, tongue and palate. The cervical glands are enlarged. Eating and drinking are painful, and the child may become dehydrated. The illness lasts about 10 to 14 days. A vulvovaginitis may result from transfer of the infection from the mouth by the child's finger.

Keratoconjunctivitis is associated with severe oedema of the eyelids and dendritic ulcers of the cornea which may lead to scarring and loss of vision. Primary infection of the skin with vesicular lesions tends to develop in older children, often at the site of trauma. In children with eczema, an extensive vesicular rash which later scabs may occur on the eczematous skin. The child may be febrile and sometimes there is generalised infection due to bloodstream spread, which is potentially fatal. Secondary infection of skin lesions is a complication.

The diagnosis of local infection is not difficult, as the vesicular lesions are characteristic. Rapid confirmation can be obtained by culture of the vesicular fluid or microscopic examination of scrapings for inclusion bodies. Topical treatment with idoxyuridine is partially effective.

Herpes simplex may cause generalised infection in malnourished children, or those with a cellular immune deficiency. It is also a relatively common cause of meningoencephalitis in apparently normal children and it can occur in the absence of skin lesions. The illness may be very severe and the mortality rate is high. Frontal and temporal lobe abnormalities are found on the electroencephalogram and a brain scan may demonstrate a 'space-occupying' lesion. A rising titre of antibody in the blood or cerebrospinal fluid confirms the diagnosis. Treatment has been attempted with drugs such as adenosine arabinoside but the results are disappointing so far. There has been some improvement in survival, but with a very high rate of chronic neurological handicap.

Recurrent herpes simplex infection is common and usually occurs as 'cold sores' round the mouth. The recurrence rate is very variable and though the lesions may be associated with respiratory infections, they may also be related to nonspecific factors such as sunshine, menstruation and emotional stress.

MUMPS

Mumps is caused by a paramyxovirus. Subclinical infection is common. A long incubation period of 16 to 21 days is followed by fever, malaise and enlargement of one or both parotid glands, which develop over a period of 1 to 3 days. The child may complain of earache and difficulty in swallowing, and the glands may be painful and tender. The submandibular glands may also be affected. The swellings settle in 7 to 10 days and there is no specific treatment. Other causes of parotitis are rare in children and distinction from cervical lymphadenopathy should not be difficult after careful examination.

Meningitis is a common complication, but is usually mild and characterised by headache, photophobia and neck stiffness. The cerebrospinal fluid contains an increased number of lymphocytes and a raised concentration of protein. Recovery is almost always complete. Epididymo-orchitis is a rare complication before puberty; pancreatitis is a recognised but uncommon complication.

Differential diagnosis of mumps and cervical adenitis

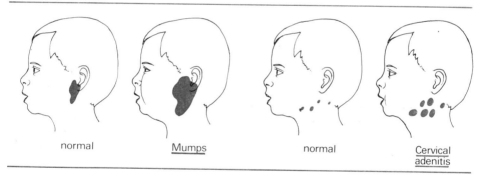

normal   Mumps   normal   Cervical adenitis

GLANDULAR FEVER

Glandular fever, infectious mononucleosis, occurs most often in adolescents and young adults, but is not uncommon in children. Infection is usually sporadic, though epidemics can occur in schools or residential homes. The Epstein-Barr virus is the cause of the infection and is excreted in nasopharyngeal secretions. Close contact is necessary for infection to be transmitted.

The onset of glandular fever is usually insidious and occurs after an incubation period of four to 14 days. The clinical features are anorexia, malaise and fever and they are usually accompanied by a sore throat and enlarged glands in most affected children. The tonsillitis may be very severe with a thick white exudate covering the tonsils and surrounding areas. Petechiae may be seen on the palate. Cervical lymph nodes are enlarged, and the spleen is often palpable. A macular rash occurs in 10 to 20 per cent of cases, especially if ampicillin has been given. Hepatitis, often with jaundice is common, but other complications such an pneumonitis and neurological disturbances are rare.

The diagnosis is supported by the presence of atypical mononuclear cells in the blood film. These large cells have an irregular nucleus and pale-staining cytoplasm containing vacuoles, and may account for 10 to 25 per cent of the total white cell count. The Paul-Bunnell test for antibodies is positive in about 60 per cent patients during the first week of the illness but the agglutinins may disappear by two to four weeks. These antibodies agglutinate sheep red blood cells and are not absorbed by guineapig kidney cells as are similar antibodies occurring sometimes in normal people. Horse red blood cells are also agglutinated, and this is the basis of the monospot test. Liver function tests are abnormal in over half the patients.

Glandular fever is a self-limiting disease for which there is no specific treatment. The lymphadenopathy and splenomegaly may persist for weeks or months, and there may be a long period of debility. The differential diagnosis when tonsillitis is severe includes streptococcal tonsillitis and diphtheria; when lymphadenopathy is prominent it includes leukaemia, toxoplasmosis and cytomegalovirus infection; and when jaundice or a rash are present, infectious hepatitis, measles or rubella may be suspected. However, the diagnosis is not difficult if the clinical features are characteristic and the appropriate laboratory tests are obtained.

PERTUSSIS (WHOOPING COUGH)

Bordetella pertussis is the cause of a prolonged respiratory illness which is particularly dangerous in infancy. After a seven-day incubation period, there is a 'catarrhal' stage lasting one to two weeks, during which the child is unwell, with signs of upper respiratory tract infection. A cough develops which becomes increasingly severe and paroxysmal. Spasms of coughing may be followed by an inspiratory 'whoop', especially in older children. Vomiting may occur, and the child can become cyanosed or apnoeic during coughing spasms and be left exhausted afterwards. Between spasms there may be no obvious respiratory difficulty and the lungs are clear on examination. This phase lasts four to six weeks, and the cough gradually improves over another two to three weeks. The causative organism is cultured in early cases from a nasopharyngeal swab using Bordet-Gengou medium, but is difficult to isolate once the cough is established. A striking lymphocytosis supports the diagnosis.

The most common complication is bronchopneumonia which is especially common in infants and accounts for most of the deaths. Bronchiectasis used to be a well-recognised sequela but is now very uncommon. Convulsions may occur due to asphyxia from severe spasms, intracranial bleeding or encephalopathy. Subconjunctival haemorrhages and facial petechiae due to raised venous pressure during spasms may be alarming but resolve spontaneously.

The treatment of pertussis is largely symptomatic and careful nursing is required. Oxygen, suction and tube-feeding may be necessary. Erythromycin given in the catarrhal stage may abort or modify the illness but the result is often disappointing. Its use in infant contacts is justifiable. No drugs prevent the spasms once the disease is established.

Immunisation against pertussis is the subject of considerable controversy at present following reports of neurological damage associated with reactions to the triple vaccine. The frequency of serious reactions is very difficult to assess as varying figures are reported. Similar neurological problems may occur in infancy unrelated to immunisation. The risk of vaccine damage has to be balanced against the risks of the disease itself. The incidence and mortality have fallen considerably, but there was an epidemic in 1977 to 1978 of about 100 affected children admitted to hospital in Nottingham during this time, almost all were infants. Seven had recurrent episodes of apnoea, one developed encephalopathy, and there was one death; so there is no doubt that pertussis is still a serious disease. A full course of immunisation reduces both the attack rate and the severity of the illness. The protection of infants depends on the state of immunity of their older siblings as maternal antibody does not cross the placenta. The first dose of vaccine is now recommended at three rather than six months of age. Present advice is that pertussis immunisation should be recommended, except where the child has had convulsions or is known to have a neurological disorder or where there is a close family history of epilepsy (Joint Committee on Vaccination and Immunisation, 1977).

A prospective study of childhood encephalopathy now in progress in the U.K. may help establish the true incidence of vaccine-related complications. If parents refuse pertussis immunisation, it is important to make sure that the child receives immunisation against diphtheria, tetanus and poliomyelitis which are normally given at the same time.

TUBERCULOSIS

Tuberculosis is no longer the 'captain of the kings of death' in Europe, but is still a major problem in many developing countries despite being both preventable and treatable. The incidence of TB in Europe fell steadily as a result of better social conditions and nutrition, and with the advent of effective chemotherapy. Most children with the disease are now contacts of asymptomatic adults, often their grandparents. The children of Asian families are at special risk of infection from recent adult immigrants.

In Nottinghamshire, 10 per cent of 12-year-old children tested in 1978 were Heaf positive, indicating that they had had a primary tuberculosis infection or had been immunised. Only three cases of TB in children under age 12 were notified in 1978 and 8 in 1977.

By contrast, 40 per cent of children in Bombay were Heaf positive by 14 years of age in 1961 to 1971, and 55 per cent by 20 years. TB was responsible for 7 per cent of total deaths in the one- to four-year-old age group, 8 to 9 per cent between 5 and 14 years and 15 to 16 per cent at 15 to 24 years.

Primary infection
Mycobacterium tuberculosis is spread by droplets, and primary infections may occur in the lung, skin or gut. Sensitivity to tuberculin develops four to eight

Primary tuberculosis

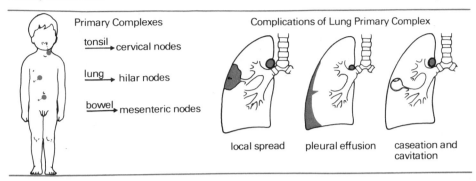

Primary Complexes

tonsil → cervical nodes

lung → hilar nodes

bowel → mesenteric nodes

Complications of Lung Primary Complex

local spread　　pleural effusion　　caseation and cavitation

weeks after infection, as shown by a positive Mantoux or Heaf test, though this may be absent if there is severe malnutrition or overwhelming infection. Sensitivity reactions such as erythema nodosum (red, shiny lumps on the shins), or phlyctenular conjunctivitis appear in a few cases. Local infection develops and spreads to lymph nodes, together these constitute the primary complex. Usually this heals slowly by fibrosis and may calcify, the process taking 12 to 18 months. In some children, complications may arise from local progression of the primary complex or from bloodstream spread. Children at special risk are the very young, malnourished or those suffering from an intercurrent infection such as measles or whooping cough.

Lung complications of tuberculosis. Miliary lesions are due to blood spread. The tubercles might be seen in the retina. Always suspect tuberculous meningitis

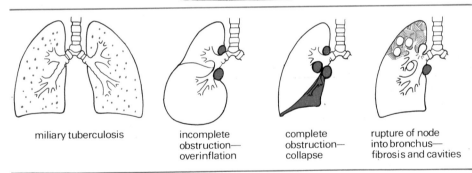

miliary tuberculosis

incomplete obstruction— overinflation

complete obstruction— collapse

rupture of node into bronchus— fibrosis and cavities

Pleural effusion may develop as a sensitivity reaction to the primary infection and is most common in children over five years of age. Empyema, caseation and cavitation occur more often in malnourished children from developing countries. Unless the lesion cavitates into a bronchus, children with primary TB do not cough up sputum, and are not infectious. General malaise, fever and loss of weight may occur but there may be little or no cough. The enlarged mediastinal glands may also cause problems. Adult pulmonary TB, characterised by cavitation, occurs later as the result of a new infection or breakdown of the primary complex.

Gastrointestinal lesions

A primary focus in the tonsillar region may present with cervical adenitis. This is usually due to human tuberculosis. Infection with the bovine strain due to infected milk may cause a primary lesion in the neck or bowel. Occasionally, the latter leads to malabsorption, stricture formation and peritonitis. Cervical adenitis may also follow infection with atypical mycobacteria.

Miliary TB and meningitis

Bloodstream spread is most common in young children, especially in developing countries, and almost always occurs within one year of infection. It accounts for at least 70 per cent childhood deaths due to TB. The child presents with fever, anorexia and loss of weight. The liver and spleen are usually enlarged and choroidal tubercles may be seen on examining the fundus. Chest auscultation may be normal or scattered crepitations may be heard. The chest X-ray shows generalised mottling. There may be associated meningitis which develops insidiously, with gradual progression of lethargy, headache, convulsions and coma. A tuberculoma of the brain, presenting as a space occupying lesion, is much commoner in developing countries than in Europe. The cerebrospinal fluid in TB meningitis is opalescent with increased lymphocytes and protein but low sugar. Adhesions may occur and hydrocephalus is an important complication. Other neurological damage is unfortunately common in survivors.

Tuberculosis of the bones and joints also develops as a result of bloodstream spread, usually within three years of infection. Renal infection may become apparent after five or more years.

Treatment

Chemotherapy, rifampicin and isoniazid for nine months, is advisable for all children found to have a primary complex, mainly to prevent miliary disease and meningitis. Treatment should also be given to children under five years with a positive Heaf test only, but over this age it is not necessary provided the child is kept under regular supervision and the chest X-ray is repeated after three months. Rifampicin may cause hepatitis, in which case ethambutol may be a suitable substitute. In TB meningitis streptomycin is also given for 6 to 12 weeks by intramuscular infection; in severe cases it may be given intrathecally as well. Rifampicin is very effective but it is expensive. In developing countries, tuberculosis is treated with isoniazid alone or in combination with thiacetazone for 18 months. If possible with this regimen an initial course of streptomycin should be given.

Prevention

It is essential to trace contacts of newly diagnosed patients and perform a Heaf test and chest X-ray. If the Heaf test is negative, it should be repeated after six weeks. If still negative, the contact should be offered BCG vaccination.

BCG vaccination essentially involves producing a highly modified primary infection with attenuated organisms. It has been shown to give 80 per cent protection against TB and in particular to protect completely against miliary spread. In this country, it is offered to 12-year-old school children who are Heaf negative, and to the newborn infants of Asian families. In countries with a high incidence of TB, routine neonatal vaccination is advisable after an initial campaign to reach as many of the population as possible. Initial Heaf testing is not essential; BCG can be given safely to positive reactors who produce an accelerated response. Following BCG, the Heaf test will become positive though not strongly so and it may revert after some years. Natural infection occurring after BCG vaccination will give a strongly positive reaction and difficulties with diagnosis are unlikely.

MALARIA

Malaria is endemic in many parts of the world. As a consequence of the increase in international travel more children suffering from malaria are seen in non-endemic countries. 'Where have you been?' is now an important question to ask of children presenting with an unexplained high fever.

   Characteristically, the fever is intermittent and the spleen enlarged, but these signs are not always present. There may be associated vomiting and rigors. The treatment is chloroquine by mouth in the appropriate dose. In certain parts of the world *Plasmodium falciparum* strains may be resistant to chloroquine. If the illness is due to *Plasmodium vivax*, a two week course of primaquine should also be given to eliminate the parasites from the liver and to prevent a subsequent relapse unless the patient has a glucose-6-phosphate dehydrogenase deficiency.

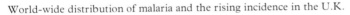

World-wide distribution of malaria and the rising incidence in the U.K.

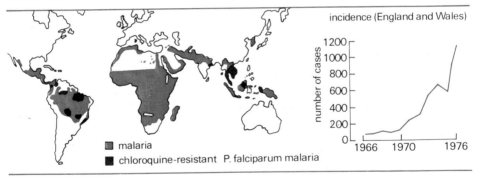

POLIOMYELITIS

The introduction of successful immunisation against poliomyelitis has been one of the greatest success stories of modern medicine. A dreadful disease has been virtually eradicated.

   In most people, the poliomyelitis virus produces a mild illness with fever, sore throat, headache and vomiting, lasting up to three days. In about one third of affected children this is followed by improvement for one to seven days and then a recurrence of more severe symptoms with pain and stiffness in the neck, back and legs. As in other types of viral meningitis, the cerebrospinal fluid contains increased lymphocytes and protein. Paralysis may develop in association with muscle pain and tenderness. This is due to anterior horn cell damage, is usually asymmetrical, and varies considerably in extent, in the severe forms causing

The clinical course of poliomyelitis

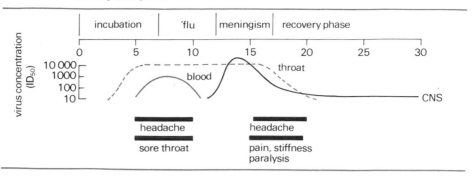

respiratory failure and bulbar paralysis. Once the fever subsides, the spread of weakness and paralysis is halted and there is then a slow improvement over a period of about 18 months. After this time any residual paralysis is likely to be permanent.

IMMUNISATION

Protection against some of the infectious diseases is available in the form of immunisation which is given at various stages throughout childhood and early adulthood. Immunisations for different diseases are scheduled in an attempt to balance the risks of the disease with the child's ability to produce a good immunological response. Immunisation should not be given if the child is unwell, and at least three weeks should elapse between each immunisation.

  Pertussis vaccine should not be given to children with a history of convulsions or neurological damage or to those with a close family history of epilepsy? *degree relative* Living attenuated virus vaccines, that is poliomyelitis, measles, rubella, BCG, should not be given to children with immune deficiency states, including those on corticosteroids and cytotoxic drugs, because of the risk of severe generalised infection.

Recommended immunisation programme for U.K.

Age	Immunisation		
Neonatal	BCG		Infants of Asian mothers or with family history of tuberculosis
3 months	Diphtheria Pertussis Tetanus Poliomyelitis	DPT	1st dose
5 months	DPT Poliomyelitis		2nd dose
10 months	DPT Poliomyelitis		3rd dose
1 year	Measles		
5 years	DT Poliomyelitis		
11 years	Rubella (girls) BCG		(Heaf negative)
15–19 years	Tetanus toxoid Poliomyelitis		

Incidence of whooping cough in the U.K. In the last few years immunisation rates have fallen. Note the recent increase in incidence

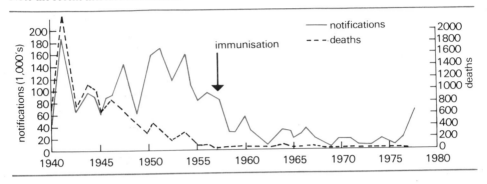

IMMUNE DEFICIENCY

Contact with infecting organisms is one of the major challenges that face the newborn infant as he establishes an independent existence. Cellular immunity is present at birth, and although the neutrophil count is relatively low the infant is able to respond to bacterial infection with a leucocytosis. Humoral immunity is not well developed in infancy, but the infant is protected initially by maternal IgG antibodies which cross the placenta, and IgA which he receives in colostrum and breast milk. IgM does not cross the placenta, but the infant is capable of producing it in response to infection.

Maternally provided IgG globulins are progressively catabolised so that the infants circulating immunoglobulins fall to a minimal level at two to three months. The subsequent rise parallels endogenous production as a result of exposure to environmental antigens. IgM concentrations reach normal adult levels earliest followed by IgG and then IgA.

Sometimes there is a delay in synthesis of immunoglobulins, especially in preterm babies. Low levels of IgA are particularly common and may persist for years. IgA is important in the protection of mucosal barriers and its absence predisposes to recurrent respiratory infection.

Most children with recurrent infections are normal, but immunological investigation should be undertaken when recurrent bacterial or fungal infections occur.

Examples of diseases due to defects in the body defences

Immune deficiency	Pathogens	Disease	Treatment
Humoral	Bacteria, pneumocystis	Agammaglobulinaemia	Gammaglobulin
Cellular	Viruses, tuberculosis, candida	DiGeorge's syndrome (absent thymus)	Thymus graft
Stem cell	Bacteria, pneumocystis, viruses, tuberculosis, candida	Combined immune deficiency syndrome	Bone marrow graft
Complement deficiency	Bacteria		Antibiotics
Neutrophil disorders	Bacteria	Chronic granulomatous disease	Antibiotics

There are a number of rare inherited disorders of the immune mechanisms, the immune deficiency syndromes. However, immunological deficiencies may also occur in association with systemic illness, for example transient immunosuppression occurs during viral infections, especially measles, and the resulting susceptibility to infection contributes to malnutrition which in turn impairs defence mechanisms. Susceptibility to infection also occurs in relapsed nephrotic syndrome which limits the available immunoglobulins. Corticosteroid and cytotoxic therapy also reduces immunological competence.

BIBLIOGRAPHY

Jelliffe D B, Stanfield J P 1978 Diseases of children in the sub-tropics and tropics. Arnold, London
Krugman S, Ward R, Katz S L 1977 Infectious diseases of children. Mosby, St Louis
Morley D 1973 Paediatric priorities in the developing world. Butterworth, London

Bruton - agammaglob → bact   x rec

Swiss type   "   - ↓ L-cytes also   Autorec.
                also viral, fungal inf! →↑
            (Gitlin's similar) - x link/autorec.

Ig A. defic   resp, sinus inf⁵   Auto rec
                                 enteropathy

Wiskott - Aldrich   Thrombocytopaenia
                                eczema   x-link rec
                                Ig M defic
                                egotitis media

7
Hazards

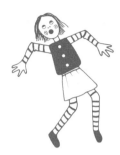

Accidents are by far the commonest cause of death in children over the age of a year. Recently in the U.K. the number of deaths due to accidents has declined but still approximately 1000 children between the ages of one and 14 years die each year as a result of an accident. Road accidents are by far the commonest cause of childhood accidental fatalities, followed by drowning and burns. For every child who is killed, many are seriously injured and many more receive minor injuries. Again in the U.K. about 150 000 children each year have to be admitted to hospital following an accident; this represents nearly a fifth of all paediatric admissions and one child in 80 of the whole child population. As many as one child in six attends a hospital casualty department each year with an injury and a similar number seek advice from their general practitioner. As well as killing and injuring children, accidents are also expensive!

How do accidents in childhood differ from those affecting adults? Three factors are important in any accident: the causative agent or situation, for example a car or a swimming pool; the circumstances in which it took place, for example the degree of parental supervision; and most important of all, the child himself. The type of accident is related to the age, sex, intelligence, social circumstances and

Accident rates in England and Wales, 1960 to 1976

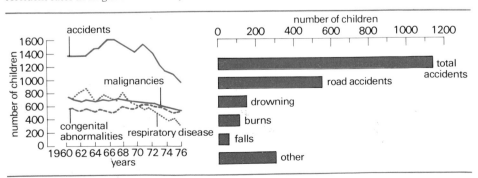

Causes of accidents at home

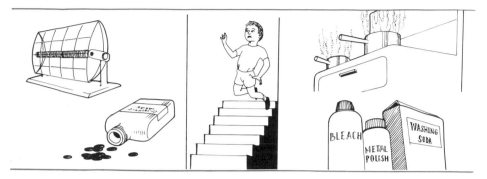

personality of the child. Physical and mental development is particularly important. The toddler is fearless and inquisitive, but spends most of his time indoors, so that he is susceptible to falls, burns and self-poisoning. The child who has just started school is impulsive but inexperienced, and therefore likely to be knocked down by a car. The older school child is vigorous and adventurous, he is likely to fall and injure himself while climbing or to drown in a quarry or canal.

An understanding of the cause of accidents may lead to prevention. A young toddler cannot be reasoned with and therefore he must be protected by those around him and by those who design his house and its contents. The young school child can be actively taught about the dangers of traffic, but equally those who design schools, playgrounds and streets must take account of his inexperience. The older child can scarcely be prevented from taking risks and resents adult interference. He must learn to come to terms with himself and the amount of risk he can safely take. Most minor accidents are unavoidable and it is both unrealistic and possibly undesirable to seek ways of avoiding them altogether for they are all part of a child's experience, part of his education. But it is surely the duty of planners and educators to try to reduce the number of *serious* accidents which cause death or severely damage children to an absolute minimum.

INJURIES

Road traffic accidents

Nearly a half of all accidental deaths are a result of road accidents. As in most

Road accidents

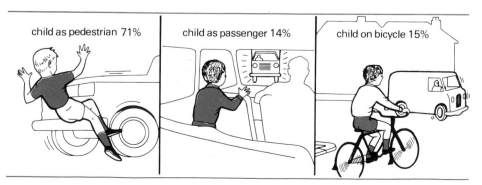

child as pedestrian 71%   child as passenger 14%   child on bicycle 15%

accidents, it is predominantly boys who are killed or injured. Most road accidents occur when the child is on foot and is hit by a moving vehicle. In a minority of instances the child is either riding a bicycle or a passenger in a car. The management consists of dealing with the multiple injuries in order of priority.

Falls

Children frequently suffer slight head injury as a result of falling out of beds, cots or windows, down stairs or from trees, climbing frames and so forth. While such injuries are not usually fatal, they are a common cause of hospital admission.

Head injury

In western societies, head injury is a common cause of death in childhood and many who survive are left with severe and permanent brain damage. However, of all children who are thought to merit admission for observation, only 5 per cent will prove to have major brain injury.

Indications for admission. As most children with head injuries are conscious when seen in the accident and emergency department, it is often hard to know whether or not to admit them for observation. A child should be admitted if the blow was or may have been severe, or if he momentarily lost consciousness or had a period of impaired consciousness. The presence or absence of a skull fracture should not be regarded as the deciding factor: extensive brain damage can be present and is indeed more likely in a child *without* fracture. Extreme pallor and vomiting are common in young children, even after a very minor bump, but if they are marked or persistent then they obviously merit admission. Certain features in a conscious, rational child are obviously absolute indications for admission; blood or c.s.f. from the nose or the ear, conjunctival haemorrhage without a definable limit, a scalp wound with a underlying fracture, and a fracture crossing the groove of the middle meningeal artery. Many children can be allowed home if instructions regarding observations are given to the parents, and it is felt that these will be carried out.

Skull X-rays need not be carried out for every minor bump on the head, but they are essential where the trauma has been severe or where there is scalp injury. Cervical spine X-rays should also be performed where the trauma has been severe.

The most frequent important complication of head injury is cerebral oedema. It

Management of head injuries

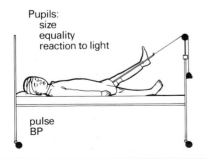

Pupils:
 size
 equality
 reaction to light

pulse
BP

Level of consciousness:
 1. drowsy but responding to command
 2. unconscious but responding to minimal stimuli
 3. unconscious but responding to maximal painful stimuli
 4. unconscious and unresponsive

Focal neurological signs:
 paralytic squint
 hemiplegia

is more common in children than in adults because of their soft easily distorted skull. In an adult the kinetic energy is absorbed by the occurrence of a fracture whereas in a child, the skull distorts and all the kinetic energy is transmitted to the brain. The resulting pressure waves and stresses within the brain cause extreme pallor, impaired consciousness and severe vomiting, usually lasting only a few hours but sometimes two to three days. During this period it is important to be sure that the child is ventilating well since a high pCO_2 causes a rapid increase in cerebral oedema.

Less commonly, intracranial bleeding occurs. This may be extradural, usually from the middle meningeal artery and therefore rapid in onset, or else subdural from cerebral veins and of slower onset. The head-injury observations of level of consciousness, pulse, BP and pupil size and reactivity are intended to make early detection of these relatively uncommon occurrences possible. The presence of intracranial blood or a sudden increase in cerebral oedema, perhaps because of hypoventilation, is indicated by a fall in the level of consciousness, a falling pulse rate, rising blood pressure, and alterations in the size and reactivity of the pupils. If the intracranial lesion is unilateral so will be the pupillary changes.

If intracranial bleeding is suspected, three exploratory burr holes are made on each side of the head, in the frontal, temporal and parietal regions. If blood clot is found it is washed out, visible bleeding points are coagulated and the wound is closed with drainage. Often no blood is found only a swollen brain. A child with a skull fracture is unlikely to develop a clot under tension because it will often decompress via the fracture.

It is often asked whether intravenous fluids should be given to a child with a head injury: there is no doubt that a period of relative dehydration is of some benefit; on the other hand, if a child's condition is worrying, the presence of an i.v. line is comforting; indeed, it may be essential for some other injury. If it has been introduced for the head injury alone only sufficient fluid should be given to keep the line open, that is 5 to 10 ml/h.

DROWNING

Most drowning accidents occur in inland waters, swimming pools and baths. About a quarter occur in the sea. Again, boys are more commonly involved than girls. Swimming and life saving lessons at school, wearing life-jackets on boats and having supervision at pools and beaches are important preventive measures. Occasionally, children play the game of hyperventilation before a dive so that they may stay under the water for a long time. This can be dangerous and should be discouraged.

Children die during drowning either as a result of laryngeal spasm, when the cause of death is cerebral anoxia (dry drowning), or else water may enter the lungs, rapidly leading to respiratory failure with cardiac arrest (wet drowning). In either situation, the child may respond well to immediate cardiac massage and artificial ventilation once the airway has been cleared. Sometimes, if the water is muddy or polluted, the child may be revived only to die later with progressive pneumonia and pulmonary oedema (secondary drowning).

BURNS AND SCALDS

Most accidents involving burns and scalds occur at home, particularly in poorer families. The inquisitive toddler is fascinated by matches and by flames. He knocks over paraffin heaters, goes too close to the open fire and sets light to his clothes, grasps a saucepan of boiling water by the handle and pulls it over himself or pulls a boiling electric kettle by the flex. Burns outside the home involving bonfires and fireworks tend to happen to older children.

The immediate treatment is to relieve the pain, ensure an adequate airway, and then assess the extent of the burns. If more than 10 per cent of the child's surface area is burned, intravenous fluids (plasma and saline) are necessary. If more than 50 per cent of the child's surface area is affected, the chances of survival are poor. Large quantities of fluid, blood and protein are lost from the burned areas and have to be replaced. A careful eye must be kept on the child's urine output and haematocrit. Tetanus toxoid and antibiotics are frequently used. Skin grafting may well necessary at a later date. Children who have been burned are often also psychologically adversely affected.

Supervision of toddlers in the home is the most important aspect of prevention of burns and scalds. The diminishing use of open fires and paraffin heaters, and the increased use of central heating has resulted in a decline in the incidence of burns in children in the last 20 years.

POISONING

Few children die as a result of poisoning, but many thousands are admitted to hospital each year for observation. Occasionally a child may intentionally ingest a poison, but in most cases the self-poisoning is accidental. Children may also be poisoned deliberately by their parents or inadvertently by their doctors. Most children who ingest a poison are fearless, inquisitive toddlers attracted by the appearance of tablets, medicines, household and garden substances, berries, seeds or fungi. They will eat almost anything, regardless of taste. It has been shown that a child is particularly likely to ingest a poison when the family is under some sort of stress, presumably because of decreased supervision.

The management of a poisoned child consists of removal of the poison, followed by observation for the expected symptoms and signs. Treatment is generally

Age of children admitted to hospital after accidental poisoning

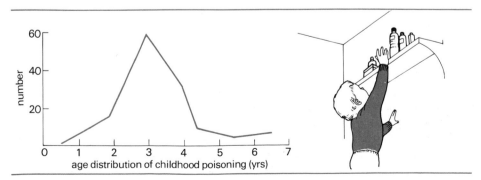

age distribution of childhood poisoning (yrs)

Some poisonous toadstools

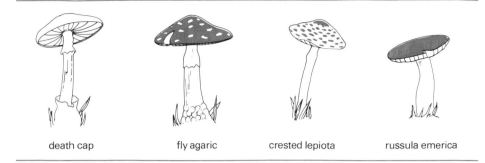

death cap   fly agaric   crested lepiota   russula emerica

symptomatic and nonspecific. Vomiting is induced to remove the poison from the stomach by giving the child syrup of ipecacuanha. Gastric lavage is rarely necessary, but emetic administration is obviously inappropriate for the unconscious child and in such cases the stomach should be emptied by lavage, but only after intubation with a cuffed endotracheal tube. Induced vomiting serves little purpose if more than four hours have passed since the ingestion, although there are exceptions, for example in cases of ingested aspirin and atropine, which delay gastric emptying. Vomiting is also to be avoided after ingestion of corrosive substances, or volatile agents such as paraffin or turpentine which are likely to be inhaled and may cause lung damage.

If the side effects of a poison are not known, information can be obtained at any time of day or night from one of the regional poison centres. Children likely to have ingested a toxic agent are admitted to hospital for observation. If respiratory failure develops, mechanical ventilation is necessary. If cardiovascular shock occurs, intravenous plasma or saline should be given.

Specific poisons

Aspirin is a respiratory stimulant and a cell poison. When taken in large quantities it produces nausea, vomiting, tinnitus and dehydration. Hyperventilation with deep sighing respirations is a consequence of both metabolic acidosis and respiratory alkalosis. Hypoglycaemia, hyperglycaemia and an

Some poisonous berries

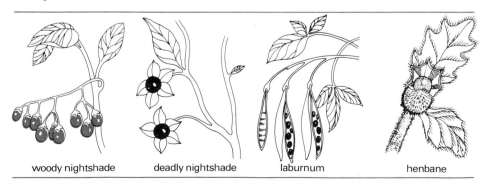

woody nightshade   deadly nightshade   laburnum   henbane

increased prothrombin time may occur in cases of severe poisoning. Fortunately children do not usually ingest sufficient amounts of aspirin to develop symptoms. If they do, then active steps should be taken to hasten the excretion of aspirin. When blood levels of salicylate are high, excretion should be enhanced by inducing a diuresis and reducing tubular reabsorption of the drug by making the urine alkaline. As with most poisons, there is no specific antidote.

Iron tablets are frequently swallowed by toddlers because they are likely to be available (for example, iron tablets are routinely prescribed throughout pregnancy) and because they look like sweets. A small child can be fatally poisoned by as little as 2 grams of iron. The progress of a poisoned child can be divided into four phases. Firstly, within an hour of the ingestion the child develops severe gastrointestinal symptoms, diarrhoea, vomiting, haematemesis and melaena. These symptoms may gradually subside so that the child seems well. However, some hours later, the serious third phase may develop with iron encephalopathy manifested by coma and fits, liver damage and circulatory collapse. Finally, a child who survives this may develop scarring of the stomach and pylorus as a consequence of local irritation. Iron ingestion is an indication for gastric lavage. The iron chelating agent desferrioxamine is useful. It can be left in the stomach to prevent further absorption of iron and it can be administered parenterally to enhance iron excretion and lessen the severity of the poisoning.

Tricyclic agents such as amitriptyline and imipramine are among the commonest and most dangerous drugs consumed by young children. They may be available because one of the parents is taking them for depression or because a child in the family is being treated for bed-wetting. The effects of poisoning include respiratory and cardiovascular depression, as well as cerebral stimulation leading to irritability, excitation, hallucinations and fits, with exaggerated tendon reflexes. They have a marked atropine-like action, with fixed dilated pupils, a dry, red skin, sinus tachycardia, urinary retention and paralytic ileus. Finally, their most serious effect is on heart rhythm, resulting in atrial and ventricular tachycardias, fibrillation or heart block. There is no specific antidote, but after removal of the poison the atropine-like symptoms may be improved by anticholinesterase drugs and the cardiac arrythmias may respond to β-adrenergic blocking agents.

Child-resistant containers

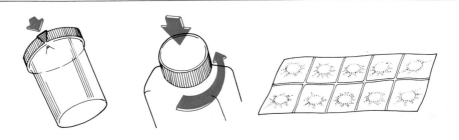

Important recent developments have lead to a decrease in the incidence of severe accidental poisoning in children. Child-resistant containers have been developed which can only be opened by lining up an arrow on the lid with an arrow on the bottle or by pushing the lid down and twisting it open at the same time. In the U.K. it is compulsory for all aspirin and paracetamol tablets to be prescribed in this way, and pharmacists are encourage to disperse other dangerous tablets in this form too. 'Blister packs' are also helpful. It takes the child a long time to eat sufficient tablets to cause symptoms, and he frequently loses interest or is discovered in the act.

OTHER HAZARDS

The risk of a noxious agent producing permanent damage is highest in the earliest phase of development, embryogenesis. A number of such agents have been identified as being associated with a high incidence of congenital abnormalities.

Environmental factors after birth are less easy to identify because so many children are exposed to potential hazards, and the ill effects may be quite subtle, making an association difficult to prove. Two hazards will be considered here, one physical, the other chemical.

Smoking
The harmful effects of smoking on those who actually smoke are well known. Chronic bronchitis, lung cancer and coronary heart disease are three common conditions whose incidence is greatly increased in smokers. Many school children now smoke regularly and are therefore at risk. It is obviously important to try to dissuade children from taking up smoking by appropriate health education in schools. It is also known that the children of smoking parents have a higher incidence of bronchitis and pneumonia; this applies particularly to babies and young children. Presumably the passive inhalation of tobacco smoke by the children at home is the important factor.

Lead
Lead is an environmental element which is undoubtedly harmful. If it is ingested or inhaled in large quantities it can produce a serious illness which may be lethal or result in brain damage. Less certain, however, is the effect that chronic exposure to environmental lead has on mental development. There are several sources of lead. It used to be present in paint, so that children who chewed painted surfaces were liable to be poisoned. Water in lead pipes may contain sufficient lead to cause poisoning. Lead fumes produced by burning car batteries may produce toxic symptoms. Asian families use lead salts ('surma') in cosmetics applied regularly to the conjunctivae of the child and this may cause poisoning. More recently, there has been concern about atmospheric lead. Lead is present in exhaust fumes from vehicles and blood lead levels are higher in urban children and in those living close to major motorways. It has been suggested, but not proven, that this chronic exposure to moderate amounts of atmospheric lead may produce permanent intellectual impairment.

A child who has ingested lead may show symptoms of encephalopathy, with irritability, drowsiness, convulsions and eventually coma. Papilloedema may be present. Colicky abdominal pain is common and an abdominal X-ray may actually show radio-opaque lead fragments in the gastrointestinal tract. The diagnosis is made on the clinical picture, a history of exposure to a source of lead and investigations. Blood lead levels can be measured and are a guide to severity of poisoning. Lead affects many enzyme systems, but particularly those involved in haem synthesis. Measurement of blood levels of haem precursors forms the basis of a screening test for early lead poisoning which can be carried out in children who are at risk. In chronic poisoning, lead interferes with the growing ends of bones producing the X-ray sign 'lead lines'.

The treatment of a poisoned child is directed at removing lead from the body. This is achieved by using lead-chelating agents which increase lead excretion. In severe cases with encephalopathy, calcium edetate (EDTA) and dimercaprol (British Anti-Lewisite, BAL) are given parenterally. In less severe cases oral D-penicillamine is used. If there are signs of raised intracranial pressure, cerebral oedema can be lessened by intravenous mannitol or dexamethasone. The source of the lead must obviously be identified and removed. Severe lead poisoning carries a high mortality and survivors are often neurologically handicapped.

BIBLIOGRAPHY
Jackson R H 1977 Children, the environment and accidents. Pitman, Tunbridge Wells

8
Airway and Lungs

Acute respiratory problems are the commonest reason for a child visiting a doctor and are responsible for approximately 50 per cent of all patient-doctor contact. More serious respiratory illness leads to about 30 per cent of hospital admissions and respiratory disease appears to be an important factor in some 30 per cent of children who die. The preschool child has on average, six to eight respiratory infections per year, ranging from mild colds to severe bronchiolitis. Lower respiratory infections are commonest in the first year of life and then fall in incidence, presumably because of increasing resistance.

These impressive statistics are not surprising as the need to breathe air in and out of the lungs makes the respiratory tract particularly susceptible to infection. In the upper airways there are elaborate defence mechanisms and most of the infections that do occur are confined to this area. The majority of infections are viral with rhino, respiratory syncytial, influenza, para-influenza and adenoviruses being most prevalent. Though less common, bacterial infections still produce serious illness sometimes with residual damage. The bacteria which invade the respiratory tract include the β-haemolytic streptococcus, the pneumococcus, *Haemophilus influenzae* and the coagulase positive staphylococcus. In infants and those with impaired resistance the gram negative bacilli including *E. coli* and pseudomonas are also found.

Incidence of disease in childhood

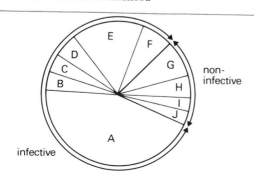

A. respiratory disease
B. whooping cough
C. staphylococcal infections
D. alimentary infections
E. infectious diseases
F. other infections
G. accidents
H. urticaria
I. environmental—developmental
J. other non-infective

UPPER RESPIRATORY TRACT

Coryza (common cold)

Coryza is usually a mild illness characterised by nasal obstruction and discharge usually due to one of the many rhinoviruses. There may be associated constitutional symptoms. It can be troublesome in infants under three months of age who are obligate nasal breathers, when feeding can become a major problem. There is also a suggestion that mild viral upper respiratory tract infections may be an important factor in some infants who die suddenly at home, cot deaths. Treatment with anti-pyretics and nasal decongestants may help feeding and reduce irritability. Antibiotics are not indicated unless there is good evidence to suggest secondary bacterial infection.

Pharyngitis and tonsillitis

These infections can occur at any age but are seen most frequently in children aged 4 to 7 years. The majority are caused by one of the many viruses which invade the respiratory tract but β haemolytic streptococcal infections do occur and may have important systemic reactions, for example scarlet fever, rheumatic fever and acute glomerulonephritis. On examination, the feverish child will have swelling and inflammation involving his tonsils and pharyngeal mucosa. If an exudate is not visible, the infection is almost certainly viral. The presence of pus suggests, but is by no means diagnostic of, bacterial infection. Confirmation by culture of throat swabs is an ideal which is seldom possible in general practice but it does provide a scientific basis for eradicating streptococcal infection in the child and close contacts. Streptococcal infections require treatment with oral penicillin for 10 to 14 days. If, as is often the case, the tonsillitis is associated with abdominal pain and vomiting, the initial dose should be given parenterally. The other disease which regularly produces an acutely inflamed throat with exudate is glandular fever. In this condition there are often punctate haemorrhages at the junction of the soft and the hard palates.

Tonsillectomy and adenoidectomy

Children who have recurrent infections in the upper respiratory tract are often considered for adenoidectomy and tonsillectomy. These operations are not without their problems and occasionally lead to death. As children on average get

Upper airway infections

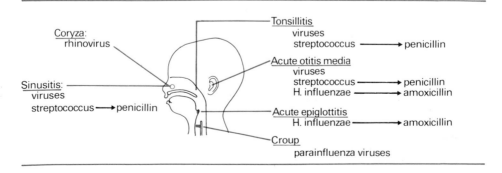

tender

7+ ? C . lymphadenopathy.

six to eight infections per year, recurrent tonsillitis alone is not sufficient reason for proceeding to operation. The indications for tonsillectomy are frequent attacks of tonsillitis which interfere with development or schooling, and peri-tonsillar abscesses. Enlargement of the tonsils is not of itself an indication unless they are so massive that they obstruct the airway. Tonsillar tissue shrinks spontaneously in later childhood. The adenoids should be removed if they are so large as to obstruct the Eustachian tube with resultant recurrent otitis media, if there is persistent nasal obstruction or if they interfere with speech.

risks of op: haem, cardiac arrest, pneumonia

Otitis media

Earache is very common in children and is often associated with upper respiratory tract infection. This does not necessarily mean that the infection involves the middle ear, for the pain may be due to pressure changes resulting from obstruction to the Eustachian tube. The diagnosis of acute otitis media is based on ear pain with fever, associated with a bright red, bulging drum. Infants too young to complain of earache are irritable, restless and scream. Examination of the tympanic membrane is an essential part of the routine examination of any child with fever. The pathogens include viruses, the pneumococcus, the β-haemolytic streptococcus, and *Haemophilus influenzae*. Treatment with a 7- to 10-day course of penicillin is indicated in the older child. Those under the age of three years should be given a broad spectrum antibiotic (amoxycillin) as at this age *Haemophilus influenzae* infections predominate. Relief of pain can be accelerated by giving analgesics and decongestants to help drainage through the Eustachian tubes. Myringotomy is rarely required.

Before antibiotics, otitis media was followed by many complications including acute mastoiditis. Fortunately these are now rare, but recurrent ear infections still lead to a chronic exudative otitis media ('glue ear'), with subsequent conductive hearing loss. The parents may not be aware how much the child's ears have been involved in respiratory infections and his problems only come to light because of inattention at school. If this condition does not respond to simple treatment with decongestants, surgical drainage of the middle ear may be required. *adenoidect grommets.*

Acute sinusitis

Viral infections may spread to the para-nasal sinuses. There may also be secondary bacterial infection in the maxillary sinuses, associated with fever, local tenderness and pain. As the frontal sinuses are not fully developed in early childhood, sinusitis is rarely a cause of frontal headache in the first ten years of life. On X-ray, the maxillary sinuses are usually completely opaque due to the presence of pus. The antibiotic of choice is penicillin but broad spectrum antibiotics such as amoxycillin should be prescribed if the child fails to respond. Recurrent or chronic infection can lead to post-nasal drip and a recurrent chronic cough with little or no evidence of local tenderness over the sinuses.

Acute laryngo-tracheobronchitis (Croup)

Croup tends to occur in epidemics particularly in autumn and early spring. It is almost exclusively viral in origin, commonly the influenza, para-influenza or respiratory syncitial virus. The larynx, trachea and bronchi are all involved in the inflammatory process. Symptoms start with a mild fever and runny nose. In the older child this progresses to sore throat, dysphagia and a dry, irritant cough. The younger child has a relatively small laryngeal airway and the resulting oedema and secretions can cause severe upper airway obstruction. The clinical features include a barking cough and a respiratory noise, particularly on inspiration (croup) which often start in the middle of the night. The natural tendency for the laryngeal airway to collapse on inspiration is increased by the child's desperate attempts to overcome the obstruction, thus exacerbating the situation. This effect is likely to be greater if parental anxiety is added to that of the child.

All children who are cyanosed or who have intercostal recession need to be admitted to hospital for observation. Many improve rapidly when they reach a warm, confident atmosphere but the occasional child has progressive airways obstruction which can only be relieved by tracheostomy or intubation. This intervention may be essential to prevent hypoxial brain damage or death. There is no evidence that putting the child in a cold mist tent or prescribing antibiotics or corticosteroids are of any value. It is of greater importance to reassure the child and to observe him carefully for signs of deterioration, measuring pulse rate, respiratory rate and looking for signs of hypoxial restlessness, cyanosis and deterioration in level of consciousness. If the child is showing evidence of these features or is becoming exhausted the obstruction must be relieved, preferably by tracheal intubation. This is a difficult procedure when the larynx is swollen and considerable skill will be required. If this fails, the obstruction must be relieved by tracheostomy.

Acute epiglottitis

This is a rare specific infection caused by *Haemophilus influenzae* Type B and produces sudden rapid oedema of the epiglottis and aryepiglottic folds. Lethal airway obstruction can develop within hours. The children are likely to be toxic and may, by the time they come into hospital, be semiconscious. The throat may be intensely sore, and occasionally the swollen, cherry red epiglottis can be seen welling up into the pharyngeal space. Attempts to get a good view with the help of a tongue depressor have led to fatal acute total obstruction and this examination should only be performed when facilities for immediate intubation or tracheostomy are available.   Lat XR.

Once the diagnosis is suspected the child must be admitted to hospital, nursed

Airway collapse occurs during inspiration in children with upper airway obstruction.

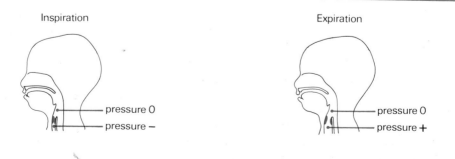

Inspiration

pressure 0
pressure −

Expiration

pressure 0
pressure +

in a humid atmosphere, propped up on pillows and given intravenous ampicillin (300 to 400 mg/kg/day). An alternative is chloramphenicol with an initial dose of 50 mg per kg intravenously followed by 50 mg/kg per day.

Despite adequate antibiotic therapy, many of these children develop such severe obstruction that intubation or tracheostomy is unavoidable.

Persistent stridor

There is a small group of children who have inspiratory stridor at birth which persists for many months. When this presents in the first weeks of life and follows a benign course, it is referred to as congenital floppy larynx, laryngomalacia or congenital laryngeal stridor and is presumably an exaggeration of the normal tendency for the larynx to collapse on inspiration. These infants often only have signs when excited or upset. No treatment is effective and fortunately intubation is rarely required. The stridor becomes less noticeable as the child grows and usually disappears by the age of one to two years. Symptoms are likely to get worse whenever the infant has an upper respiratory tract infection.

Persistent stridor may also be produced by pressure on the trachea from without, either by a mediastinal tumour or by a vascular ring due to a double aortic arch or anomalous origin of a large artery. This will be shown on barium swallow X-rays as the oesophagus also lies within the area of compression. Stridor can also result from lesions within the trachea including papillomas, haemangiomas and tracheal stenosis. Occasionally, a stridor present from birth is due to vocal cord palsy usually secondary to birth trauma but may also result from abnormality of the central nervous system including hydrocephalus.

If the child has stridor and recession while at rest, the investigations should include a barium swallow and direct laryngoscopy.

LOWER RESPIRATORY TRACT

Acute bronchitis

Upper respiratory viral infections frequently spread down the airway to involve the mucosa of the bronchi. The child has a troublesome cough which is initially dry but becomes productive after a few days. There is little to find on examination apart from a mild pyrexia. Towards the end of the attack the increased production of secretion may result in coarse rales and low pitched rhonchi. If the child is obviously wheezing, this is almost certainly an asthmatic attack precipitated by a viral infection in a susceptible subject. Primary bacterial bronchitis, with the exception of whooping cough, is rare in childhood and antibiotics are not indicated unless secondary infection is suspected. Night time cough suppressants are useful particularly in the early stages of the illness.

Acute bronchiolitis

This is the commonest of the severe acute infections and, like laryngo-tracheobronchitis, occurs in epidemics, usually in the winter months. It affects infants and toddlers. The respiratory syncitial virus is responsible for the majority but outbreaks can also be caused by the para-influenza, influenza, rhino- and adenoviruses.

Lower airway infections

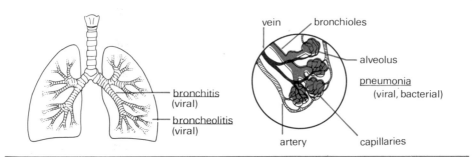

The inflammation predominantly affects the bronchioles whose calibre ranges from 75 to 300 μm leading to loss of cilia with oedema and necrosis of the epithelial cells and obstruction of the lumen by cellular debris and thick secretions. Typically, the child begins with coryzal symptoms and develops an irritable cough with rapid breathing and feeding difficulty within the next two to three days. If the illness is mild the child may then improve but in some it progresses with increasing breathlessness and cyanosis. In addition to the rapid, laboured respirations, the babies have tachycardia and often gross hyperinflation of their lungs, producing a barrel-shaped chest, prominent neck veins and downward displacement of the liver. Widespread crepitations can be heard over the lung fields, often with high-pitched rhonchi, particularly on expiration. The chest X-ray confirms the marked hyperinflation of the lungs but the picture is often complicated by areas of collapse produced by retained secretions.

The principles of management are similar to those of acute laryngo-tracheobronchitis; there is no specific measure that will alter the course of the disease. Confident supportive care with added oxygen in a carefully monitored setting is currently the best approach. Antibiotics are not indicated unless there is evidence of secondary bacterial infection which occurs rarely, and extensive clinical trials have demonstrated that corticosteroids do not modify the course of the disease. Physiotherapy should not be used in the early phase but may be helpful when the child is improving. Monitoring for apnoea and bradycardia are important as some of these children have recurrent attacks of apnoea even when not critically ill and appropriate stimulation early in the attack is usually successful. Should the baby's breathing become critical, artificial ventilation can be given but this requires considerable skill and inexperienced staff may do more harm than good attempting the exercise.

Pneumonia

Consolidation of the lung due to secondary infection is common in any child who is seriously ill. Patches of collapse and consolidation are not infrequent in a wide range of respiratory infections but should not influence the overall management of the child. Babies with feeding problems not infrequently inhale and produce patchy collapse and consolidation. In these instances physiotherapy is probably

Features seen on chest X-ray

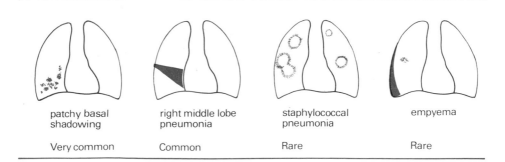

patchy basal shadowing	right middle lobe pneumonia	staphylococcal pneumonia	empyema
Very common	Common	Rare	Rare

more important than seeking an organism which might be responsible for a secondary infection.

Viral pneumonias. Primary viral infections can spread down the respiratory tract and into the lungs and should be suspected in any child, particularly those in the first year of life, in whom a respiratory infection has produced a serious illness with marked constitutional effects and circulatory failure. Respiratory syncitial virus, influenza, para-influenza and adenoviruses are among those most commonly implicated. Clinical examination of the child's respiratory system often gives little clue to the patchy shadowing which is demonstrated on a chest X-ray. Although the infection is supected to be viral, a broad spectrum antibiotic such as amoxycillin is likely to be given.

Mycoplasma pneumonia affects older children, particularly those between 5 and 15 years of age and can produce a wide range of respiratory tract infections. The picture most commonly seen is that of generalised malaise, anorexia with headache, fever and sore throat, followed by the development of a cough producing mucoid sputum occasionally tinged with blood. Fine crepitations may or may not be heard on examination. The chest X-ray may show either widespread diffuse shadowing or, on occasions, lobar or segmental consolidation. The diagnosis is made by culturing the organism or finding specific antibodies in the serum. The infection responds most readily to erythromycin.

Pneumococcal pneumonia. *Streptococcus pneumoniae* is a common secondary pathogen in the lung but occasionally produces a dramatic primary disease characterised by lobar or segmental consolidation. The child often appears very ill and drowsy and gives no clue to the site of the infection. Indeed, the headache and drowsiness with associated neck stiffness may lead to the child having a lumbar puncture before a chest X-ray. If the pneumonia involves the lower segments of the lung then referred abdominal pain may be the presenting symptom and the child is seen first by the surgeons. Localising signs, dullness to percussion, bronchial breathing and fine crepitations, are easy to miss in the young child even when the diagnosis is known but a chest X-ray will resolve the problem showing segmental or lobar consolidation. If the diagnosis is suspected a lateral X-ray is necessary in addition to an antero-posterior view to avoid missing consolidation at the posterior segment of the upper lobes. The organism may be grown on blood culture as well as from the upper respiratory tract. Parenteral penicillin remains the antibiotic of choice.

Staphylococcal infections. In debilitated children or weakly infants the coagulase positive *Staphylococcus aureus* can invade the lungs, producing widespread consolidation with abscesses. Affected babies are usually under 12 months of age and present with an acute illness often with peripheral shock due to an associated septicaemia. They have been colourfully described as 'near cot deaths'. Other infants have less constitutional reactions despite showing massive lung involvement on X-ray. The children sometimes have signs of lung over-inflation. More striking are the widespread coarse crepitations often with areas of dullness to percussion and bronchial breathing. The chest X-ray may show scattered areas of consolidation throughout the lung fields. More commonly there is a large dense area with one or more abscess cavities. Pleural effusions or empyemas also occur. These children need careful monitoring, as respiratory failure and circulatory collapse can occur with frightening rapidity, often secondary to a tension pneumothorax. Active treatment with circulatory and respiratory support and parenteral antibiotics effective against the coagulase positive staphylococcus, for example cloxacillin and gentamicin can give gratifying results.

Other organisms including β-haemolytic streptococcus group A and *Haemophilus influenzae* type B can cause pneumonia. In the newborn period *E. coli*, pseudomonas and klebsiella infections may also occur and for this reason gentamicin is probably the antibiotic of choice.

Bronchiectasis

In bronchiectasis there are cystic changes involving the bronchi particularly in the lower segment of the lungs leading to chronic abscesses with purulent smelly sputum, often complicated by haemoptyses. This used to be a common complication of respiratory illnesses particularly whooping cough, measles and bacterial pneumonias. Fortunately, with improvements in general nutrition and wider use of antibiotics, it is now rarely seen except as a complication of cystic fibrosis and in children with immune deficiency states. Regular physiotherapy with courses of antibiotics for exacerbations of infection provides the best means of control.

CYSTIC FIBROSIS

Cystic fibrosis is the commonest cause of chronic suppurative lung disease in children in the U.K., and is also the commonest cause of pancreatic insufficiency. It occurs in about 1:2000 births and is inherited as an autosomal recessive condition, the carrier rate being 1 in 25 of the population. The basic defect is unknown. Many exocrine and mucus secreting glands are affected. Abnormal secretions are produced by the sweat glands, salivary glands and pancreas, resulting in duct obstruction which leads to gradual pancreatic fibrosis, biliary cirrhosis and infertility in males. No chemical abnormality has been detected in

Mode of presentation and age at diagnosis of 75 children with cystic fibrosis

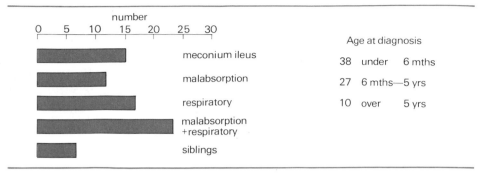

bronchial mucus, but there may be a defect in ciliary mechanisms leading to recurrent infection.

Clinical features

The children may present with meconium ileus soon after birth, failure to thrive in the first months of life or recurrent and persistent chest infections. The majority of patients are diagnosed in infancy, but a significant number with relatively mild symptoms are first recognised in later childhood. The diagnosis is made by finding increased sodium and chloride levels in sweat obtained by pilocarpine iontophoresis.

Meconium ileus is a form of neonatal small bowel obstruction, due to thick viscid meconium. Perforation and peritonitis may have occurred before birth. Treatment is surgical, though milder cases may respond to a gastrografin enema.

Recurrent lung infections The lungs are normal at birth, but the child has a tendency to frequent and prolonged infections with cough and wheeze. There is gradual progression of the disease, with the development of a chronic cough and sputum often associated with chest deformity, clubbing and poor growth, but the severity and rate of progression both vary considerably. Early chest X-rays are usually normal but they may show overdistension of the lungs and

Cystic fibrosis: severity of lung disease by age group

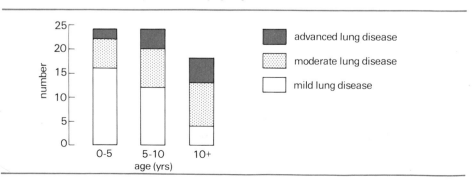

peribronchial thickening. Later dilatation of the bronchi with widespread mottling and large opacities may occur. Pseudomonas and *Staphylococcus aureus* are the usual pathogens grown from the sputum. Pulmonary function tests correlate well with X-ray changes, demonstrating airflow obstruction and increased lung volumes, but ultimately a fall in vital capacity.

Malabsorption due to pancreatic insufficiency is present in almost all children and presents with loose, offensive stools, failure to thrive and sometimes rectal prolapse. It also varies in severity. Microscopy of the stool for fat globules is a useful screening test but detailed pancreatic function tests are unnecessary as a rule.

Management

Respiratory problems are minimised by regular postural drainage which the parents are taught so they can do it at home. Antibiotics are given when the child has an infection, or exacerbation of cough. The long term use of antibiotics is sometimes advised, but has not been shown to influence the prognosis and will encourage the emergence of pseudomonas infections which are virtually impossible to eradicate and affects prognosis adversely.

Immunisation against measles and influenza is advised as viral infections can cause as much trouble as bacterial infections. Inhalation of mists with or without mucolytics, bronchodilators and antibiotics may be helpful.

Malabsorption is improved, but not cured, by giving pancreatic enzyme supplements with meals. The diet should be low in fat but high in calories and proteins, with added vitamins.

If cystic fibrosis is diagnosed before serious lung damage has occurred, treatment along these lines may lead to considerable improvement. Many children have years of active life, and are able to attend normal schools. Over the years the prognosis has improved greatly. Unfortunately, older patients may develop cirrhosis and diabetes.

A chronic disease of this nature puts great stress on the family, and the child himself may have considerable emotional problems, particularly in adolescence. Genetic counselling is essential as 1 in 4 siblings will be affected. At present, antenatal diagnosis is not possible but hopefully this may be developed in the future. Screening of all newborn infants is being undertaken in Germany and

Postural drainage

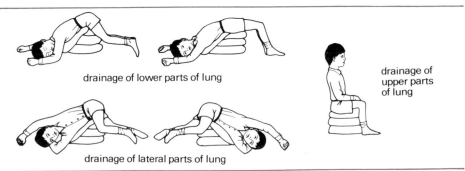

drainage of lower parts of lung

drainage of upper parts of lung

drainage of lateral parts of lung

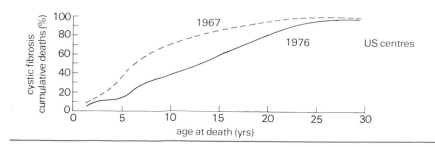

other places, using a test for increased protein in meconium. This test is not completely reliable, yielding both false positives and false negatives and therefore is not in routine use in the U.K. It has not yet been convincingly shown that neonatal screening improves the prognosis.

ASTHMA

Asthma is a disorder characterised by hyper-reactivity of the airways leading to paroxysmal attacks of airways obstruction which produce coughing, respiratory distress and wheezing. It is by far the commonest chronic respiratory disease of childhood affecting up to 12 per cent of children. There is a wide spectrum of disease ranging from single mild wheezing episodes to continuous asthma with episodic severe exacerbations. The airways obstruction is a combination of muscle spasm, mucosal oedema and increased secretions.

Clinical features

Usually episodes of coughing and wheezing appear in the latter months of the first year and as at this age the attacks are almost exclusively brought on by viral upper respiratory tract infections, a diagnosis of recurrent, wheezy bronchitis is often made. Frequently there is a history of eczema and a family history of allergic disorders. Over the next two years the pattern remains unchanged with wheezing attacks lasting several days whenever the child gets a cold. Nocturnal cough and sleep disturbance is a conspicuous complaint by the parents.

If the child is over the age of three years the parents may have noticed that prolonged exercise results in attacks of coughing and wheezing lasting for 10 to 20 minutes. Exercise induced bronchoconstriction may be an isolated disorder in a child who is otherwise free from asthmatic attacks. In others, the attacks are also induced by a variety of inhaled allergens. These foreign proteins react with IgE antibody on the surface of mast cells within the respiratory tract, leading to release of histamine, serotonin and other substances which produce smooth muscle constriction and local oedema, the so-called Type I immunological response. Many of the important allergens can be identified by taking a careful history; for example grass pollen sensitivity produces symptoms from May to June, and fungal sensitivity in the autumn. The house dust mite, *Dermatophagoides pteronyssimus*, feeds on shed skin and is found in greatest concentrations in the bed. This is probably the single most important allergen in childhood asthma and is responsible for the troublesome nocturnal symptoms. Other common sensitising substances include cat and dog fur, feathers and occasionally foods and drugs. Skin tests are helpful in providing additional evidence of suspected allergens, but many otherwise healthy children have positive skin tests. Nasal or bronchial provocation tests are probably more significant but are also more dangerous. Emotional factors are also important and enquiry about the home and school is essential in children whose asthma is difficult to control. In many children symptoms are exacerbated when the weather changes.

Children with asthma may be graded into three groups:

1. The mild group includes children whose occasional attacks are usually precipitated by infection but who have no symptoms between attacks and whose growth and pulmonary function tests are normal apart from exercise induced bronchoconstriction.
2. The intermediate or moderate group consists of those with severe, recurrent episodes but, again, they are symptom-free between attacks apart from exercise induced bronchoconstriction.
3. In the severe group, the asthmatic attacks may vary in severity but the child is never free from symptoms and the illness affects his general growth and development. Lung function tests remain abnormal at all times in this category. These children have chest wall deformity and chest X-rays show the presence of over-expanded lungs even when they are at their best.

Management
The best results are achieved by a single doctor paying attention to detail and giving the correct therapy at the appropriate time, in the optimal amount for that particular child within that particular family.

General management. The amount an asthmatic suffers from his disease is often related as much to the advice of his medical advisor and the anxiety of his parents as to the reactivity of his bronchial tree. Parents should be given a simple explanation of the nature of the disease and the purpose of the various treatments recommended. They are often the best judge of the most effective approach. In children who have recurrent severe episodes, direct admission to a ward not only allows the child to have immediate and appropriate care but it is also very reassuring to his parents. Children should be encouraged to lead a normal, outgoing existence and the parents should be encouraged to help their children to be independent and to avoid over-protection. Many who were asthmatic as children have turned out to be outstanding athletes. Indeed the prognosis for mild and moderate asthma in childhood is very good. Unfortunately severe chronic asthma tends to persist, although there may well be improvement as they enter adolescence.

Allergens

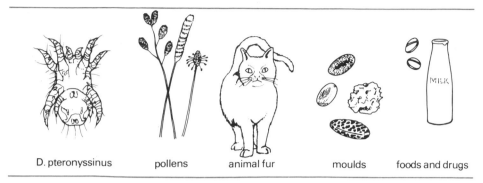

| D. pteronyssinus | pollens | animal fur | moulds | foods and drugs |

Out-patient therapy. Where possible, <u>allergens should be identified and avoided</u>. For example, the number of house dust mites can be reduced by frequent washing of bedclothes and vacuuming of the mattress and bedroom in order that the child sleeps in a relatively allergen-free environment. The child with only occasional wheezing attacks can usually lead a virtually normal life with the help of oral bronchodilator drugs. Immediate relief can be obtained if the drug is inhaled from a pressurised aerosol or as a dry powder. Those who have symptoms which are troublesome despite adequate bronchodilator therapy should be tried on sodium cromoglycate. This compound, inhaled on a regular basis either by spinhaler or, in the young child, as a nebulised solution, interferes with the IgE mediated process and prevents or reduces the frequency of asthmatic attacks in about 70 per cent of children with asthma. If the child fails to obtain sufficient benefit and is missing school, an inhaler delivering a topically active steroid, for example <u>beclomethasone,</u> should be prescribed. Long-term systemic steroids should be avoided wherever possible because of the side effects, in particular growth suppression. Short sharp courses of prednisolone given infrequently do have a part to play and may avoid the need to admit the child to hospital.

In-patient management. Admission to hospital with severe asthma indicates that the drugs used have failed. Despite this, inhalation of nebulised salbutamol

Peak expiratory flow rates measured by a Wright's Peak Flow Meter. Normal values are related to height rather than age. The serial measurements are those of a child with exercise-induced bronchospasm who responded to salbutamol.

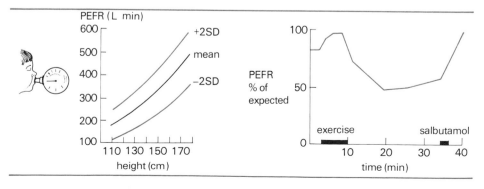

Forced expiratory volumes measured by spirometry. In children the volume exhaled in the first
0.75 of a second is used, rather than the full second which is preferred for adults. The serial
values are those of a child after bronchial provocation with house dust mite who responded to
salbutamol.

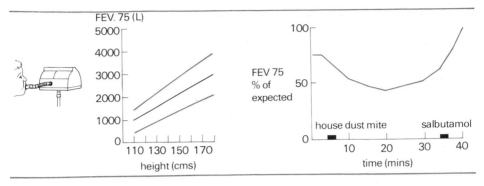

respirator solution can be very effective if this has not already been used. If the
child has not responded well to inhaled salbutamol, intravenous hydrocortisone is
indicated. Aminophylline, preferably given intravenously, is also beneficial but an
overdose can lead to vomiting, convulsions and collapse. Subcutaneous adre-
naline remains a potent form of treatment in the acute severe asthmatic attack. In
status asthmaticus the airways are often blocked with plugs of thick exudate and
desquamated cells leading to gross hyperinflation. By this stage the patients are
usually dehydrated so that they need intravenous fluids and controlled humidified
oxygen therapy. If respiratory failure develops, artificial ventilation for a period
will help. Experts disagree on the advisability of giving sedatives to children with
status asthmaticus. In some children relieving the anxiety produces dramatic
improvement. In others sedatives may precipitate respiratory failure and should
only be given when facilities for artificial ventilation are readily available.

Drugs in asthma

Type of drug	Drug	Mode of administration	
α- and β-adrenergic stimulants	Adrenaline	s.c., inhalation	
	Ephedrine	oral	
β₁ & β₂ adrenergic stimulants	Isoprenaline	inhalation	
β₂ adrenergic stimulants	Salbutamol (ventolin)	oral, i.m., i.v., inhalation	
Rimiterol - Pulmadil	Terbutaline (Bricanyl)	oral, i.m., i.v., inhalation	
Prophylactic	Sodium cromoglycate	inhalation	powder or nebulised solution
Corticosteroids Budesonide → Pulmicort	Beclomethasone	inhalation	powder or aerosol
	Betamethasone isovalerate	inhalation	aerosol
	Prednisolone	oral	
	Hydrocortisone	i.v.	

Antichol — Atrovent

RARE LUNG DISEASES

Occasionally children present with respiratory problems which do not fit into the categories already described. The commonest picture is that of an infant who has a persistently raised respiratory rate with respiratory distress, cough and failure to thrive. There are a number of causes which need to be considered which include antenatally acquired infections such as rubella and cytomegalovirus pneumonia or respiratory problems secondary to an underlying congenital abnormality. These include clefts of the larynx, a persisting tracheo-oesophageal fistula, congenital lung cysts and abnormalities of the diaphragm. Infants who have difficulty in coordinating their swallowing or those with hiatus hernias may also present with chronic respiratory infection due to recurrent chronic aspiration of milk and food. Infants and children with an immunological deficiency state frequently have severe respiratory tract infections, often due to organisms such as *Pneumocystis carinii* which are not pathogenic to the healthy child. Occasionally, an acute viral infection, particularly an adenoviral bronchiolitis can produce severe lung damage resulting in a condition known as obliterative bronchiolitis. Some infants present with respiratory distress due to congenital lobar emphysema, the aetiology of which is often obscure. Finally, there is a group of rare respiratory diseases including fibrosing alveolitis and pulmonary haemosiderosis which occur in the young as well as the old. Severe lung disease can be regarded with rather more optimism in the infant than in the adult, as alveolar budding occurs up to the age of eight years so that remarkable improvements can occur even after the most devastating illnesses.

BIBLIOGRAPHY

Clark T J H, Godfrey S 1977 Asthma. Chapman & Hall, London
Colley J R T 1976 The epidemiology of respiratory disease in childhood. In: Hull D (ed) Recent advances in paediatrics — 5. Churchill Livingstone, Edinburgh, ch 9, p221-258
Godfrey S 1974 Exercise testing in children. Saunders, Philadelphia
Kendig E L 1977 Disorders of the respiratory tract in children. Saunders, Philadelphia
Leer J A, Green J L, Heimlick E M, Hyde J S, Moffett H L, Young G A, Barron B A 1969 Corticosteroid treatment in bronchiolitis. American Journal of Diseases of Childhood 117: 495
Miller F J W, Court S D M, Walton W S, Knox E G 1960 Growing up in Newcastle Upon Tyne. Oxford University Press, Oxford
Williams H E, McNichol K N 1969 Prevalence, natural history and relationship of wheezy bronchitis and asthma in children. An epidemiological study. British Medical Journal 4: 321
Williams H E, Phelan P D 1975 Respiratory illness in children. Blackwell, Oxford
Workshop on bronchiolitis 1977 Pediatric Research 11: (3)

9

Heart

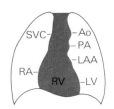

RA	right atrium
RV	right ventricle
LV	left ventricle
LAA	left atrial appendage
PA	pulmonary artery
Ao	aorta
SVC	superior vena cava

Now that rheumatic fever is rare, congenital abnormalities have become the main cause of heart disease in children. Acquired heart disease still occurs but it is not common; congenital heart defects, however, occur in approximately seven to eight infants per thousand live births and congenital heart disease thus forms the commonest single group of serious congenital abnormalities. About a quarter of affected children will die in the first year of life, the majority within the first month. These children have severe cardiac abnormalities which, in many cases, are complex and inoperable. However, the number of children with severe lesions who are now surviving beyond the first year is increasing, a tribute to the skill and ingenuity of cardiac surgeons. Ten to 15 per cent of children with congenital heart disease have more than one cardiac abnormality. Ten to 15 per cent have an associated non-cardiac abnormality; the skeletal, gastrointestinal and genito-urinary systems are the most commonly involved. There are nine common congenital heart lesions which together make up 90 per cent of all cases. The remaining 10 per cent consists of numerous rarer, more complex anomalies.

Aetiology

As with most congenital defects, the precise aetiology is unknown but both genetic and environmental factors have been identified. Family studies suggest that the mode of inheritance is polygenic, although occasionally single gene mutations occur. If a mother has a child with a congenital heart defect, the chances

The nine commonest congenital heart defects

Acyanotic	Cyanotic
Ventricular septal defect} L=> R shunt.	Transposition of the great arteries
Atrial septal defect	Tetralogy of Fallot
Patent ductus arteriosus	
Pulmonary stenosis	
Aortic stenosis	
Coarctation of aorta	
Hypoplastic left heart	

Congenital heart disease in chromosome disorders

Chromosomal Abnormality	Clinical syndrome	Type of lesion commonly seen
Partial deletion of chromosome 5	Cri du chat	VSD
Trisomy 13-15	Patau's syndrome	VSD, PDA Dextrocardia
Trisomy 18	Edward's syndrome	Complex lesions
Trisomy 21	Down's syndrome	VSD, ASD, Fallot's
XO	Turner's syndrome	Coarctation, Aortic stenosis

of a second child being affected are about three times higher than if her child had no heart defect. Children with chromosomal abnormalities have a greatly increased incidence of congenital heart disease; nearly half of all children with Down's syndrome have a cardiac lesion. Maternal rubella in the first trimester of pregnancy, maternal diabetes and drugs in pregnancy are environmental factors associated with an increased incidence of congenital heart disease.

Presentation
Congenital heart disease usually presents in one of the three following ways:

Heart murmur. This is the commonest mode of presentation. Most murmurs are detected in the first year of life, either on routine examination in the newborn period or in the child health clinics. A minority are not discovered until the child starts school.

Heart failure. A number of lesions will cause heart failure, commonly in the first year of life. The symptoms and signs are similar to those found in an adult. The baby becomes breathless, particularly after the exertion of feeding or crying. He may have difficulty completing feeds and as a consequence fails to thrive.

Heart failure in infancy

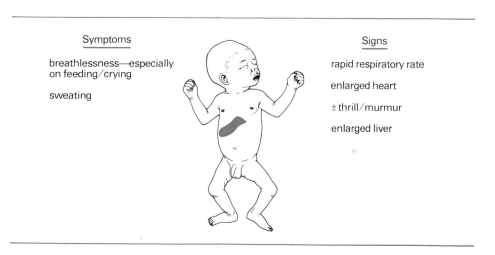

Symptoms

breathlessness—especially on feeding/crying

sweating

Signs

rapid respiratory rate

enlarged heart

± thrill/murmur

enlarged liver

Sweating is often a prominent symptom. On examination, the baby has a rapid respiratory rate and a rapid pulse rate. Heart enlargement is usually present and can be detected clinically; a thrill or murmur may be present and there is often a gallop rhythm due to a third heart sound. Invariably, the liver is enlarged due to venous congestion. Oedema of the dependent parts of the body is rarely seen, although infants in failure frequently show rapid weight gains suggesting fluid retention. Fine moist sounds of pulmonary oedema are less easily heard in babies than in adults. If frank pulmonary oedema is present, the baby may be centrally cyanosed and the cyanosis will disappear when oxygen is given.

Cyanosis ('blue baby'). If the heart defect results in unsaturated venous blood by-passing the lungs, central cyanosis will be present and is not corrected while breathing 100 per cent oxygen. This lack of response to oxygen helps to distinguish cyanosis due to heart disease from cyanosis due to severe lung disease, especially in the newborn period when this distinction can be difficult. Long-standing central cyanosis results in clubbing of the fingers and toes and secondary polycythaemia. A child with cyanotic congenital heart disease often has a reduced exercise tolerance and fails to grow normally.

Investigations

A chest X-ray and electrocardiogram are essential investigations in the assessment of a child with suspected heart disease. Cardiac catheterisation is necessary if the infant presents with heart failure or cyanosis. If the infant presents with symptoms in the first weeks of life, catheterisation is a matter of urgency and arrangements should be made to transfer the baby to a unit where this can be carried out. Catheterisation may also be performed on a child without symptoms if surgery is being considered. It enables the pressures and saturations within the chambers of the heart to be measured and, with angiocardiography following injection of radio-opaque dyes, permits precise anatomical and physiological diagnosis. Echocardiography, using ultrasound, is non-invasive and is becoming a useful investigative tool.

The innocent murmur

Many babies and children have heart murmurs without any structural abnormality of the heart. Indeed, in one reported series, a cardiologist detected a heart murmur in the majority of healthy school children on routine examination! Such murmurs are termed innocent, or functional. They are diagnosed as being innocent on the basis of their characteristics and are associated with a normal chest X-ray and e.c.g. If a murmur is obviously innocent, the parents need not be told and no follow-up is necessary. If there is uncertainty, an expert opinion should be sought as soon as possible, before the seeds of cardiac neurosis are sown. There are three types of innocent murmur:

1. Venous hum. This is a blowing, continuous murmur heard at the base of the heart, often just below the clavicles. It varies both with respiration and the position of the head, and disappears when the child lies down. It is due to blood flow through the systemic great veins and is sometimes confused with a patent ductus arteriosus.

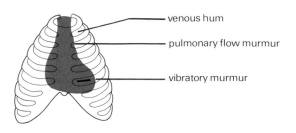

venous hum

pulmonary flow murmur

vibratory murmur

2. Pulmonary flow murmur. This is a soft, systolic ejection murmur heard in the pulmonary area (the second left intercostal space). It is due to rapid flow of blood across a normal pulmonary valve and is especially prominent when the cardiac output is high, for example after exercise, in febrile children or in cases of anaemia.

3. Vibratory murmur. This is a short, buzzing murmur heard in systole at the left sternal edge or at the apex of the heart. It is variable and changes with position.

If a murmur is pansystolic, diastolic, loud or long, associated with a thrill or with cardiac symptoms, it is not innocent.

Classification of congenital heart disease

Congenital heart disease can conveniently be classified into two groups: (1) acyanotic due to either a left to right shunt or obstructive lesion, and (2) cyanotic with either increased or diminished pulmonary flow.

ACYANOTIC LESIONS WITH A LEFT TO RIGHT SHUNT

A common type of congenital heart defect is a hole between the two sides of the heart, at the level of either the atria, the ventricles or the great arteries. In fetal life, pulmonary blood flow is small and the pressure in the right ventricle and pulmonary artery is high. With the onset of regular respirations, the pulmonary vascular resistance falls, with a consequent fall in the pressures on the right side of the heart. Since the pressure on the left side of the heart now exceeds that on the right side, blood will start to flow from the left side to the right side through the hole. The fall in pulmonary vascular resistance occurs rapidly in the first few days after birth and then more slowly over the next few weeks, so that by the age of about three months the left to right flow of blood reaches a maximum. There is therefore an additional circulation of blood from the left side of the heart to the right side, thence to the lungs and back to the left side of the heart again. This is termed a shunt. If the hole is small, the shunt may be trivial, but if it is large, it may represent the majority of the cardiac output, so that the blood flow through the pulmonary artery may be several times greater than the flow through the aorta. A large shunt imposes an added burden on the heart, with consequent hypertrophy, dilatation and sometimes failure. Because of the high pulmonary vascular resistance immediately after birth, frequently a murmur is not heard and in babies with a simple left to right shunt, heart failure is uncommon in the first few weeks of life.

A left to right shunt, if appreciable, will give rise to a number of consistent findings, regardless of the site of the hole. Clinical examination may show an enlarged heart with hypertrophy of one or both ventricles. Signs of ventricular hypertrophy will be present on the electrocardiogram. A chest radiograph will reveal an enlarged heart with a prominent pulmonary artery and an increase in vascular markings (pulmonary plethora) due to the high pulmonary blood flow.

Atrial septal defect (ostium secundum)
In the majority of atrial septal defects, the hole is in the atrial septum in the region of the fossa ovalis, the site of the foramen ovale: this is the ostium secundum defect. Because the right ventricle is less muscular and easier to fill with blood than the left ventricle, blood will flow from the left atrium to the right atrium through the defect, thence to the right ventricle and the lungs. The right side of the heart therefore takes the whole of the added burden of the shunt.

Natural history. Symptoms are rare in infancy and uncommon in childhood, even if the shunt is large. However in the third or fourth decade, heart failure, pulmonary hypertension or atrial arrhythmias may occur.

Clinical features. Because symptoms are unusual in childhood, most children with atrial septal defects present as a heart murmur. The murmur is often quite soft and frequently not detected until the child is at school. If symptoms do occur, they are of breathlessness or tiredness on exertion, or recurrent chest infections.

Atrial septal defect (ASD): anatomy, presentation, examination and investigations.

CXR	— Chest X-ray	1	— first heart sound
ECG	— Electrocardiogram	A2	— aortic component of the second heart sound
RAD	— Right axis deviation		
RBBB	— Right bundle branch block	P2	— pulmonary compenent of the second heart sound
PA	— Pulmonary artery		

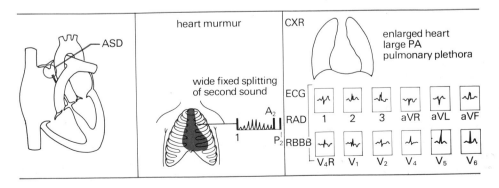

Examination. The child is well, pink and has normal pulses. The right ventricle may be easily felt. There is a systolic murmur in the pulmonary area at the second left interspace. This is due not to flow of blood across the defect, but to a high flow of blood across a normal pulmonary valve. If the shunt is large, a mid-diastolic tricuspid flow murmur may be heard too. The aortic and pulmonary components of the second sound are widely separated because the excessive filling of the right ventricle delays closure of the pulmonary valve. Furthermore, the time interval between these two sounds does not vary with respiration ('fixed splitting') because the two atria function as a single unit and respiration affects them both equally.

Investigations. The chest X-ray shows cardiomegaly with a prominent right atrium and pulmonary artery, and pulmonary plethora. The electrocardiogram shows right axis deviation, right ventricular hypertrophy and in most cases right bundle branch block. If the investigations suggest that the shunt is appreciable, cardiac catheterisation is recommended.

Treatment. If cardiac catheterisation reveals a pulmonary blood flow more than twice systemic flow, closure of the defect is advisable, using cardiopulmonary by-pass. Repair is by simple suture or by insertion of a patch.

Atrial septal defect (ostium primum)
Although less common than secundum defects, ostium primum defects are more serious. The hole is situated low down in the atrial septum and represents a failure of development of the septum primum in fetal life. The defect is just above the atrioventricular valves, and usually extends to the insertion of the anterior leaflet of the mitral valve, so that the latter is cleft and frequently incompetent. An ostium primum atrial septal defect represents the mild end of the spectrum of developmental abnormalities involving the central portion of the heart, endocardial cushion defects. In the most severe form, the defect extends from the atrial septum, through the origin of both atrioventricular valves into the ventricular septum. This is described as an atrioventricular canal defect and gives rise to a large left to right shunt and both mitral and tricuspid incompetence. The endocardial cushion defects are particularly common in children with Down's syndrome.

Natural history. Symptoms frequently arise in infancy and childhood and congestive cardiac failure is common. Severe pulmonary hypertension may develop.

Clinical presentation. Symptoms and signs of heart failure commonly occur in infancy and childhood. Death may occur if surgical correction is not undertaken.

Examination. The child is often breathless at rest, with deformities of the lower ribs (Harrison's sulci). He is pink, with normal pulses. Clinically, the heart is large with increased activity of both ventricles. In addition to the auscultatory signs of an atrial septal defect there may be an apical pansystolic murmur signifying mitral regurgitation.

Investigations. The chest X-ray shows marked cardiomegaly, prominent pulmonary arteries and pulmonary plethora. The electrocardiogram is frequently diagnostic, showing left axis deviation and right bundle branch block. Catheterisation is required to assess the size of the shunt and the degree of mitral incompetence.

Treatment. Early surgery is usually advised for children with ostium primum defects. The defect is closed and the cleft mitral valve repaired. It is a more difficult and risky operation than that for a secundum defect.

Ventricular septal defect

This is the commonest of all congenital heart lesions. In 25 to 30 per cent of affected children other heart defects are also present. Usually a single hole is found high up in the membranous portion of the ventricular septum just below the aortic valve. Occasionally several holes are present in the lower muscular part of the septum, the 'Swiss cheese' abnormality.

Natural history. There are four possibilities, as follows:
1. The hole may close spontaneously. This occurs in perhaps as many as 50 per cent of cases, usually in early childhood but sometimes in later childhood, adolescence or adult life.
2. The hole may remain the same size. Since the heart is growing throughout childhood, the defect becomes relatively smaller.
3. Stenosis of the outflow tract of the right ventricle, the infundibulum may occur. This raises the pressure in the right ventricle and steadily reduces the size of the left to right shunt. Eventually the shunt may reverse and the child will become cyanosed. The child, in effect, develops Fallot's tetralogy.
4. Progressive pulmonary hypertension may develop. If the left to right shunt is large, the torrential pulmonary blood flow irreversibly damages the smaller pulmonary vessels, giving rise to pulmonary hypertension. This makes the defect inoperable and considerably reduces the child's life span.

Clinical presentation depends on the size of the defect and whether pulmonary hypertension is present.

Small ventricular septal defect ('maladie de Roger'). Since the shunt through the defect is small, the child is symptom-free and the heart murmur is often picked up on routine examination. The child is well, pink and has normal pulses, and the heart is not enlarged. Frequently there is a thrill, at the lower left sternal border. On auscultation a harsh, pansystolic murmur is heard at the same site due to flow of blood through the defect. The heart sounds are normal.

Investigations: The chest X-ray and electrocardiogram are usually normal. Catheterisation is unnecessary.

Treatment: There is a risk of bacterial endocarditis and antibiotic prophylaxis is therefore necessary at the time of dental extractions, etc.

Moderate ventricular septal defect. Symptoms usually occur in infancy, with breathlessness on feeding and crying, failure to thrive and recurrent chest infections. As the child gets older, the symptoms tend to improve and may

Ventricular septal defect

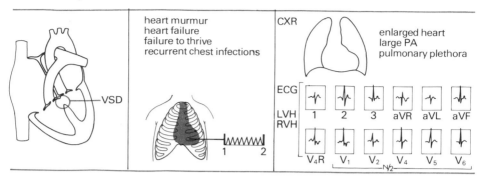

disappear altogether, because of actual or relative closure of the defect.

Examination: the baby is breathless at rest but is pink, with normal pulses. The heart is enlarged clinically with prominent activity of both ventricles. There is a systolic thrill at the lower left sternal border. On auscultation there is a loud, harsh pansystolic murmur, maximal at this site but heard all over the chest. There is frequently an apical mid-diastolic murmur, caused by an increased flow of blood across a normal mitral valve. The second heart sound is noticeably split and the pulmonary component may be louder than normal.

Investigations: the chest X-ray shows cardiomegaly, prominent pulmonary arteries and pulmonary plethora. The electrocardiogram shows biventricular hypertrophy, since both ventricles are involved in the shunt. Cardiac catheterisation should be carried out if the child does not improve with age or if there is evidence of pulmonary hypertension.

Treatment: If symptoms are prominent, digitalisation is of benefit. Surgery should be avoided because of the tendency to spontaneous improvement. Exceptions are continuing symptoms and the development of pulmonary hypertension.

Large ventricular septal defect. When the pulmonary vascular resistance falls to its lowest level at about three months of age, the shunt through a large defect is great and results in heart failure. Symptoms of breathlessness on feeding usually start earlier than this and sweating is very common. Affected babies may be severely ill with congestive cardiac failure, and they have an increased tendency to chest infections which often precipitates episodes of failure.

Examination: The baby is usually underweight, breathless and ill. If there is frank pulmonary oedema, cyanosis will be present. The heart is large clinically with increased ventricular activity and a systolic thrill. Signs of heart failure will be present. On auscultation, there is a harsh systolic murmur which is often not pansystolic because of the high right ventricular pressures. A pulmonary (systolic ejection) and a mitral (mid-diastolic) flow murmur are usually heard and the pulmonary second sound is loud.

Investigation: The chest X-ray shows very marked cardiomegaly, large pulmonary arteries and pulmonary plethora. The electrocardiogram shows biventricular hypertrophy. Catheterisation is almost always necessary, if only to

Treatment of heart failure in infancy

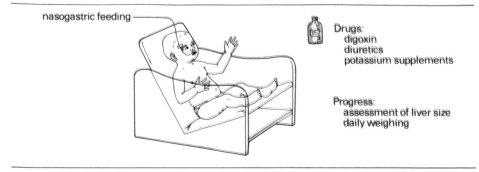

nasogastric feeding

Drugs:
digoxin
diuretics
potassium supplements

Progress:
assessment of liver size
daily weighing

confirm the diagnosis and exclude any other lesion.

Treatment: The initial treatment is medical. The infant in heart failure is nursed sitting up, in oxygen if necessary. Digoxin, diuretics and potassium supplements are given. The success of treatment can be gauged by regular weighing and by recording the size of the liver. As the heart failure responds to treatment there will be a rapid weight loss and a progressive decrease in liver size. If the baby does not respond to treatment, surgical closure is necessary. This is best done as a single stage operation, using cardiopulmonary by-pass. Such an operation in an ill baby requires the highest medical and surgical skills. An earlier alternative method of surgical treatment was to place a constricting band around the base of the pulmonary artery, thus reducing the size of the shunt. A second operation was required to remove the band and close the defect. If the baby's heart failure responds to medical treatment, then surgical closure is best delayed. It is necessary if repeat catheterisation suggests that pulmonary vascular disease is developing or if the child is chronically underweight and getting frequent chest infections. However, even the largest defects have been shown to close spontaneously, and since surgical closure carries a certain risk a conservative approach is favoured.

Patent ductus arteriosus

This is a common congenital heart lesion, either singly or in combination with other heart defects. It is particularly common in girls, in children whose mothers had rubella in early pregnancy and in babies who are born prematurely. In fetal life the ductus arteriosus, which is a large vessel with a muscular wall, diverts blood from the right ventricle and pulmonary artery into the aorta. Within the first 24 hours after birth, it closes in response to oxygenated blood. Spontaneous closure of a ductus arteriosus which remains patent after the first few days of life is unlikely. The only exception is the premature baby in whom closure of the ductus may still occur at any time in the first three months of life. As the pulmonary vascular resistance falls after birth, a left to right shunt of blood from the aorta to the pulmonary artery occurs through the ductus which is in the opposite direction to the flow in fetal life.

Natural history. If the duct is small, the only risk to the patient is from bacterial endocarditis, or more accurately, endarteritis. This is appreciable. If the

Patent ductus arterious (PDA). LVH = left ventricular hypertrophy

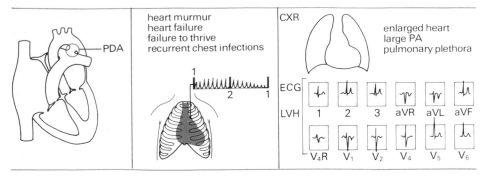

duct is larger, heart failure may occur in infancy, or may occur for the first time in adult life. Pulmonary hypertension and shunt reversal may occur.

Small ductus. The child is symptom free and a heart murmur is detected routinely or coincidentally. He is pink with normal pulses. On auscultation there is a loud, continuous murmur heard best in the pulmonary area below the left clavicle. The murmur extends through systole into diastole because the pressure in the pulmonary artery is lower than that in the aorta throughout the whole cardiac cycle. It has a rough 'machinery' quality.

Investigations: Chest X-ray and electrocardiogram are normal. Catheterisation is unnecessary.

Treatment: Surgical ligation is recommended because of the risk of bacterial endocarditis. The operation itself carries a very low risk.

Large ductus. The severity of symptoms are related to the size of the shunt. The child may be rather underweight with a reduced exercise tolerance and increased tendency to chest infections. At the other end of the spectrum, severe heart failure may develop in infancy. On examination the child is often small and thin. An increased respiratory rate is common. There is no cyanosis, but the pulses are easily felt, being full and collapsing in nature. The diastolic blood pressure is low and pulse pressure is wide. The heart is enlarged clinically with a prominent left ventricle and there is a systolic thrill in the pulmonary area. On auscultation, there is a harsh systolic murmur in the pulmonary area which may extend through the second sound into early diastole. The length of the murmur depends on the pulmonary artery pressure. This is high in large shunts so that blood only flows from left to right during systole. The pulmonary second sound is loud. A mitral (mid-diastolic) flow murmur may be heard.

Investigations: The chest X-ray shows the typical features of a left-to-right shunt. The electrocardiogram shows left ventricular hypertrophy. Catheterisation is unnecessary since the diagnosis can be made clinically.

Treatment: If heart failure is present, medical treatment is necessary. Surgical ligation should be carried out as soon as the child's condition allows.

Pulmonary hypertension

A large left to right shunt with a high pulmonary blood flow may produce an elevation of pulmonary artery pressure simply because of the increased flow (hyperdynamic pulmonary hypertension). Following surgical closure of the defect, the pulmonary artery pressure returns to normal. Persisting high pulmonary blood flow may result in permanent damage to the smaller pulmonary vessels with consequent narrowing and irreversible pulmonary hypertension. If the defect is closed under these circumstances, the pulmonary artery pressure remains elevated. When the pulmonary artery pressure reaches systemic levels the left to right shunt ceases and may acutely reverse.

Clinical features. The child becomes mildly cyanosed, with clubbed fingers and toes, but otherwise may appear remarkably well. However, exercise tolerance is usually considerably reduced. On examination, the right ventricle is prominent and heaving, and the pulmonary second sound is palpable. On auscultation there is usually a systolic ejection murmur in the pulmonary area due to blood flow through the huge pulmonary artery, not through the shunt, and sometimes an early diastolic murmur signifying pulmonary incompetence. The pulmonary component of the second sound is very loud.

Investigations. A chest X-ray shows an enlarged heart with a prominent right atrium. The pulmonary artery is greatly increased in size but its smaller branches are not seen. The electrocardiogram shows right axis deviation, right atrial hypertrophy and right ventricular hypertrophy. Cardiac catheterisation is needed to demonstrate the site of the shunt and to measure the pulmonary artery pressure.

The development of severe, irreversible, pulmonary hypertension as a result of a large left to right shunt is called the Eisenmenger syndrome. Although it was originally described in association with a ventricular septal defect (Eisenmenger complex), it may occur with a left to right shunt at any site. It is particularly likely to occur in cases of large ventricular septal defects, atrio-ventricular canal defects and transposition of the great arteries where there is a large shunt. No surgical treatment is possible and the life expectancy of affected children is considerably reduced.

OBSTRUCTIVE LESIONS

The most common examples of obstructive lesions are aortic stenosis, coarctation of the aorta and pulmonary stenosis. The chamber of the heart proximal to the obstruction hypertrophies in an attempt to overcome it. If the obstruction is severe, heart failure may result.

Aortic stenosis

This is a common congenital heart lesion which may occur in isolation or in combination with other heart defects. In the majority of cases the aortic valve itself is narrowed by congenital deformity. The deformed valve may be bicuspid instead of tricuspid and the cusps are frequently fused at the edges. The degree of stenosis may worsen as the child gets older, with thickening and calcification of the cusps. A biscuspid aortic valve may open normally in childhood, but becomes thickened and narrowed in adult life. If the aortic valve is particularly narrowed and rigid, a degree of aortic incompetence is common too.

Occasionally, aortic obstruction may be above or below the aortic valve. In supravalvular stenosis, the ascending aorta above the valve is narrowed. This is often a familial condition, associated with an unusual facial appearance, mental retardation and hypercalcaemia in infancy. In subvalvular aortic stenosis, there may be a fibrous diaphragm below the valve obstructing the flow of blood from left ventricle to aorta, or there may be excessive hypertrophy of the left ventricle and interventricular septum which obstructs the outflow tract of the left ventricle during systole, hypertrophic obstructive cardiomyopathy.

Natural history. In severe cases of aortic stenosis with heart failure in infancy there is a high mortality without treatment. There is a reduced life expectancy in the less severe cases because the stenosis may get worse and death may occur suddenly. Bacterial endocarditis is a well recognised complication.

Clinical presentation. In very severe cases a baby with aortic stenosis may develop frank heart failure. Otherwise the murmur is detected routinely. A minority of older children with severe aortic stenosis may have symptoms due to a low cardiac output; on exertion they feel dizzy, faint and may lose consciousness. Angina may occur.

Examination. The child appears well and is pink. The pulses are often small in volume, and of the slow rising, plateau type. The systolic blood pressure may be low. On palpation, the left ventricle is prominent and a thrill may be palpable at the lower left sternal border, in the suprasternal notch and in the neck over the carotid arteries. On auscultation there is a systolic ejection murmur heard at the apex and lower left sternal edge, which is conducted upwards into the neck. There is usually an ejection click immediately before the murmur. The aortic second sound is soft and delayed. If the stenosis is severe the aortic second sound may actually occur later than the pulmonary component so that there is apparent paradoxical splitting of the second sound with respiration.

Investigations. A chest X-ray may show a prominent left ventricle with post-stenotic dilatation of the ascending aorta. An electrocardiogram shows varying degrees of left ventricular hypertrophy relating to the severity of the stenosis. Cardiac catheterisation is indicated if there is clinical evidence of moderate or severe stenosis to measure the pressure gradient across the aortic valve.

Aortic stenosis. ec = ejection click

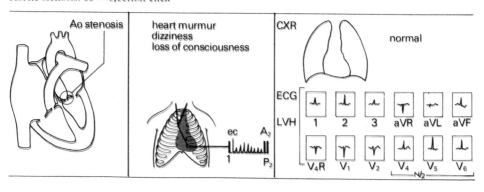

Treatment. If the gradient across the valve exceeds 70 mmHg an aortic valvotomy is indicated. Residual stenosis and incompetence are common but severe stenosis producing heart failure in infancy requires urgent surgery. Aortic stenosis is the one congenital heart lesion in which strenuous activity should be avoided because of the risk of sudden death. Prevention of bacterial endocarditis is important.

Coarctation of the aorta

This is a localised narrowing of the descending aorta, close to the site of the ductus arteriosus and usually distal to the left subclavian artery. Arterial blood by-passes the obstruction reaching the lower part of the body through collateral vessels which become greatly enlarged. The left ventricle hypertrophies to overcome the obstruction and heart failure may result. The systolic blood pressure in the upper part of the body is usually elevated.

Clinical presentation. If the narrowing is severe, heart failure may occur in the first few days or weeks of life. In most cases, however, the diagnosis is made on routine or coincidental examination, either because a murmur is heard, or the femoral pulses cannot be felt or because of the discovery of hypertension. Occasionally, a child or adult may present with a complication such as a subarachnoid haemorrhage from rupture of a berry aneurysm or bacterial endarteritis.

Examination. The child is well and pink. The brachial and radial pulses are normal but the femoral pulses are either absent or weak and delayed. There is usually systemic hypertension and the left ventricle may be prominent. On auscultation, a systolic ejection murmur is usually heard over the left side of the chest, especially at the back. Collateral arteries are often palpable over the scapulae.

Investigations. A chest X-ray may show a prominent left ventricle. In older children rib notching may be seen where the enlarged intercostal arteries have eroded the under side of the ribs. An electrocardiogram may show left ventricular hypertrophy.

Treatment. In most cases surgery is recommended when the child reaches school age. The narrowed segment of aorta is resected and the two ends sewn

Coarctation of the aorta

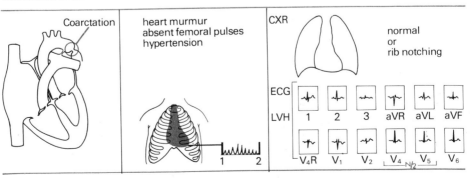

together. Sometimes a patch of Dacron is necessary to bridge the gap. Earlier surgery is more effective in permanently treating the hypertension but as the child grows there is a risk that relative narrowing at the site of the coarctation will occur again, requiring further surgery.

Hypoplastic left heart

In this condition, the left ventricle is underdeveloped, frequently with hypoplasia or atresia of the mitral valve, aortic valve and arch of the aorta. The ductus arteriosus is patent and blood therefore by-passes the left sided obstruction. Affected babies present in the first few days after birth with severe progressive heart failure, usually with cyanosis. They are pale and shocked, with very weak pulses. Unfortunately it is a relatively common condition for which there is no treatment. Death occurs within the neonatal period.

Pulmonary stenosis

The pulmonary valve is congenitally deformed, thickened and narrowed. The right ventricle hypertrophies in an attempt to overcome the obstruction. The muscular outflow tract of the right ventricle, the infundibulum, also hypertrophies and this may increase the degree of obstruction.

Clinical presentation. If the stenosis is severe, the infant presents with right-sided heart failure. There may be cyanosis from a right to left shunt of blood through the foramen ovale. In mild and moderate cases a heart murmur is heard on routine examination Symptoms are rare in childhood. However, in cases of moderate stenosis, dysfunction of the right ventricle and arrhythmias are liable to occur in adult life.

Examination. The child is well, pink, and has normal pulses. Right atrial hypertrophy produces a large 'a' wave in the jugular venous pulse. The right ventricle is heaving and a systolic thrill is palpable in the pulmonary area. On auscultation, there is usually an ejection click followed by a systolic ejection murmur caused by blood flowing across the narrowed valve. The murmur is heard in the upper part of the left chest anteriorly and not conducted to the neck. The pulmonary component of the second sound becomes softer and more delayed as the stenosis increases.

Pulmonary stenosis (PS). RA = right atrium. RVH = right ventricular hypertrophy

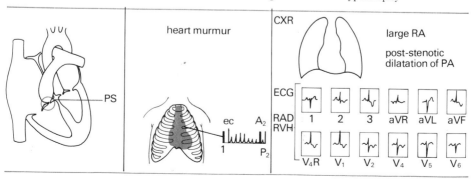

Investigations. A chest X-ray shows post-stenotic dilatation of the pulmonary artery. An enlarged right atrium and right ventricle are seen in severe cases. An electrocardiogram shows varying degrees of right axis deviation, right atrial hypertrophy and right ventricular hypertrophy, according to the severity of the stenosis. Catheterisation is indicated to measure the gradient across the pulmonary valve if signs suggest that the stenosis is moderate or severe.

Treatment. If the gradient across the valve exceeds 70 mmHg, a pulmonary valvotomy is indicated.

CYANOTIC CONGENITAL HEART DISEASE

A minority of babies or children with congenital heart disease are centrally cyanosed because unsaturated blood is by-passing the lungs. An affected child may be quite well at rest, even though he may be grossly blue. However, when the body's demand for oxygen increases during exercise, he becomes very easily tired and breathless. Even though the arterial oxygen saturation may be very low, the child's intelligence is usually normal. Secondary polycythaemia follows chronic hypoxia. This is to the child's advantage at first since it increases the actual amount of oxygen that can be transported in the blood. However, when the packed cell volume exceeds a certain limit, the viscosity of the blood increases with a resultant tendency to thrombosis, particularly cerebral. Embolism from thrombosis and haemorrhage from consumption coagulopathy are also well recognised complications of cyanotic heart disease.

Cyanotic heart disease can be subdivided into two types. In the first type the lungs are under-perfused with blood as the right to left shunts by-pass the lungs. Fallot's tetralogy is the commonest example. In the second type, the lungs are normally filled or even over-perfused with blood, but cyanosis results because there is inadequate mixing of the systemic and pulmonary circulations. Transposition of the great arteries is the commonest example.

Fallot's tetralogy

The two essential features of this condition are a large ventricular septal defect, usually sited high up in the membranous part of the septum beneath the aortic valve, and stenosis of the pulmonary valve or infundibulum. There is therefore resistance to the flow of blood through the pulmonary valve with a consequent shunt of blood from the right to left ventricle and thence to the aorta. In fact, since the septal defect is just below the aortic valve, the aorta appears to override the right ventricle and the shunt is directly from the right ventricle to the aorta. Pulmonary or infundibular stenosis leads to right ventricular hypertrophy. The overriding of the aorta and right ventricular hypertrophy, in combination with the ventricular septal defect and pulmonary stenosis make up the tetralogy originally described by Fallot. The main pulmonary artery is small and in the most severe cases may not be patent (pulmonary atresia with a ventricular septal defect).

Clinical features. Affected children are usually pink in the newborn period, although a heart murmur due to blood flow through a narrowed infundibulum or pulmonary valve may be detected. Cyanosis develops and increases over the next

Fallot's tetralogy. RAH = right atrial hypertrophy

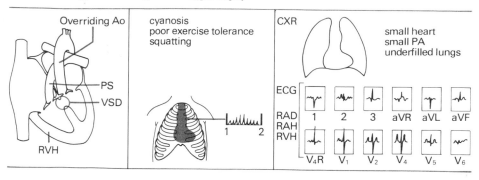

few weeks or months. Sometimes the baby may be quite pink when at rest, only becoming cyanosed with the exertion of crying or feeding. Sometimes cyanotic 'attacks' or 'spells' occur. An affected baby is relatively well most of the time but is prone to attacks during which he becomes extremely cyanosed and pale often with loss of consciousness. Such spells are thought to be due to spasm of the muscular infundibulum, increasing the right to left shunt and preventing blood from reaching the lungs. As the children become older, cyanosis at rest becomes more obvious, exercise tolerance is reduced and the typical squatting may occur. The latter is a manoeuvre to gain symptomatic relief after exercise in which the child squats down on his haunches with his knees up to his chest. It traps unsaturated venous blood in the legs preventing it from returning to the heart and also raises aortic pressure by obstructing the femoral arteries, with consequent reduction in size of the right to left shunt.

Heart failure is extremely rare in Fallot's tetralogy but the thromboembolic complications of polycythaemia, bacterial endocarditis and cerebral abcess may occur.

Examination. The affected child may be cyanosed at rest with clubbing of the fingers and toes. The heart is not enlarged clinically but the right ventricle is easily felt and there may be a systolic thrill in the pulmonary area. On auscultation, there is a systolic ejection murmur in the pulmonary area and a single second heart sound. No murmur arises from blood flow through the septal defect because the pressures in the two ventricles are similar.

Investigations. The chest X-ray shows a normal size heart with the apex above the left diaphragm but the left heart border is concave because the main pulmonary artery is small and the heart is said to look like a boot. The lung fields are oligaemic. The electrocardiogram shows right axis deviation, right atrial hypertrophy and right ventricular hypertrophy. The haemoglobin and packed cell volume are elevated and cardiac catheterisation is essential.

Treatment. This is usually surgical, although use of β-adrenergic blockers such as propranolol may lessen infundibular spasm and prevent cyanotic spells. Severely affected infants require a palliative operation to improve their symptoms until they are old enough to have a total repair of their defect. A shunt operation is performed, creating a communication between the aorta and pulmonary artery, so that sufficient blood can enter the lungs. A Blalock operation, in which the subclavian artery is joined to the pulmonary artery on either the left or right side, or a Waterston operation, in which the ascending aorta is joined to the right pulmonary artery, are the most commonly used procedures. Alternatively, pulmonary valvotomy and infundibular resection (Brock's operation) may give symptomatic improvement. When the child approaches school age, total correction of the defects is carried out using cardiopulmonary by-pass. The results of such surgery are excellent.

Transposition of the great arteries

In this heart lesion, the aorta and pulmonary arteries are 'transposed' so that the aorta arises from the right ventricle and the pulmonary artery from the left ventricle. This means that there are now two isolated circulations, pulmonary and systemic, working in parallel. Obviously this would not be compatible with life were it not for the fact that there must be some mixing between the two circulations. In fetal life, the baby is in no difficulty because the pulmonary blood flow is very small. After birth however, as the ductus arteriosus and foramen ovale begin to close, progressive cyanosis develops. The severity of the symptoms depends on the degree of mixing of the two circulations through these fetal channels. In some cases, a large ventricular septal defect or a large patent ductus arteriosus may be present, in which case there is a high pulmonary blood flow and only slight cyanosis. In the simple form however, progressive cyanosis develops in the first hours or days after birth. Without treatment, few children survive the first year of life.

Clinical features. Progressive cyanosis develops within the first few hours or days of life. The affected baby becomes increasingly blue and acidotic. Breathlessness and heart failure may follow.

Examination. Cyanosis is the major physical sign and persists even if the baby is given 100 per cent oxygen. There are usually no heart murmurs but the second sound is loud because the transposed aorta lies anteriorly, close to the chest wall.

Investigations. The chest X-ray is often typical. The heart is slightly enlarged and is said to look like an egg lying on its side. The vascular pedicle of the heart is

Transposition of the great arteries

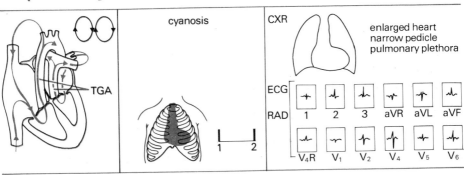

narrow because the aorta and pulmonary artery lie one in front of the other. The lung fields are normally filled or plethoric. The electrocardiogram shows the normal neonatal pattern of right sided dominance, which persists as the child gets older. Catheterisation is essential and should be performed urgently. It demonstrates that the aorta arises from the right and the pulmonary artery arises from the left ventricle.

Treatment. A shunt between the systemic and pulmonary circulations is urgently needed. This can be created at the time of catheterisation without recourse to surgery by performing a balloon atrial septostomy (Rashkind's procedure). A special double lumen catheter is passed via the inferior vena cava, right atrium and foramen ovale into the left atrium. A balloon near the tip of the catheter is then inflated using contrast medium and the catheter and inflated ballon are pulled sharply back through the atrial septum, tearing it and creating a large septal defect. The effect is usually dramatic; the baby, who is often desperately ill, becomes moderately pink. The shunt is usually large enough to enable him to thrive until a definitive procedure can be performed, usually at about the age of one year. The commonest definitive procedure is Mustard's operation which provides a physiological, although not anatomical, correction. The atrial septum is excised and the two venous returns diverted using a patch of pericardium or Dacron. The systemic venous blood from the venae cavae is diverted into the left ventricle and the pulmonary artery. The pulmonary venous blood is diverted into the right ventricle and thus to the aorta. Sometimes an anatomical correction is possible, whereby the aorta and pulmonary arteries are re-attached to their appropriate ventricles.

CARDIAC ARRHYTHMIAS

Children often have cardiac arrhythmias which are of no clinical significance; sinus arrhythmia is the most common example. A number, however, have symptoms which are a direct result of an abnormality of heart rhythmn.

Paroxysmal supraventricular tachycardia

This is a regular, rapid rhythm at the rate of 240 to 300 beats per minute. It is due to a 'circus' movement of impulses originating in the atrio-ventricular node re-

The ECG of supraventricular tachycardia

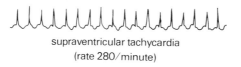

supraventricular tachycardia
(rate 280/minute)

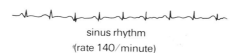

sinus rhythm
(rate 140/minute)

entering the atria via an accessory pathway and thus exciting the atrio-ventricular node prematurely. Since the heart rate is so rapid, diastolic filling of the ventricles is impaired and cardiac failure arises. The younger the patient, the less well is the rapid heart rate tolerated and the earlier heart failure develops. The tachycardia is paroxysmal and frequently recurs. About a quarter of the children with this disorder have an underlying cardiac defect, either congenital or acquired.

Clinical features. Paroxysmal tachycardia may be noted *in utero* or occur at any time in infancy, childhood or adult life. As the heart rate suddenly becomes rapid, the baby may go pale, start to breathe quickly and vomit. After a few hours, symptoms of heart failure occur and death may result if no treatment is given. Older children can usually recognise the onset of the tachycardia by describing palpitations. Paroxysms may occur spontaneously or be precipitated by illness. Return to sinus rhythm produces a diuresis.

Examination. The child looks pale but may be otherwise well. A baby is more likely to show obvious signs of heart failure. The pulse is weak, rapid, regular and does not gradually slow when carotid sinus or eyeball pressure is applied.

Investigations. The electrocardiogram shows a heart rate in excess of 240 per minute. The P waves may be present, abnormal, or absent, and the QRS complexes are normal. Between paroxysms, the electrocardiogram shows normal sinus rhythm. A number of children show the Wolf-Parkinson-White syndrome, an electrocardiographic abnormality comprising a short P-R interval and slurring of the beginning of the QRS complex.

Treatment. In some cases an attack can be terminated by vagal stimulation, for example, carotid sinus or eyeball pressure may be tried in older children. Ice packs applied to the face may be effective in babies. If this fails, digitalisation is effective but may take some time to work even if given intra-muscularly. Conversion to sinus rhythm using DC shock may be necessary if the baby is desperately ill. Recurrent attacks can be prevented or suppressed by regular digoxin or propanolol.

Complete heart block

Complete heart block with atrio-ventricular dissociation may occur in otherwise normal children or in children with underlying congenital or acquired heart disease. It is usually congenital and is sometimes suspected before birth. The ventricular rate of contraction is in the region of 50 per minute and may increase with exercise. Many affected children lead normal, healthy lives and remain symptom-free. A minority have classical Stokes-Adams attacks in which they fall to the ground and lose consciousness. The latter require treatment and this can either be given with drugs, such as long-acting isoprenaline or by insertion of an artificial pacemaker.

RHEUMATIC FEVER

There has been a dramatic fall in the incidence of this disease which used to cause much illness in children and permanent valvular damage in adults. The decline of

Clinical features of rheumatic fever

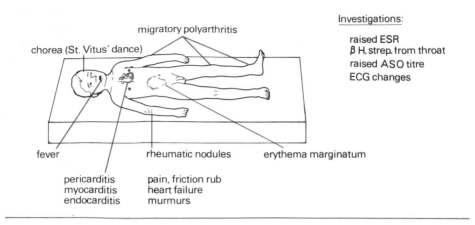

chorea (St. Vitus' dance)

migratory polyarthritis

fever

rheumatic nodules

erythema marginatum

pericarditis
myocarditis
endocarditis

pain, friction rub
heart failure
murmurs

Investigations:

raised ESR
β H. strep. from throat
raised ASO titre
ECG changes

the disease is probably the result of diminished virulence of the β-haemolytic streptococcus, the introduction of antibiotics and improved social conditions. Rheumatic fever may represent an abnormal immunological response to the β-haemolytic streptococcus, an organism commonly responsible for sore throats and tonsillitis. It is thought that the body confuses its own heart antigens with those of the organism, thereby causing an autoimmune reaction.

Rheumatic involvement of the heart causes a pancarditis (involving all three tissues of the heart), with infiltration by lymphocytes and plasma cells. In a number of cases this inflammation heals by scarring, leading in later life to manifestations of valvular heart disease, particularly of the aortic and mitral valves.

Clinical features. One to three weeks after a throat infection, the child (usually of school age) develops an acute migratory polyarthritis involving the medium-sized joints. Skin rashes occur, particularly erythema marginatum. The child is usually febrile and unwell. Rheumatic nodules may be felt subcutaneously over the occiput or on the extensor surfaces of elbows, wrists and fingers. Carditis occurs in a proportion of children. Pericarditis is detected by hearing a friction rub. Myocarditis is likely if there are arrhythmias or if the heart is enlarged clinically. Endocarditis is suggested by the presence of a heart murmur. This may be either an apical systolic murmur with or without a mid-diastolic murmur, suggesting mitral incompetence; or an early diastolic murmur at the left sternal border, suggesting aortic incompetence. Chorea is a neurological manifestation of rheumatic fever.

Investigation. The erythrocyte sedimentation rate is raised. Evidence of recent streptococcal infection should be sought, bacteriologically or serologically. The electrocardiogram may be helpful. In cases of rheumatic carditis, the P-R interval is frequently greater than 0.2 seconds, first degree heart block. Non-specific QRS and T wave changes also occur. If there is pericarditis, concave elevation of the S-T segment is seen.

Treatment. This is symptomatic only; the child is rested in bed and aspirin is given in doses sufficient to relieve the arthritis. A course of penicillin is given to eradicate the streptococcus. The disease, including cardiac involvement, is self-limiting but the process of healing can be speeded up by giving corticosteroids although this does not reduce the incidence of rheumatic heart disease in later life. Since rheumatic fever tends to recur, children who have had it should be given penicillin prophylactically, probably for an indefinite period. The risk of permanent heart damage is much greater after a second attack of rheumatic fever.

Subacute bacterial endocarditis

This is a well recognised complication of congenital as well as rheumatic heart disease. The risk is highest with those lesions which result in a turbulent jet of blood, such as ventricular septal defects, coarctation of the aorta, patent ductus arteriosus and aortic stenosis. The endocardium becomes infected in the presence of a bacteraemia or septicaemia, the commonest source of infection being the teeth. *Streptococcus viridans* is the usual infecting organism.

Clinical features. An affected child shows signs of infection with fever, malaise and anorexia. Clubbing of the fingers and an enlarged spleen may be noted. Embolic manifestations occur, either to the body or to the lungs depending on the site of the heart defect. The physical signs of the heart defect may alter as the endocarditis produces increasing damage to one of the heart valves.

Investigations. The diagnosis is made on the basis of the clinical picture and a positive blood culture.

Treatment. Sometimes this has to start before the diagnosis has been confirmed by blood culture. Bacteriocidal antibiotics are given, parenterally at first, for at least six weeks. Benzylpenicillin and streptomycin are an effective combination against *Streptococcus viridans*.

Prevention. This is always better than cure. Any child known to have a congenital heart lesion should carry a card to show to his doctor or dentist. This should state that the child has a heart lesion and that in the event of dental treatment (e.g. scaling, fillings or extractions), oral surgical procedures (e.g. tonsillectomy) or a sore throat or middle ear infection, prophylactic penicillin

Clinical features of subacute bacterial endocarditis

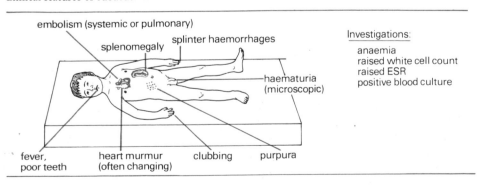

should be given, starting with an injection shortly before the procedure and continuing with oral treatment for the next three days at least.

HYPERTENSION

Unfortunately blood pressure measurement is often overlooked when assessing a child's problems. This attitude arises from the difficulties of making accurate measurements in a restless young child with equipment which is designed for adults and also because the yield of abnormal readings is very low. With attention to correct technique using suitable cuff sizes and making repeated attempts in a relaxed atmosphere, reliable measurements can be made using a mercury sphygmomanometer. In infants and young children the Doppler method is more reliable. Blood pressure increases with age, height and weight although it should be remembered that the fat arm may give an artificially high reading. Too narrow a cuff in a normal arm also causes this error. There is no precise definition of hypertension in childhood and although the figure 130/85 mmHg is often used, this overlooks those children who fall in the top 5 per cent of the blood pressure distribution for age. A proportion of these high rankers, particularly those with a family history of hypertension, become the adult population at risk from symptomatic hypertension, ischaemic heart disease and cerebrovascular disease. It must be emphasised that no child should be regarded as having an abnormal blood pressure until this has been confirmed on several occasions.

Causes of hypertension in childhood

age (yrs)	mean mm. Hg systolic	diastolic	mean +2 SD systolic	diastolic
0-2	95	55	110	65
3-6	100	65	120	70
7-10	105	70	130	75
11-15	115	70	140	80

Normal blood pressure values

conditions causing hypertension
%0   20   40   60   80   100%

renal parenchymal disease
coarctation disease
renovascular disease
Cushing's syndrome
phaeochromocytoma
other disorders

Surveys in several countries have demonstrated that the majority of children with mild asymptomatic hypertension fall into the primary or essential category. In contrast 70 to 90 per cent of those with severe symptomatic hypertension have some underlying cause, most commonly renal parenchymal disease. Greater attention to blood pressure measurement will bring these underlying problems to attention more promptly and may avoid life threatening complications. Hypertension may manifest itself as persistent headache, dizziness, disturbed vision, unexplained irritability, convulsions, and other neurological signs. Naturally, blood pressure should always be measured in the presence of cardiac and renal disorders. Paroxysmal episodes of palpitation and sweating raise the possibility of a phaeochromocytoma.

HYPERLIPOPROTEINAEMIA

The morbidity and mortality arising from atherosclerosis has reached such epidemic proportions in industrial societies that paediatricians can no longer evade their responsibilities in this direction. Fatty streaks are already present in the aortas of children aged 10 to 11 years and the coronary arteries start to show involvement in the early twenties. Both genetic and environmental factors contribute towards atheroma. Currently there is great interest in preventive measures. Some measures, such as antismoking campaigns, the prevention of obesity and the provision of facilities for regular physical exercise are well validated although not always easy to implement; others such as the widescale modification of diet in infants and young children, must be approached with caution.

Hyperlipidaemia and in particular hypercholesterolaemia has been convincingly linked to the development of atheroma. The majority of serum cholesterol is transported as β-lipoprotein, a low density lipoprotein.

Hyperbetalipoproteinaemia (familial hypercholesterolaemia)

This is an autosomal dominant condition in which homozygote individuals have a severe disease in which they develop tuberous and tendon xanthomata in early childhood and die of ischaemic heart disease in the second or third decade. The heterozygote condition is relatively common, affecting approximately 1 in 280 in England and Wales. 51 per cent of heterozygote males and 12 per cent of heterozygotes females have a heart attack by the age of 50 years. There are obviously grounds for detecting this disease in early childhood but serum cholesterol determination is not reliable in the first year partly because normal breast fed infants tend to have considerably higher cholesterol levels than those fed on polyunsaturated fat formulae. There is certainly no basis for assuming that this is a case against breast milk! In older children, the diagnosis can be confirmed by measuring serum cholesterol and β-lipoprotein. Long term treatment schedules consisting of low fat intake and where necessary drugs such as cholestyramine are currently being assessed.

Diet and hypercholesterolaemia

The majority of hypercholesterolaemia in affluent society is not due to a single, genetically-inherited disorder but reflects the impact of a high animal fat diet on a polygenically susceptible population. Within families there is a significant correlation between the serum cholesterol concentrations of children and those of their parents. The family history should include details of the occurrence and age of onset of ischaemic heart disease so that advice can be offered in an attempt to safeguard at-risk children. It is obviously sensible to reduce the fat intake, particularly from dairy products, but there is still insufficient evidence for the radical exclusion of cholesterol. Children tend to acquire the tastes of their parents and habituation to high fat or salt diets or smoking may well contribute to the future toll of atherosclerosis.

BIBLIOGRAPHY

Nadas A S, Fyler D C 1972 Paediatric cardiology. Saunders, Philadelphia
Scott O, Jordan S C 1973 Heart disease in paediatrics. Butterworth, London.

10
Gut

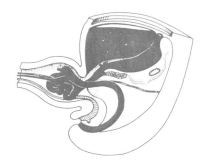

Normal function of the gastrointestinal tract depends on a carefully regulated balance between motility, sphincter tone, exocrine secretion and integrity of the absorptive surfaces. These functions begin to evolve early in fetal life: digestive enzymes and primitive swallowing movements are first detectable in the 12-week fetus and regular flow of amniotic fluid into the gut occurs from 20 weeks; by term this amounts to approximately 500 ml per day or half the total amniotic volume.

Gut function must undergo abrupt adjustment and maturation with birth and the onset of intermittent oral feeding. There is a marked increase in small intestinal mucosal surface area and this is at least partially mediated by gut hormones such as gastrin which are released in response to milk feeds. Digestive enzymes show a varied pattern of maturation, lactase activity being fully developed at term whereas trypsin takes 12 months to reach maximal levels. Although the gut is probably sterile at birth, it is rapidly colonised by bacterial entry through the mouth and anus. A normal microflora contributes to the available supply of vitamin K, folic acid and biotin. Immunological protection is provided to the newborn by secretory IgA antibodies in the maternal milk and by the transplacental passage of IgG antibodies. Endogenous IgA is produced in the first three to four weeks and is a major component of the barrier against bacteria and other antigens. Infants with immunological deficiencies are liable to develop gastrointestinal symptoms after three months of age when the reserve of maternal IgG is exhausted.

ACUTE ABDOMINAL PAIN

In children the 'acute abdomen' is a common and testing problem. Surgical conditions which require prompt diagnosis and treatment have to be distinguished from a large number of medical disorders. Careful general examination and urinalysis is essential.

Acute appendicitis
Appendicitis is the commonest acute surgical emergency of childhood. Three or

Causes of acute abdominal pain

Surgical	Medical (relatively common)	Medical (rare but important)
Acute appendicitis	Mesenteric adenitis	Lead poisoning
Intussusception	Constipation	Diabetes
Intestinal obstruction secondary to congenital anomalies	Gastroenteritis	Sickle cell crisis
	Lower lobe pneumonia	Acute porphyria
Torsion of ovary or testis	Acute nephritis	Pancreatitis
Hydronephrosis	Acute pyelonephritis	Primary peritonitis
Renal calculus	Henoch Schönlein purpura	
	Hepatitis	

four children in every 1000 have their appendix removed each year. It can occur at any age but is usually seen in children over five years of age. The characteristic triad of clinical features seen in adults, abdominal pain, low grade fever and tenderness with guarding in the right iliac fossa, is seen in the older child but in infants pain may not be a feature; they are more likely to present with a history of a recent respiratory infection followed by anorexia, vomiting, irritability and a high fever. This often leads to diagnostic confusion and delay so that the incidence of perforation with resulting peritonitis or abscess formation is higher in the younger child. The course of the disease in the young child is extremely rapid: a two-year-old can progress from apparent normality to perforation in six hours. There is no place therefore for prolonged observation in the young patient.

Mesenteric adenitis

Vague central or generalised abdominal pain commonly accompanies viral upper respiratory tract infections. It is due to non-specific inflammation in the mesenteric lymph nodes which provokes a mild peritoneal reaction and stimulates painful peristalsis in the terminal ileum. It is usually possible to distinguish mesenteric adenitis from acute appendicitis, but if there is any doubt four to six

Features which distinguish appendicitis and mesenteric adenitis

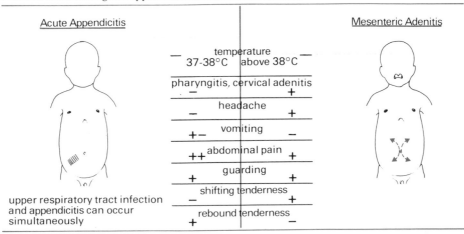

Acute Appendicitis			Mesenteric Adenitis
	temperature		
	37-38°C —	above 38°C —	
	pharyngitis, cervical adenitis		
	−	+	
	headache		
	−	+	
	vomiting		
	+−	−	
	abdominal pain		
	++	+	
	guarding		
	+	+	
	shifting tenderness		
upper respiratory tract infection and appendicitis can occur simultaneously	−	+	
	rebound tenderness		
	+	−	

hours after the child is first seen, and in all cases where there is persisting local tenderness the child must be surgically explored.

Malrotation

The midgut loop of the developing embryo elongates by herniating out into the umbilical cord from the sixth to the fourteenth intrauterine weeks. The apex of the loop communicates with the yolk sac by the vitelline duct, and this is the site of a possible Meckel's diverticulum. While still in the extra-embryonic coelom a counter clockwise rotation of 270° round the superior mesenteric artery occurs. At about 14 weeks the gut starts to return to the abdominal cavity, the proximal jejunum leading and lying in the left upper abdomen. The caecum is the last portion of the gut to re-enter the abdomen and it initially lies in the subhepatic position. This state of affairs is the most common abnormality seen clinically and to be accurate it should be called arrested caecal descent, not *mal*rotation. It can cause neonatal duodenal obstruction due to Ladd's bands, and partial recurrent volvulus in the older child due to the narrow mesenteric attachment between caecum and the duodenojejunal flexure. Often it is asymptomatic but causes severe technical difficulty if the patient develops acute appendicitis.

Maldescent and malrotation

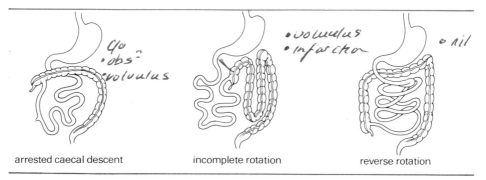

| arrested caecal descent | incomplete rotation | reverse rotation |

The second anomaly causing clinical problems is correctly called incomplete rotation of the gut, and again is not malrotation. Here rotation in the extra-embryonic coelom only amounts to 90° counter-clockwise, and the colon and caecum return first to the abdomen and occupy the left side. The small bowel fills the right side. The whole small bowel is suspended by an extremely narrow 1 cm mesenteric attachment between duodenojejunal flexure and caecum, and volvulus in the early days of life is extremely likely. Total small bowel infarction can result.

Extremely rarely a true malrotation can occur, if embryonic rotation is 90° clockwise instead of 270° counterclockwise. In this case, the duodenum will be anterior to the transverse colon. Clinical problems are rare.

Meckel's diverticulum

This diverticulum is a remnant of the vitellointestinal duct. It arises from the antimesenteric border of the terminal ileum and usually gives no trouble, but very rarely it may become inflamed and then the symptoms and signs mimic acute appendicitis. More commonly the diverticulum causes an intussusception, or a volvulus, or it contains ectopic gastric mucosa and peptic ulceration results in rectal bleeding or perforation. A technetium scan may help to identify ectopic mucosa.

Primary peritonitis
Primary peritonitis, usually due to pneumococcus, is considerably rarer than peritonitis secondary to appendicitis. Patients with nephrotic syndrome and immune deficiency states are susceptible.

Intussusception
Intussusception is an invagination of bowel into an adjacent lower segment. The usual origin is the terminal ileum or ileo-caecal valve resulting in an ileocolic intussusception. Although uncommon (2:1000 live births), it is the most frequent cause of intestinal obstruction in the first two years of life. It presents as paroxysmal pain sometimes with reflex vomiting and a sausage shaped mass is palpable in the right upper abdomen. If there is delay in diagnosis the child will develop fever, a distended abdomen and will pass bloodstained mucus rectally. The diagnosis is clinical and X-rays are not indicated in an ill child. Immediate surgery is arranged since bowel viability is rapidly lost. If the history is for less than 24 hours and there are no signs of fever, tenderness or blood rectally, the intussusception can sometimes be reduced hydrostatically by barium enema. This only has a 75 per cent success rate in suitable cases and the remaining 25 per cent have to go to theatre thereafter. Surgery has the advantage of establishing underlying causes such as a Meckel's diverticulum but such a cause is found in only 5 to 7 per cent. Recurrence is more frequent following barium enema reduction. A barium enema is useful in the diagnosis of chronic recurrent non-obstructive intussusception.

Intussusception

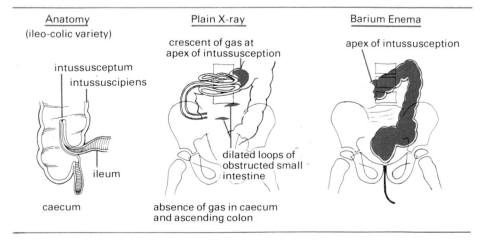

| Anatomy (ileo-colic variety) | Plain X-ray | Barium Enema |

Anatomy (ileo-colic variety): intussusceptum, intussuscipiens, ileum, caecum

Plain X-ray: crescent of gas at apex of intussusception, dilated loops of obstructed small intestine, absence of gas in caecum and ascending colon

Barium Enema: apex of intussusception

RECURRENT ABDOMINAL PAIN

This is a common problem affecting at least 10 per cent of school children. Although no organic cause is found in over 90 per cent, it is essential to identify those with an organic condition promptly. This enables specific management of the problem and confident counselling of children with functional disorders. Ideally, the children should be assessed when they have the pain as well as between episodes.

Renal tract infection

Renal tract infection must be excluded by urine culture and microscopy. Loin pain in the absence of urinary abnormality may still be an indication for an intravenous pyelogram, for it may reveal a hydronephrosis.

Peptic ulcers

Peptic ulcers are now being diagnosed more often in school children. This diagnosis should be suspected if there is a family history of ulceration. Duodenal ulcers occur eight times more frequently than gastric ulcers. The pain may be vague and not have the characteristics found in adults, although it is usually relieved by alkali. Conservative management including dietary advice and alkalis is usually sufficient. The long term use of cimetidine in children has still be be assessed. Gastroscopy provides a higher yield of positive results than barium meals.

Chronic recurrent pancreatitis

This is rare. There may be a family history. Clinical suspicion may be confirmed by finding calcification of the pancreas on abdominal X-ray.

Crohn's disease

Crohn's disease is rare in children but its incidence is thought to be on the increase. The diagnosis is often delayed because the symptoms are confused with those of the periodic syndrome. The usual features are recurrent abdominal pain with anorexia, diarrhoea, fever and growth impairment. Rarely perianal lesions, finger clubbing, arthritis and an abdominal mass occur. Diffuse involvement of the jejunum and ileum makes surgical resection difficult. Recurrence is common.

Features of 200 children with recurrent abdominal pain (from Apley 1975)

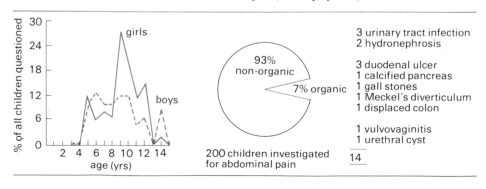

Features pointing to an organic cause for recurrent abdominal pain

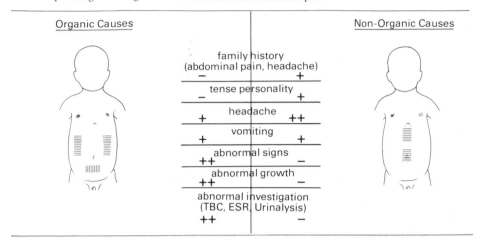

Organic Causes		Non-Organic Causes
	family history (abdominal pain, headache)	
−		+
	tense personality	
−		+
	headache	
+		++
	vomiting	
+		+
	abnormal signs	
++		−
	abnormal growth	
++		−
	abnormal investigation (TBC, ESR, Urinalysis)	
++		−

Corticosteroids and sulphasalazine together with dietary and vitamin supplementation are used in medical treatment but up to 90 per cent require surgery. It is sometimes difficult to distinguish Crohn's disease from ulcerative colitis although the latter seldom causes recurrent abdominal pain.

Ulcerative colitis
This is a condition in which there is mucosal ulceration of the distal large bowel. In children, total colon involvement is relatively more common than in adults. The child usually presents with diarrhoea, the stool containing both mucus and blood. Anaemia and growth failure are common, and arthritis, erythema nodosum, recurrent mouth ulceration and pyoderma gangrenosum may also occur. In the initial stages it is important to exclude bacterial infection and to define the extent of the disease by means of endoscopy and barium enema. Ulcerative colitis is a life-long condition and is very disruptive to the young person. Initial control of the disease is by means of dietary measures, iron supplements, sulphasalazine and corticosteroids. The long-term risk of carcinoma of the colon eventually necessitates colectomy and ileostomy formation. If possible these drastic procedures are delayed until after puberty, but disturbed schooling and growth failure favour earlier surgery.

GASTROENTERITIS

Although gastroenteritis is usually a mild disease in western countries, it is still reputed to be the fifth commonest cause of death in children under age one year in England and Wales. Epidemics of *E. coli* gastroenteritis may be particularly serious in neonatal units. In developing countries infectious diarrhoea and vomiting is an enormous health problem. In India, at least 1.5 million children die each year from this disease. Early weaning and mulnutrition create a vulnerable population of infants.

Bacterial gastroenteritis may be due to either invasive or non-invasive organisms

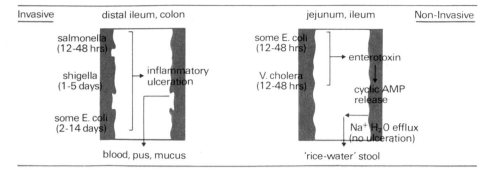

Bacterial gastroenteritis

Salmonella, Shigella, *E. coli* and *Vibrio cholerae* may be classified as invasive or noninvasive but enterotoxin producing. The traditional serotyping of *E. coli* does not relate directly to pathogenecity as strains may fall into either category. Some asymptomatic infants harbour invasive pathogenic serotypes while others are ill due to enterotoxin producing strains which do not belong to a pathogenic serotype. Fever is usual in bacterial gastroenteritis and in shigella infection, pyrexial convulsions and marked meningism may precede overt enteric symptoms. Food poisoning may be due to the ingestion of the exotoxin produced by coagulase positive staphylococcus.

Viral gastroenteritis

Viral infection is responsible for 50 to 60 per cent of acute gastroenteritis in children under the age of five years. A group of RNA viruses have been identified and variously called reo-like, orbivirus or rotavirus. Characteristically, viral gastroenteritis causes winter epidemics. Vomiting may be the only obvious presenting feature as diarrhoea may not occur for several hours and even then a watery stool is liable to be confused with urine in the wet napkins. Colicky abdominal pain with ill-defined tenderness and exaggerated bowel sounds is common. It is important to remember that vomiting and diarrhoea may be the presenting symptoms of surgical conditions, for example appendicitis, Hirschsprung's disease and intussusception. They also result from non-gastrointestinal disorders such as upper respiratory tract infections, renal infections and meningitis.

Dehydration

The water loss associated with gastroenteritis places a relatively greater stress on the young infant for he has a higher percentage of body water (80 per cent at term and 60 per cent at 12 months), a higher metabolic rate and a larger surface area to volume ratio. The assessment of dehydration relies upon a series of clinical signs which reflect changes in body tissues and circulatory status. The tissue changes are more easily recognised in thin than in overweight infants. A recent reliable weight is the best guide to body fluid loss. The clinical estimate indicates the percentage of the expected body weight which requires to be replaced, so that 10

Clinical assessment of dehydration

Sign	5% dehydration	10% dehydration
Skin	Loss of turgor	Mottled, poor capillary return
Fontanelle	Depressed	Deeply depressed
Eyes	Sunken	Deeply sunken
Peripheral pulses	Normal	Tachycardia, poor volume
Mental state	Lethargic	Prostration, coma

Features which differentiate isotonic and hypertonic dehydration

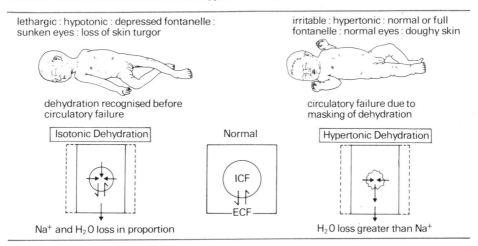

lethargic : hypotonic : depressed fontanelle : sunken eyes : loss of skin turgor

irritable : hypertonic : normal or full fontanelle : normal eyes : doughy skin

dehydration recognised before circulatory failure

circulatory failure due to masking of dehydration

Isotonic Dehydration   Normal   Hypertonic Dehydration

ICF

ECF

Na$^+$ and H$_2$O loss in proportion   H$_2$O loss greater than Na$^+$

per cent dehydration in a 5 kg infant indicates a replacement volume of 500 ml. It is also necessary to assess the type of dehydration; hypotonic, isotonic or hypertonic (also termed hypernatraemic when the serum sodium is above 150 mmol/l).

Mild dehydration (under 5 per cent) can be treated in the home by a regime of clear fluids for at least 24 hours followed by the gradual re-introduction of the normal diet. Standardised electrolyte powder sachets for solution are available. Carefuly daily assessment and weighing is essential.

Moderate to severe dehydration (over 5 per cent) requires intravenous therapy and this is especially urgent when there are signs of peripheral circulatory failure. Appropriate management demands an understanding of normal maintenance requirements as well as an assessment of the deficit. Acidosis may accompany

Maintenance requirements (above) and commonly prescribed electrolyte solutions for intravenous use (below)

age months	H$_2$O ml/kg	Na mmol/kg	K mmol/kg
0–6	150	2.5	2.5
6–12	120	2.5	2.5
12–24	100	2.5	2.5
Over 24	80	2.0	2.0

dehydration and if severe is treated by providing about half the calculated deficit as sodium bicarbonate:

deficit (mmol) = weight (kg) $\times$ 0.6 $\times$ 24 $-$ observed plasma bicarbonate (mmol/l).

Antibiotics are not indicated unless systemic spread of bacterial infection is likely. Anti-diarrhoeal agents should also be avoided as they slow transit time and encourage the persistence of an abnormal bowel flora.

Principles of intravenous therapy

	maintenance	0.2N Saline in 4.3% dextrose plus KCl
Total fluid requirements =	deficit	N saline plus KCl
	ongoing loss	0.5 N saline plus KCl

Scheme
1 0–½ h Treat shock immediately
        Plasma or N saline 20 ml/kg body weight
2 ½–4 h Initial replacement (awaiting serum electrolyte results) 0.5N or N saline 10 ml/kg/hour
3 4–24 h Continuing replacement
        (a) Serum Na under 150 mmol/l
            0.2N saline in 4.3% dextrose plus KCl 30–40 mmol/l
            Plan total correction by 24 h
        (b) Serum Na above 150 mmol/l
            0.2N saline in 4.3% dextrose plus KCl 30–40 mmol/l
            Restrict fluids to 150 ml/kg body weight in first 24 h and plan total correction over
            48 h

Solution	Na	K	mmol/l Ca	Cl	Lactate
Normal saline (0.9%)	155	—	—	155	—
0.5 N saline in 5% Dextrose	77	—	—	77	—
0.2 N saline in 4.3% Dextrose	31	—	—	31	—
Ringer's lactate solution (Hartmann's solution)	130	5	4	112	27

Complications

Post gastroenteritis diarrhoea is relatively common in young infants. A short

Complications of gastroenteritis and its treatment

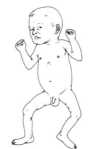

Convulsions
  fever
  hypo-, hypernatraemia
  hypoglycaemia
  hypocalcaemia

Cerebral damage
  hypotension
  vascular thrombosis

Pulmonary oedema
  fluid overload

Oliguria
  prenatal failure (urine urea ↑, urine Na⁺ ↓)
  renal failure   (urine urea ↓, urine Na⁺ ↑)
  —renal vein thrombosis
  —medullary necrosis

Protracted diarrhoea
  secondary lactose intolerance
  secondary cow's milk protein intolerance
  bacterial overgrowth

period of lactose free milk may be required. Refractory cases require careful evaluation.

MALABSORPTION

Enzymatic degradation of the major nutrients occurs within the gut lumen, at the microvilli and in the cytoplasm of the columnar epithelial cells. Disorders in the lumen may be due to failure of exocrine secretion, for example pancreatic insufficiency in cystic fibrosis, or disrupted bile salt circulation as in cholestatic liver disease. The mucosa may suffer non-specific epithelial damage in a variety of conditions, including coeliac disease and post-gastroenteritis. Other more specific inherited disorders interfere with individual pathways in the epithelium, for example primary congenital alactasia and familial chloride diarrhoea. Malabsorption may also occur due to obstruction of lymphatics in the intestinal wall as in congenital lymphangectasia.

Investigation of malabsorption is relatively complex and must not be initiated until it has been established that the child is failing to gain weight on a normal diet, does not have other systemic diseases and is being cared for in an adequate environment. Stool microscopy may reveal abundant fat globules. Three-day stool fat collections provide a more exact measure of steatorrhoea, an abnormal fat content being greater than 10 per cent of intake but it is a demanding and often unsuccessful investigation. A sweat test to exclude cystic fibrosis and a

Digestion and absorption

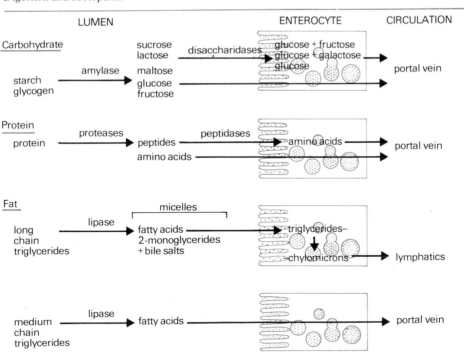

barium meal to detect anatomical malformations may be indicated. Peroral jejunal biopsy is a valuable diagnostic tool when appropriate care in patient selection is exercised.

Coeliac disease

Coeliac disease is the permanent inability to tolerate dietary wheat or rye gluten. Exposure to gluten results in morphological and functional abnormality of the proximal small intestine which can be reversed by exclusion of gluten. The incidence is about 1 in 2000 in the United Kingdom and as high as 1 in 300 in West Ireland. It is becoming less common in Europe. There is evidence that affected children have a susceptibility to an abnormal immune response to the gliadin fractions of gluten. The majority of children with coeliac disease present before the age of two years. The weight record may show progressive growth failure dating from the introduction of gluten-containing solids. In a few, overt malabsorption may not occur for many years. The one hour xylose absorption test in which 5 grams of xylose is given while fasting and the blood level measured after 1 hour, is of help in screening for coeliac disease. The jejunal biopsy is essential for definitive diagnosis. There are other causes of a flattened mucosa in childhood such as post-gastroenteritis, cow's milk protein intolerance and giardiasis so that repeated biopsies with and without dietary gluten are usually necessary to make a precise diagnosis. Coeliac disease has life-long implications. There is a risk of intestinal lymphoma which may be reduced by strict adherance to a gluten free diet. Infants with bowel upsets may display a temporary gluten intolerance.

Normal and abnormal jejunal mucosa, and the clinical features of gluten enteropathy

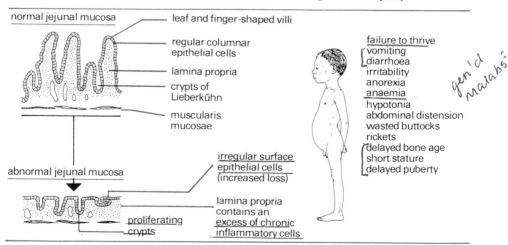

normal jejunal mucosa — leaf and finger-shaped villi

— regular columnar epithelial cells

— lamina propria

— crypts of Lieberkühn

— muscularis mucosae

abnormal jejunal mucosa

irregular surface epithelial cells (increased loss)

lamina propria contains an excess of chronic inflammatory cells

proliferating crypts

failure to thrive
vomiting
diarrhoea
irritability
anorexia
anaemia
hypotonia
abdominal distension
wasted buttocks
rickets
delayed bone age
short stature
delayed puberty

gen'd malabs:

Sugar intolerance

Sugar intolerance results from failure to absorb particular sugars, most commonly lactose. The osmotic load of the undigested sugar results in explosive watery diarrhoea and the intraluminal fermentation produces an excess of lactic acid and carbon dioxide. The fluid stools are acid (pH less than 5.5) and contain reducing substances which can be demonstrated using clinitest tablets.

Lactose intolerance is a common sequel of gastroenteritis or coeliac disease. It also occurs in premature infants; as a rare inherited disorder in Caucasians (autosomal recessive) and as a frequent finding in non-Caucasians after early childhood (autosomal dominant).

Sucrase-isomaltase deficiency. This can occur after severe mucosal damage or be inherited in an autosomal recessive mode.

Galactose-glucose malabsorption is extremely rare, and results in severe persistent diarrhoea from birth.

Cow's milk protein intolerance
This is a mainly clinical diagnosis which is made when either acute or chronic symptoms appear to be related to cow's milk ingestion. Acute reactions after small amounts of milk include vomiting, diarrhoea, urticaria, stridor and bronchospasm, and when this happens the association with milk intake is fairly readily established. It is more difficult to confirm that chronic effects such as failure to thrive, rectal bleeding, anaemia and hepatosplenomegaly are due to a reaction to milk protein. Immunological studies indicate a variety of mechanisms. Susceptible infants may have enhanced absorption of antigenic quantities of β-lactoglobulin in early infancy and this may in turn be related to transient IgA deficiency or follow gastroenteritis. Jejunal biopsy shows variable villous flattening. The disorder is usually temporary and can be managed by dietary adjustments. Protein is given in the form of casein hydrolysate, chicken meat or soya protein.

Chronic non-specific diarrhoea
Persistent diarrhoea in a thriving child is a very common complaint. The most frequent explanation is an exaggerated gastrocolic reflex repeatedly provoked by frequent snacks and cold drinks. Simple measures such as restricting fluid intake to meal times obviates the need for antidiarrhoeal preparations of dubious therapeutic value.

Acrodermatitis enteropathica
This is a rare genetic disorder recently recognised as being linked to a defect of zinc metabolism. The infants develop severe diarrhoea and failure to thrive with a characteristic rash over the mucocutaneous junctions and pressure areas. There is also alopecia and nail dystrophy. The onset is delayed if the child is breast fed. Without appropriate therapy it is a fatal condition, and until the recognition of the value of zinc supplements the disease was controlled by the use of dihydroiodoquin.

Intestinal parasites
These are common causes of malabsorption, anaemia and chronic diarrhoea in developing countries.

Threadworm and roundworm

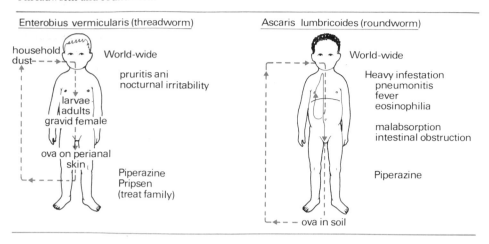

Giardia lamblia is a flagellate protozoon transmitted by contaminated food and water. Infection may be asymptomatic or result in malabsorption due to jejunal mucosal damage. Metronidazole is the treatment of choice.

Ascaris lumbricoides (roundworms) infection follows ingestion of the eggs. The larvae migrate via the portal system to the lungs where they ascend the bronchial tree to re-enter the gut. Heavy infestation may result in pneumonitis and eosinophilia during the larval phase. Gut symptoms are rare but include pain, obstruction and appendicitis. Piperazine treats the adult phase.

Ankylostoma (hookworm) is a major cause of iron deficiency in hot, humid climates. Bephenium hydroxynaphthoate is an effective treatment.

Toxocara canis and catis may have their migratory larval phase in children who are in close contact with animal excreta. Infection produces eosinophilia, hepatomegaly and bronchospasm. The larvae may encapsulate in the eye

Hookworm and toxocara

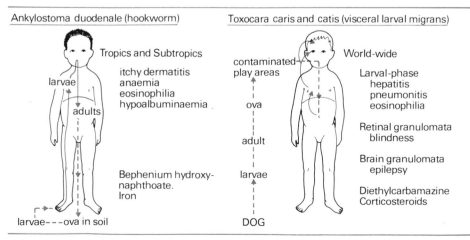

producing retinal granulomata, or in the brain acting as potential epileptogenic foci.

Taenia saginata (beef tapeworm) and Taenia solium (pork tapeworm). The adult worms inhabit the intestinal canal of man. It is also possible for man to be infected by the larval phase of *T. solium* as a result of consumption of inadequately cooked pork. The larvae or cysticerci may encapsulate and calcify in the tissues. The adult tapeworms may be killed by either niclosamide or dichlorophen.

Enterobius (threadworm). Infestation is seldom symptomatic other than by causing pruritis ani. The entire family must be treated with piperazine.

CONSTIPATION

Constipation is a frequent complaint in all age groups and reflects a common obsession with regular bowel function. It is valid to differentiate the problem of infrequent hard stools from the less worrying complaint of infrequent normal stools. Healthy infants show a considerable variation in the pattern of bowel frequency depending on their diet, and indeed mother's diet if breast fed. They may also show alarming colour changes and vigorous abdominal contractions during defaecation which may be interpreted by mother as straining. Genuine hard stools may result from an inadequate milk intake, hunger stools, or from over strength artificial feeds where the free water is diverted to facilitate renal solute excretion. The change from an artificial milk formula or breast milk to cow's milk is accompanied by production of smaller, harder and less frequent stools. Their passage may require more effort and resulting anal irritation may provoke withholding, and a pattern of behaviour which can evolve into troublesome constipation. Constipation may accompany more generalised disorders but it is seldom the chief complaint. Hypothyroidism, idiopathic hypercalcaemia and neuromuscular problems fall into this category.

In older children, acute constipation is a common accompaniment of febrile illnesses and the resulting hard stools may cause an anal tear which in turn initiates the cycle of faecal retention and chronic constipation. The prompt use of gentle laxatives and abundant fluids facilitates healing of the traumatised anal margin and helps the child to regain confidence in his toilet activities. It is sad that so

Chronic constipation

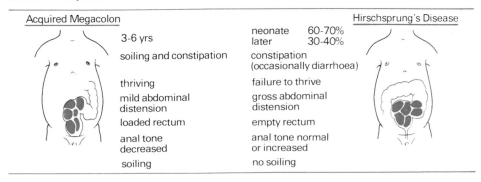

Acquired Megacolon				Hirschsprung's Disease
	3-6 yrs	neonate 60-70% later 30-40%		
	soiling and constipation	constipation (occasionally diarrhoea)		
	thriving	failure to thrive		
	mild abdominal distension	gross abdominal distension		
	loaded rectum	empty rectum		
	anal tone decreased	anal tone normal or increased		
	soiling	no soiling		

many of these children are allowed to develop chronic constipation with all its attendant problems. These include abdominal pain, anorexia, vomiting, failure to thrive, and a predisposition to urinary tract infections. The accumulation of hard stool in the rectal ampulla leads to an acquired megacolon. The distention of the rectum results in relaxation of the internal sphincter so that the child must continually call on the external sphincter and the levator ani, which are voluntary muscle groups, in order to resist stool passage. Eventually this effort fails and the external sphincter is no longer able to prevent constant leakage of faecal matter. The soiling is often the dominant complaint and the families become desperate in their attempts to cope with this unsocial problem. Examination confirms the presence of the indentable faecal mass, the perianal soiling and the firm stool just within the internal sphincter.

Treatment requires an enthusiastic but relatively simple approach. The main objectives are to dislodge the faecal mass, overcome withholding behaviour and promote a regular bowel habit. Success revolves around the child regaining confidence in being capable of painless easy defaecation. A short course of liquid paraffin or mineral oil with the unpleasant taste suitably disguised is an effective means of dislodging the faecal mass. More refractory cases may require a brief course of enemas but the oral approach is more satisfactory for both child and therapist. This is followed by a programme of copious fluids, a high roughage diet and Senokot at a dosage sufficient to amplify the gastrocolic reflex. The child must learn to take advantage of the latter by spending 5 to 10 minutes on the toilet after breakfast and the evening meal. It is worth checking that the child has firm foot support so that he can obtain the optimal mechanical advantage while sitting on the toilet. The use of laxatives and in particular liquid paraffin may cause the soiling to be worse during the initial period of treatment and parents must be warned about this. In most children, the physical and emotional problems improve in parallel with the recovery of normal bowel function. In a minority there are more profound behavioural problems which warrant a careful psychiatric evaluation.

Although chronic constipation can usually be overcome by this regime, in some children the possibility of short segment Hirschsprung's disease arises. If the problem persists in spite of anal dilatation under general anaesthetic, re-evaluation is necessary.

Hirschsprung's disease

Hirschsprung's disease must be considered if constipation presents in infancy. In Nottingham it accounts for about 10 per cent of neonatal intestinal obstruction, but it may also present in the older child. It results from failure of migration of ganglion cells to the submucosal and myenteric plexuses of the large bowel. The aganglionic segment, which remains tonically contracted and aperistaltic, invariably involves the internal sphincter. Sometimes there is a very short segment, but 80 per cent involve the recto-sigmoid colon and 15 per cent extend to more proximal colon. In one large series 85 per cent developed difficulties in the first month of life and 95 per cent by the end of the first year. The typical infant fails to pass meconium within the first 24 hours of life, develops progressive abdominal distention, refuses to feed and finally has bilious vomiting. A severe form of enterocolitis with perforation and septicaemia may complicate this picture and has a high mortality rate. The older child suffers with intermittent bouts of intestinal obstruction from faecal impaction, failure to thrive, hypochromic anaemia and hypoproteinaemia. Soiling is extremely unusual but not unknown in Hirschsprung's disease. On examination, the upper abdomen is distended with gas as well as faeces, the costal margin is flared and the umbilicus is displaced downward. Characteristically, the anal canal and rectum are free of faeces and may feel narrow and grip the finger. The diagnosis may be confirmed by barium enema of an unprepared colon, rectal biopsy and ano-rectal manometry. The latter demonstrates an absence of the normal reflex inhibition of the internal anal sphincter on rectal distention. Surgical treatment often entails an initial colostomy to relieve the obstruction. The subsequent definitive operation is designed to bypass the aganglionic segment and bring normal bowel down to the anus.

LIVER DISEASE

Hepatomegaly
Liver disease presents with hepatomegaly, jaundice, metabolic disturbance or intestinal bleeding either singly or in combination. The normal liver has a soft, smooth, non-tender edge 1 to 2 cm below the costal margin. An enlarged liver may be a transient finding accompanying acute disorders like infectious hepatitis or glandular fever, or it may be long-standing, requiring detailed investigation.

Persistent neonatal jaundice
Jaundice persisting beyond the second week is abnormal and in considering the possible cause, a distinction must be made between conjugated and unconjugated hyperbilirubinaemia.

Breast milk jaundice is a relatively uncommon problem, and is due to a complex steroid in the milk which inhibits hepatic glucuronyl transferase. It is seldom necessary to advise against breast feeding in this condition as it resolves spontaneously. It is often confused with jaundice due to fluid deprivation.

Crigler-Najjar syndrome is a rare, autosomal recessive condition in which hepatic glucuronyl transferase is deficient or absent. The most severe form causes neonatal kernicterus and is incompatible with life. A milder variety may respond to long-term phototherapy.

Neonatal hepatitis is not a discrete entity but is the end result of a range of injurious processes which produce a similar histological picture, hepatocellular necrosis and inflammatory cell infiltrates in the portal tracts and lobules. Infants with conjugated hyperbilirubinaemia must be investigated for the known infective, genetic and metabolic causes, and it has to be appreciated that neonatal hepatitis is part of a spectrum of hepatic injury which overlaps with biliary atresia.

Biliary atresia is the end stage of a sclerosing process in an initially patent biliary tree. With few exceptions the prognosis was uniformly dismal until the recent introduction of early laparotomy and porto-enterostomy, the Kasai

Causes of persistent neonatal jaundice

Unconjugated hyperbilirubinaemia	Conjugated hyperbilirubinaemia
Infection, e.g. urinary tract	(a) Neonatal hepatitis syndrome
Hypothyroidism	Congenital infection, e.g. rubella, cytomegalovirus, toxoplasmosis
Haemolytic anaemia	Metabolic
High gastrointestinal obstruction	alpha-1 antitrypsin deficiency
Breast-milk jaundice	galactosaemia
Transient familial hyperbilirubinaemia	tyrosinosis
Crigler-Najjar syndrome	cystic fibrosis
	storage disorders
	(b) Duct obstruction or obliteration
	Extrahepatic biliary atresia
	Intrahepatic biliary hypoplasia
	Choledochal cyst

procedure. This operation is followed by bile flow in approximately 25 per cent of children and has provided a stimulus to the early diagnosis and selection of those infants who might benefit from surgery. The longer term outcome has still to be assessed.

Percutaneous liver biopsy and iodine[131] rose bengal excretion studies are useful in separating the majority of infants with biliary atresia from those with neonatal hepatitis syndrome. The latter may deteriorate if subjected to inappropriate surgery, and if no specific therapy is indicated by the investigations, a trial of phenobarbitone and cholestyramine may promote recovery. In a prospective study of the neonatal hepatitis syndrome in S.E. England, homozygous α_1 antitrypsin deficiency was the single most commonly identifiable cause but the majority of cases had no demonstrable aetiology.

Prolonged neonatal jaundice

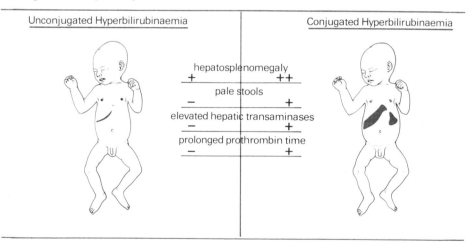

Unconjugated Hyperbilirubinaemia		Conjugated Hyperbilirubinaemia
hepatosplenomegaly	+	++
pale stools	−	+
elevated hepatic transaminases	−	+
prolonged prothrombin time	−	+

Infectious hepatitis

Hepatitis A infection (incubation 15 to 50 days) is the commonest cause of jaundice in older children. It spreads by the oral route and is usually mild or subclinical. Fever, vomiting and abdominal pain may precede the jaundice. Elevation of serum transaminase levels is the first biochemical abnormality and they remain raised for up to three weeks in most cases. Passive immunisation with pooled immunoglobulin provides protection and may be indicated for family and other close contacts. There are no readily available specific tests for hepatitis A and alternative causes of jaundice must be considered in isolated cases.

Hepatitis B (incubation 50 to 180 days) seldom infects healthy children but can be transmitted by carrier mothers to newborn infants. It is usually self-limiting but is capable of causing chronic hepatitis. Infectious mononucleosis (EB virus) and cytomegalovirus can also cause hepatitis.

Wilson's disease (hepato lenticular degeneration)
This is a rare and potentially very damaging disease which merits prompt consideration in any child with unexplained liver disturbance. The pathognomic appearance of copper at the periphery of the cornea (Kayser-Fleischer rings) requires slit lamp examination but is often absent in the young. The majority of cases have low serum levels of copper and caeruloplasmin. Oral penicillamine facilitates removal of the excess body copper. The disorder is inherited as an autosomal recessive and siblings must be screened for low caeruloplasmin levels.

Chronic aggressive hepatitis
Chronic aggressive or active hepatitis is an autoimmune disorder and is relatively more frequent in adolescent girls. The majority have an insidious onset with fever, acneiform rashes, erythema nodosum, colitis, jaundice and hepatomegaly but a significant number have an initial illness resembling infectious hepatitis. Disturbed liver function tests, an elevated ESR and positive antinuclear factor tests favour the diagnosis but it is essential to confirm it by percutaneous liver biopsy. The natural history is one of progressive fibrosis with the development of cirrhosis. Prolonged corticosteroid therapy combined with azathioprine may control this grave development.

Causes of hepatomegaly and clinical signs which may aid the diagnosis

Causes		Signs

• Systemic infection
  infectious hepatitis
  glandular fever
		mental retardation
		<u>mucopolysaccharidoses</u>

• Primary liver disease
  chronic hepatitis
  polycystic disease
  hepatocellular carcinoma
		Kayser-Fleischer rings:
		<u>Wilson's disease</u>

• Other neoplasia
  leukaemia
  reticulosis
  nephroblastoma
  neuroblastoma
		spider naevi:
		liver palms:
		finger clubbing
		<u>chronic liver failure</u>

• Metabolic storage +enzactic.
  glycogenoses   galac
  lipidoses
  mucopolysaccharides fruc. utol
		splenomegaly
		collateral veins
		ascites
		<u>portal hypertension</u>

• Cardiac		bone lesions <u>lipidoses</u>

Causes and clinical features of cirrhosis in childhood

Causes		Clinical Features
Genetic (metabolic/storage) cirrhosis		Portal hypertension
eg. α_1-antitryspin deficiency Wilson's disease galactosaemia cystic fibrosis		oesophageal varices splenomegaly hypersplenism ascites
Post-necrotic cirrhosis	biopsy	Hepatic failure
eg. neonatal hepatitis chronic aggressive hepatitis drugs, toxins, poisons venous congestion		failure to thrive fatigue, anorexia spider naevi finger clubbing liver palms
Biliary cirrhosis		
eg. extrahepatic biliary atresia intrahepatic biliary hypoplasia choledochal cyst	regenerating nodules broad bands of fibrosis	

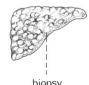

Childhood cirrhosis

Cirrhosis may result from inherited metabolic disorders or from acquired disease of the liver or biliary tract. In the majority of affected children no specific therapy is available and treatment is directed towards combating the resultant malabsorption, bleeding problems and ascites.

Portal hypertension

This usually presents as intestinal bleeding and splenomegaly, but the spleen may not be palpable immediately after a severe haemorrhage. The majority of cases are due to thrombosis of the portal vein; either idiopathic or secondary to sepsis of the umbilical vein and portal system in infancy. Hepatic cirrhosis and congenital hepatic fibrosis may also cause portal hypertension. The exact cause needs to be established by selective angiography of the coeliac axis and by a liver biopsy. If portal vein thrombosis is diagnosed, the long-term management should be as conservative as possible as splenorenal shunts are technically difficult and seldom successful before the age of ten years. There is a tendency for bleeding from the oesophageal varices to improve with age.

Congenital hepatic fibrosis

Congenital hepatic fibrosis may be either sporadic or familial and is diagnosed by liver biopsy which shows marked portal fibrosis but retention of the normal hepatic lobular architecture. It may be associated with polycystic disease of the kidneys.

LIVER ENZYME DEFICIENCIES

Glycogen storage diseases

Enzyme deficiencies with their resulting disorders have been recognised for each of the steps in the pathways of glycogen synthesis and degradation. They enter into the differential diagnosis of recurrent hypoglycaemia, hepatomegaly, muscle weakness with cramps, and congestive cardiac failure.

Type I: Glucose-6-phosphatase deficiency is a serious disorder, usually presenting in infancy, and manifest by hepatomegaly, hypoglycaemia and a metabolic acidosis. The enzyme deficiency prevents the normal glycaemic response to intramuscular glucagon and can be confirmed by liver biopsy. Frequent glucose feeds and restriction of galactose and fructose intake are helpful in treatment.

Type III: Debranching enzyme deficiency and type VI: liver phosphorylase deficiency present in a similar although milder fashion and can be diagnosed by measurement of leucocyte enzyme levels.

Type II: Acid maltase deficiency (Pompe's disease) results in excessive glycogen deposition in both liver and muscle, with cardiac muscle expecially involved. The majority of affected infants present soon after birth with poor feeding, weakness, tachypnoea and cardiac failure. Muscle or leucocyte enzyme analysis confirm the diagnosis but treatment is supportive only and the child will survive only for a matter of months.

Galactosaemia

Galactosaemia is a very rare, recessively inherited disorder but its importance lies in the disastrous consequences of being overlooked. It results from deficiency of the enzyme, galactose-1-phosphate uridyl transferase, which is essential for galactose metabolism. Affected infants are normal at birth but shortly after the commencement of milk feeds the majority develop jaundice, vomiting, diarrhoea, and fail to thrive. If the disorder remains unrecognised liver disease, cataracts and mental retardation will result. The urine contains galactose and is characteristically clinitest positive but clinistix negative, the latter being specific for glucose. Specific enzymatic techniques confirm the diagnosis and establish the necessity of a lactose-free diet.

Hereditary fructose intolerance

This is another rare enzyme deficiency in which prompt recognition can prevent the onset of life-threatening complications. The low activity of aldolase B not only results in the accumulation of fructose-1-phosphate but also causes a secondary inhibition of hepatic pathways responsible for maintaining normoglycaemia. In susceptible children, fructose-containing foods provoke abdominal pain, nausea, vomiting and symptoms of hypoglycaemia. In the longer term hepatomegaly, growth failure and liver failure occur. A detailed dietary history reveals normal health until the introduction of sucrose into the diet, and suspicion may be substantiated by a fructose tolerance test or by liver enzyme analysis. Therapy simply involves the elimination of all fructose containing items from the diet.

Benign or essential fructosuria is an asymptomatical deficiency of the enzyme fructokinase.

BIBLIOGRAPHY

Apley J 1975 The child with abdominal pains. Blackwell, Oxford
Anderson C M, Burke V 1975 Paediatric gastroenterology. Blackwell, Oxford
Harries J T 1977 Essentials of paediatric gastroenterology. Churchill Livingstone, Edinburgh
Mowat A P 1979 Liver disorders in childhood. Butterworths, London

11

Urinary Tract and Testes

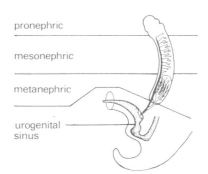

pronephric

mesonephric

metanephric

urogenital sinus

Renal function undergoes a major transition with the onset of extrauterine life and the demands of water conservation and electrolyte homeostasis. The nephrons at birth are still relatively immature both morphologically and physiologically so that young infants are susceptible to hypernatraemia, hyperphosphataemia, hypocalcaemia and metabolic acidosis if given inappropriate feeds. The already restricted glomerular filtration rate, only 25 per cent of the mature value, is very dependent on the extracellular volume and is liable to fall if stressed by dehydration.

Renal function matures considerably in the first two years of life out of proportion to the actual increase in renal mass. The tubular capacity to concentrate urine rises from a maximum of 800 milliosmoles per kg in the first week of life to the adult range of 1200 to 1400 milliosmoles per kg by three months of age.

RENAL FUNCTION TESTS

Proteinuria

Albustix provide a rapid assessment of proteinuria but register positive with levels which are often insignificant. Transient positive readings are common during febrile illness possibly representing the deposition of soluble immune complexes in the kidney. The finding of proteinuria does not necessarily mean that the urine is infected.

Microscopy

Microscopy is a useful guide to urinary tract infection but must always be linked with urine culture, preferably using a dipslide or slope technique. Microscopy of fresh urine should normally demonstrate no casts, less than 5 white blood cells, and less than 2 red blood cells per mm³. Motile bacteria can usually be seen in uncentrifuged infected urine.

Urine microscopy

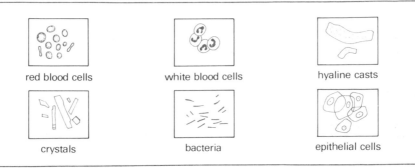

red blood cells   white blood cells   hyaline casts

crystals   bacteria   epithelial cells

Urine osmolality and pH

A second morning void after fasting overnight provides a useful screening test of renal concentration, normal values are above 900 milliosmoles per kg, and of acidification, normal pH less than 5.3.

Glycosuria and aminoaciduria

Glycosuria and aminoaciduria may be secondary to elevated serum levels or due to tubular defects.

Glomerular filtration rate (GFR)   CREATININE.

Derived from 24 hour urine volume and measurement of plasma creatinine, this is very liable to error in young children because of difficulty of collection techniques. The approximate GFR can be derived from the plasma creatinine using the equation:

$$\text{GFR}/1.73\,\text{m}^2 \text{ surface area} = 38 \times \text{height (cm)}/\text{plasma creatinine } (\mu\text{mol/l}).$$

Renal growth and the development of glomerular function

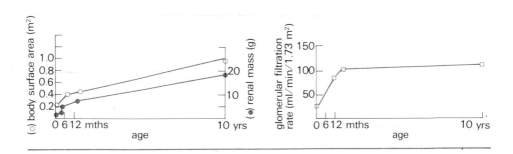

The rate of fall in blood concentration of an injected isotope (chromium[51] EDTA) is used for more precise measurement.

URINARY TRACT MALFORMATIONS

These are relatively common but most are functionally insignificant. A small proportion are fatal and may have important genetic implications.

Renal agenesis or Potter's syndrome

This is incompatible with survival, 75 per cent are associated with oligohydramnios. The majority are sporadic but there is an autosomal recessive variety.

Potter's syndrome

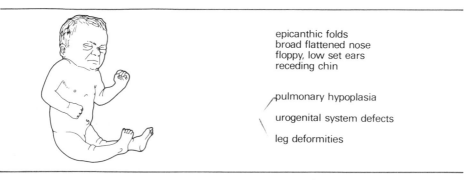

epicanthic folds
broad flattened nose
floppy, low set ears
receding chin

pulmonary hypoplasia

urogenital system defects

leg deformities

Unilateral renal hypoplasia

Unilaterial renal hypoplasia is often associated with dysplastic development. There is an interesting association between ear abnormalities and ipsilateral kidney malformation.

Polycystic kidneys

Infantile polycystic disease results in grossly enlarged spongy kidneys and cystic changes in the liver and other viscera. The bilateral kidney enlargement is conspicuous at birth or in early infancy. There are several varieties each with an autosomal recessive inheritance. The adult form, with autosomal dominant inheritance, can also present in early life although most survive to be young adults and are therefore capable of transmitting the lethal gene.

Obstructive malformations

These produce either unilateral or bilateral hydronephrosis.

Pelvi-ureteric junction obstruction is the most common cause and may be produced by intrinsic stenosis, functional obstruction or by compression from a vessel or band. Bilateral hydronephrosis suggests either a neurogenic bladder, as occurs in spina bifida, or urethral obstruction such as with post-urethral valves.

Horseshoe kidneys produce a characteristic IVP picture. Hydronephrosis due to pelvi-ureteric junction obstruction may occur. Treatment is by pyeloplasty.

Ureteric duplication and ectopia. Ureteric duplication, unilateral or bilateral is extremely common, so much so that most radiologists regard it as a variant of normal anatomy. In a duplex ureteric system, the ureters usually enter

Renal tract abnormalities liable to obstruction

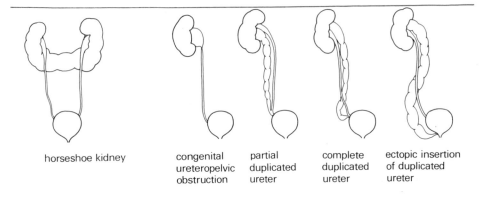

| horseshoe kidney | congenital ureteropelvic obstruction | partial duplicated ureter | complete duplicated ureter | ectopic insertion of duplicated ureter |

the bladder by a single orifice, but they may enter separately in which case the ureter from the upper moiety of the kidney enters the bladder abnormally low, and the ureter from the lower moiety enters in the normal position. Obstruction and reflux, separately or together, are relatively common complications affecting the upper moiety ureter. Ectopia of a duplex ureter sufficient to cause incontinence is very unusual. Bilateral ectopia of single ureteric systems is extremely rare. In girls it is associated with total bladder neck incompetence and failure to develop any bladder capacity. Diversion is usually necessary. In boys, reconstruction of the bladder neck and reimplantation of the ureters may be successful.

Posterior urethral valves. Valvular obstruction of the posterior urethra is the most common cause of severe bladder outflow obstruction in the male child. Most cases present during the first year of life, at least half during the first three months. An infant with severe obstruction fails to pass urine after birth, has a distended bladder, palpable kidneys and rapidly goes into renal failure. A slightly older infant with incomplete obstruction presents with failure to thrive, vomiting, abdominal distension, diarrhoea, and a distended bladder with overflow dribbling.

Urethral valves. Mortality and survival rates in 55 boys classified according to age at presentation (after Johnston)

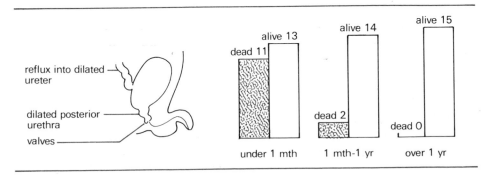

The kidneys show secondary hydronephrosis bilaterally due to vesicoureteric reflux. Diagnosis is by micturating cystourethrogram; treatment is by diathermy of the valves under general anaesthesia. Temporary proximal diversion may occasionally be necessary. The mortality from renal failure is high, especially in those presenting in the newborn period.

In children in whom the valves are successfully obliterated, the reflux will often spontaneously resolve with improvement in the degree of hydronephrosis.

Bladder exstrophy. This results from failure of midline fusion of the infra-umbilical midline structures. Males are affected more commonly than females. Clinically, the bladder mucosa is present as a small contracted circular plaque in the low abdomen, the umbilicus is abnormally low, the penis up-turned and epispadic, the pubis unfused and the lower limbs therefore apparently externally rotated, and the testes abnormally descended. In girls the genital tract is normal although vaginal stenosis may need surgery in early adult life. Bladder and especially bladder neck reconstruction is extremely difficult and many children are treated by urinary diversion.

Urachal remnants may persist producing blind tracts or cysts in the lower abdominal wall. Complete patency between the bladder and umbilicus is exceptionally rare.

URINARY TRACT INFECTIONS

This is a common paediatric problem; 1 to 2 per cent of schoolgirls and 0.2 per cent of boys have asymptomatic bacteriuria. In the newborn period, males are more commonly affected but the total incidence is less well established (0.1 to 3 per cent). The pre-school child with an associated renal abnormality, obstruction or vesico-ureteric reflux is most at risk, as the kidney is especially vulnerable to scarring in the first three years of life.

In the newborn, prolonged jaundice, excessive weight loss or a septicaemic episode may be secondary to urinary tract infection. The young child may also present with relatively non-specific symptoms; poor weight gain, irritability, fever, vomiting and diarrhoea. Urinalysis and culture must always be considered in a sick child. Apparently typical symptoms of urinary frequency and dysuria may be confusing in an older child as there is often no bacteriological confirmation of infection; the so-called acute urethal syndrome associated with acute vulvitis or balanitis. This may reflect poor hygiene, perineal candidiasis or contact sensitivity with nylon pants.

Organisms derived from bowel flora are the commonest infecting agents. Careful urine collection by clean catch or supervised use of a urine bag combined with dipslide technique allows bacteriological confirmation. Suprapubic aspiration is normally reserved for clarifying equivocal results or for use in infants.

Management
Management of an acute infection combines analgesia, copious fluids and

antibacterial therapy; sulphonamides, co-trimoxazole, nitrofurantoin, amoxicillin or naladixic acid according to bacteriological sensitivity. Suspected septicaemia merits intravenous gentamicin and ampicillin. A ten-day course is usually curative but has to be monitored by urine cultures. 75 per cent of cases relapse within two years.

All proven urinary tract infections require radiological evaluation with an IVP. A micturating cystourethrogram should also be performed in children under the age of three, where the IVP is abnormal or where there are recurrent urinary tract infections. A family history of renal malformation is a further indication. Approximately 50 per cent of both symptomatic and asymptomatic cases are found to have an underlying abnormality, most commonly vesicoureteric reflux.

X-ray abnormalities detected in children with bacteriuria (after Smellie and Normand). A classification of vesicoureteric reflux

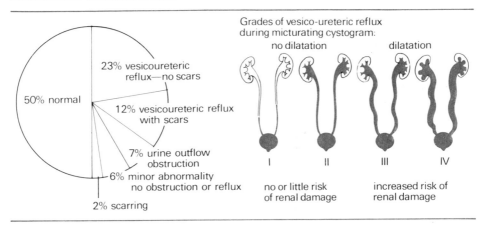

The priorities must be to deal with surgically amenable problems, for example mechanical obstruction or calculus, and to prevent further infection in scarred kidneys during growth. Vesico-ureteric reflux ceases spontaneously in 60 to 80 per cent of ureters. Ureteric reimplantation is considered where reflux is gross, is accompanied by fresh renal scarring and poor renal growth, or refractory infection.

Drugs commonly used in the treatment of urinary tract infection

Drug	Dose	Comments
Cotrimoxazole	2 mg/kg trimethoprin twice daily	Useful in prophylaxis Good compliance. Side effects — rashes, vomiting
Amoxycillin	125 mg three times a day	Less useful in prophylaxis. Side effects — rashes, diarrhoea
Nitrofurantoin	2 mg/kg three times a day	Useful in prophylaxis. Side effects — nausea, vomiting
Nalidixic acid	15 mg/kg three times a day	Useful in boys with proteus infection. Side effects — rashes
Gentamycin	1 mg/kg three times a day	Parenteral use only. Side effects — nephrotoxic, ototoxic

Long term prophylaxis is indicated in cases of recurrent symptomatic infection and to optimise renal growth in the presence of reflux. Continuous low dosage co-trimoxazole or nitrofurantoin maintains sterile urine while not inducing resistance in the bowel flora. It may be required for one to two years or until renal growth ceases. Additional preventive measures include hygiene, double micturition and a regular bowel habit.

Screening

Extensive surveys have attempted to monitor the impact of detection, investigation and treatment of asymptomatic bacteriuria in schoolgirls aged 5 to 12 years. The results suggest that such screening is not worthwhile and that kidney damage associated with infection generally occurs before five years. Screening the preschool child is time consuming and the yield of treatable abnormalities is small.

HAEMATURIA

Haematuria may occur as an isolated symptom or may be accompanied by signs of a systemic disorder, e.g. Henoch Schönlein purpura, acute glomerulonephritis; by renal colic, e.g. clot, calculus, obstructive malformation; or a loin mass, e.g. Wilms' tumour or hydronephrosis. The presence of red blood cells in urine will exclude haemaglobinuria, beeturia or false alarms due to confectionery dyes. Red cell casts and significant proteinuria establish glomerular lesions while pyuria and bacteriuria point to infection. An emergency IVP is indicated if renal tract pathology is suspected. A cystoscopy is seldom required unless the blood staining is prominent at the start or finish of the stream. Renal biopsy is reserved for children whose haematuria is accompanied by persisting proteinuria or impaired renal function.

Primary recurrent haematuria is the probable diagnosis if alternatives have been excluded and the haematuria is unaccompanied by proteinuria, obvious casts or an elevated plasma creatinine. It is relatively common in boys and is often provoked by upper respiratory tract infections or vigorous exercise.

Hereditary nephritis. A positive family history and the detection of nerve deafness suggests Alport's syndrome.

Macroscopic haematuria: causes in 120 children presenting with this complaint. Derbyshire Children's Hospital, 1964 to 1979

Benign recurrent haematuria	76
Urinary infection	14
Glomerulonephritis	10
Trauma	9
Tumour — Wilms'	3
Hydronephrosis	2
Balanitis	2
Calculus	1
Cyclophosphamide cystitis	1
Haemophilia	1
Papillary necrosis	1

Acute haemorrhagic cystitis may occur with viral infection, notably adenovirus 11, or as a complication of cyclophosphamide therapy.

ACUTE NEPHRITIC SYNDROME

Post-streptococcal glomerulonephritis

Acute glomerulonephritis occurs predominantly in school children. Although it characteristically occurs 7 to 14 days after a group A β-haemolytic streptococcal throat infection, an increasing percentage appear to have another, possibly viral explanation. Only certain serotypes of streptococcus are responsible and the detection of streptococcal antigen in the glomerular mesangium supports the concept of acute soluble complex injury. Reduced serum complement levels also indicate an immunological pathogenesis.

Glomerular histology in poststreptococcal nephritis; proliferation of endothelial and mesangial cells, oedema and infiltration with polymorphs

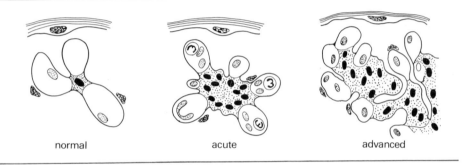

normal   acute   advanced

Many affected children are asymptomatic. Typical complaints include malaise, headache, and vague loin discomfort but it may be the smoky urine which at first causes alarm. Oedema tends to collect around the orbits and on the backs of the hands and feet. Urine microscopy shows gross haematuria with granular and red cell casts. Proteinuria is also present. In the majority of cases oliguria is only mild but severe fluid retention can occasionally produce acute hypertension, with encephalopathy and seizures, or heart failure.

Management. The confirmation of post-streptococcal glomerulonephritis establishes a benign prognosis, and therefore all cases should have an anti-streptolysin titre determination as well as a throat swab. The remainder of the family should also have throat swabs.

Treatment includes eradication of streptococcal infection with a ten-day course of phenoxymethyl penicillin. Hospital admission is required if there is any suggestion of oliguria, fluid overload or hypertension. The reduced GFR should be assessed by a plasma creatinine estimation and serial progress monitored by daily weight and fluid balance. Oliguria requires rest, salt restriction and water intake balanced against insensible loss (20 to 25 ml/kg/day), plus the previous day's urine output. More aggressive management with diuretics and hypotensive drugs may be needed to control hypertension.

The normal course is for the GFR to return to normal in 10 to 14 days. If oliguria persists or progresses, a renal biopsy is justified to define the nature of the glomerular lesion. Rapidly progressive glomerulonephritis with scarring and deteriorating renal function is fortunately rare in the young.

The long term prognosis of post-streptococcal glomerulonephritis is assumed to be excellent, 92 to 98 per cent achieving resolution. There is still some caution about the eventual status of the non-streptococcal group.

Henoch Schönlein purpura

Although approximately 70 per cent of children with Henoch Schönlein purpura have haematuria and or proteinuria, the glomerulonephritis is usually asymptomatic and non-progressive with an eventual mortality of less than 1 to 3 per cent. This grave complication is, however, responsible for 15 per cent of children entering renal dialysis programmes. Children presenting with an acute nephritic syndrome or rapidly progressing to a nephrotic syndrome have an ominous future. Normal renal function two years after the initial insult is unlikely to deteriorate but there are exceptions. Renal histology is some guide to prognosis, the glomerular lesions varying from minimal change to focal or diffuse mesangial proliferation with crescents, and in the most advanced stages, sclerosis. There is no specific therapy for this nephritis and management is symptomatic. Children with urinary abnormalities after Henoch Schönlein purpura should have urine examinations and blood pressure measurements for five years, those without may be safely discharged.

NEPHROTIC SYNDROME

Proteinuria in an otherwise normal child may have an innocent explanation.

Postural or orthostatic proteinuria

This can be readily confirmed by demonstrating a normal overnight urine protein content. It is probably a benign condition.

Asymptomatic persistent proteinuria

If unaccompanied by haematuria, abnormalities on IVP, or elevated plasma creatinine, this has an excellent prognosis and does not warrant renal biopsy. Associated haematuria demands fuller investigation.

Idiopathic nephrotic syndrome of childhood

The nephrotic syndrome occurs when there is gross protein loss resulting in hypoproteinaemia and oedema. It is uncommon, with a prevalence of 6 per 100 000 children, and a peak age incidence between one and five years. Males are more commonly affected than females, 2.5:1. The cause is unknown.

Peri-orbital or dependent oedema and abdominal ascites are usually noticed first. There may also be abdominal pain, vomiting and diarrhoea. Hypovolaemia and circulatory collapse is a danger in the early phase of the illness while fluid shifts from the intravascular to the extracellular space, and it may be exacerbated by the vomiting and diarrhoea. A careful review of pulse, blood pressure and

Incidence and cortiscosteroid responsiveness of nephrotic syndrome in young children and adolescents

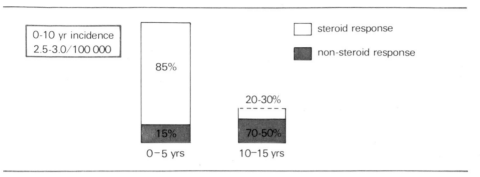

haematocrit must be maintained until the situation stabilises. Intravenous plasma replacement may be necessary. These children are also susceptible to infection, particularly pneumococcal peritonitis and urinary tract infection. Fever in the presence of ascites justifies a diagnostic ascitic fluid tap for microscopy and culture.

Pathology. The term minimal change nephrotic syndrome is derived from light microscopy appearance. Electron microscopy shows fusion of the epithelial cell foot processes, a non-specific consequence of proteinuria. An immunological basis is probable but has yet to be confirmed. Renal biopsy is not required if the clinical picture matches minimal change nephrotic syndrome and there is a definite reponse to corticosteroids.

Glomerular histology in nephrotic syndrome: minimal change, the glomeruli are essentially normal on light microscopy; membranoproliferative, irregular thickening of the glomerular basement membrane and proliferation of mesangial cells; focal segmental sclerosis, varying degrees of glomerular sclerosis involving part or all of the glomerular tuft

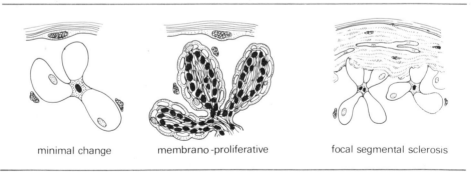

Management. Diuretics should be used with care as they promote hyponatraemia and may further reduce the intravascular volume. Salt poor albumin infusion temporarily restores the circulating volume but is required in only a minority of children. Rest and a high protein but salt-restricted diet are the main measures other than corticosteroids. Prophylactic penicillin should be given during the oedematous phase. The recovery is monitored by daily weights and Albustix.

A scheme for the management of childhood nephrotic syndrome

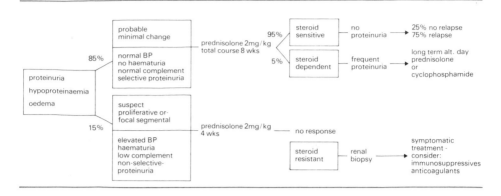

Frequent relapses may be controlled by alternate-day prednisone, but if corticosteroid toxicity occurs there may be a case for a brief course of cyclophosphamide. Concern about the long-term gonadal effects of cytotoxic therapy restricts its usage.

Congenital nephrotic syndrome
Congenital nephrotic syndrome is very rare and either presents at birth with placental oedema or develops in the first year. It may be familial with autosomal recessive inheritance, and is more common in Scandinavia.

ACUTE RENAL FAILURE

Acute renal failure is an uncommon but important problem in which the kidneys are no longer able to maintain biochemical homeostasis. Oliguria, less than 200 to 250 ml per m² surface area per day, is usually present. The possible causes fall into three main groups; pre-renal, renal, and post-renal.

Management
In practical terms the priorities are to distinguish pre-renal from established renal failure, and to exclude obstruction and pre-existing renal disease (acute on chronic renal failure). The presenting illness, gastroenteritis or septicaemic

Classification of acute renal failure

Pre-renal	Renal	Post-renal
Hypovolaemia	Acute tubular nephropathy	Obstructive
e.g. burns and acute haemorrhage	e.g. ischaemia, nephrotoxins	lesions
Circulatory failure	Acute interstitial nephropathy	
e.g. septicaemia, heart failure	e.g. septicaemia, urinary infection	
	Acute glomerulonephritis	
	Haemolytic-uraemic syndrome	
	Renal vein thrombosis	

Investigations which determine the cause of oliguria

Measurement	Pre-renal	Renal
Urine osmolality (mos/kg)	Above 500	Less than 400
Urine: plasma osmolar ratio	Above 1.3	Less than 1.1
Urinary sodium (mmol/l)	Under 10	Above 20
Urinary urea (mmol/l)	Above 250	Under 100

shock, may be very suggestive of circulatory failure and a pre-renal cause, but if oliguria has developed there is a risk that tubular nephropathy has already occurred. The examination of urine and plasma makes the distinction as normal kidneys will concentrate urinary urea and reabsorb sodium. Proteinuria, cells and casts also suggest a renal lesion.

Pre-renal failure demands urgent vascular volume expansion and careful monitoring of fluid and electrolyte replacement. *Renal failure* may respond to intravenous, high-dosage frusemide but preparations should be made for peritoneal or haemodialysis, especially if the picture is complicated by hypertension, pulmonary oedema or worsening biochemistry. Gentamicin and other drugs with a primarily renal excretion should be used with caution. *Potentially reversible obstruction* must not be overlooked and high dose IVP with tomography, micturating cystourethrograms, ultrasound, and radioisotopic procedures play a role.

Acute renal failure of childhood has a generally good outlook if dealt with expertly. Thirty-seven of 72 children referred to Guy's Hospital Renal Unit recovered completely.

Manifestations and management of acute renal failure

	Complication		Therapy
	water overload	hyponatraemia	fluid restriction, twice daily weight
	sodium overload	hypertension, oedema	salt restriction
pre-renal →	potassium overload	cardiac arrhythmias	cation exchange resin dietary restriction
renal —	metabolic acidosis		cautious administration of sodium bicarbonate
post-renal —	nitrogen retention ↑ hypercatabolic metabolism ↑ burns, sepsis		high calorie intake balanced 1st class protein

Haemolytic uraemic syndrome

This disease of pre-school children is rare in the U.K. but occurs as epidemics in South America. Typically an episode of vomiting and diarrhoea is followed by pallor, convulsions, haematuria and scanty urine as acute renal failure supervenes. A blood film shows haemolytic anaemia and thrombocytopenia. Treatment follows the principles outlined above; the additional use of anticoagulants and thrombolytic agents is still controversial. Almost one third of patients die and survivors may be left with renal insufficiency.

CHRONIC RENAL FAILURE

Children with chronic renal failure are a small group, 80 to 100 per annum in the U.K., but they make considerable demands on medical expertise and technical resources. They also raise major ethical issues when decisions relating to chronic dialysis and transplantation have to be made.

Symptoms do not usually develop until 60 to 80 per cent of renal function is lost. There may be an insidious onset with growth failure, anorexia and nocturia, or an acute on chronic crisis may be precipitated by superimposed infection. Urinary tract infection or salt wasting may cause a rapid deterioration in renal function while extra-renal infection with increased catabolic demands and vomiting may cause an acute decline in GFR. More regular measurement of blood pressure in children will also enable earlier detection of chronic renal disease.

Aetiology of chronic renal failure (European Dialysis and Transplant Association)

Cause of renal failure	%
Chronic glomerulonephritis	38
Chronic pyelonephritis	18
Congenital hypoplasia	11
Hereditary nephropathies	8
Cystic kidney disease	5
Tubular necrosis	2
Other causes	18

Manifestations and management of chronic renal failure

Effect	Cause	Therapy
growth failure	poor caloric intake deranged biochemistry –acidosis anaemia salt and fluid loss	high calory intake, balanced 1st class protein sodium bicarbonate with caution salt supplements
renal osteodystrophy	phosphate retention defective Vit D metabolism secondary hyperparathyroidism	phosphate binders (Aludrox) Vit D
anaemia	nutritional reduced erythropoeitin blood loss	blood transfusion as indicated iron supplements
hypertension	sodium retention renal disease/renin release	sodium restriction, diuretics antihypertensives nephrectomy

Optimal care is essential, both to prolong the period of adequate conservative management as well as to prepare the child for possible dialysis and transplantation. Correct dietary management must overcome the anorexia and inadequate nutrition by emphasis on a high calorie diet without necessarily enforcing any major restriction of protein. An adequate intake of first class protein is one of the main goals.

In end-stage renal failure, home dialysis and transplantation can provide a worthwhile outcome in appropriate children; usually those over the age of five and with adequate family support. Recent figures show that five-year survival rate with home dialysis is 92 per cent, with a live donor kidney transplant 75 per cent, and with a cadaver transplant 68 per cent.

Renal tubular disorders; a schematic representation of the renal tubule indicating defects, associated conditions and clinical manifestations

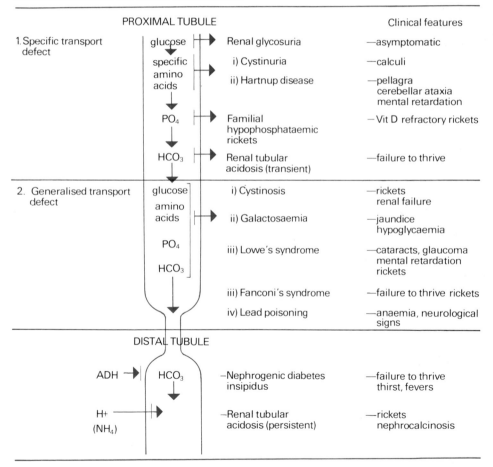

THE TESTES

Undescended testes

Testes which fail to reach the scrotum are divided into two groups; the maldescended or ectopic testes, and the truly undescended testes. Fortunately, for several reasons, about 80 per cent of testes fall into the first group, 20 per cent into the second. The maldescended or ectopic testis passes normally through the inguinal canal and emerges from the superficial ring. Thereafter, it follows an abnormal course. The sites of ectopia in order of frequency are superficial inguinal, femoral, perineal and pubic. All ectopic testes are easily palpable on clinical examination. The testis appears entirely normal in most cases at operation, although absence of the vas is sometimes coexistent. A hernial sac is present in some cases. Orchidopexy is easy because the cord is of good length. Spermatogenesis is usually approaching normal with or without operation, since even in the unoperated case the organ is lying subcutaneously.

The truly undescended testis follows a normal line of descent but stops prematurely. Its position may be abdominal, canalicular, emergent or high scrotal. Only the latter two positions will be palpable on examination. Such a testis often appears quite grossly abnormal at operation, being small, soft and with a dissociated epididymis. Virtually all are accompanied by a very large hernial sac. Spermatogenesis is poor, but is probably not significantly altered by early operation. Orchidopexy is difficult, and is carried out via an abdominal retro-peritoneal approach with dissection of the testicular vessels to the kidney under direct vision. Sometimes no testicular tissue can be found. If there is evidence of vessels or vas then presumptively neonatal torsion has taken place; if there is *no* evidence of vessels, vas or seminal vesicles then the case is that of testicular agenesis. An IVP may be done to determine whether there is also ipsilateral renal agenesis.

Testicular malignancy in the fourth decade of life is known to occur more frequently in individuals born with their testes outside the scrotum. Orchidopexy does not diminish the incidence of malignancy but it does bring a previously impalpable testis into a palpable position.

In unilateral failure of normal testicular descent, there is an increased risk of impaired spermatogenesis and malignancy on the apparently normal side. For these reasons, predictions regarding ultimate fertility should be guarded. Reasons for advising orchidopexy include cosmetic, psychological, increased risk of torsion, increased risk of trauma, the presence of a hernial sac and the increased risk of malignancy. Most paediatric surgeons now operate at two to three years of

Maldescent and undescent of the testes

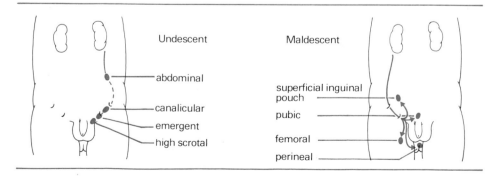

Features which distinguish maldescent and undescent of the testes

	Maldescent	Undescent
Frequency of occurrence	80% of cases	20% of cases
Presence of hernia	Some cases	100% of cases
Prognosis for fertility	Good	Poor
Technique of orchidopexy	Inguinal approach	Abdominal approach
Likelihood of getting testis into scrotum	Easy in all cases	Unpredictable
Normality of testis naked eye and histology	Normal	Abnormal
Risk of torsion	Increased	Slightly increased
Risk of malignancy	Slightly increased	Increased
(*Both* sides in unilateral presentation)		

age, but sometimes, because of a hernia or a perineal ectopic position, operation is carried out at a much earlier age.

Torsion of the body of the testis
This occasionally occurs in the neonatal period, either intra- or very shortly postpartum and almost always necessitates orchidectomy. The opposite testis should be fixed at a second procedure. Thereafter torsion is uncommon until ten years of age after which the incidence increases. It is quite common however in superficial inguinal ectopic testes.

Torsion of the hydatid of Morgagni
This is very common and can usually be distinguished from torsion of the testis because the pain is less severe, and as a consequence the history is usually longer than six hours. Sometimes it is possible to feel the torted hydatid and to demonstrate it by transillumination.

Varicoceles
Varicoceles occur infrequently in children. They do not usually need treatment during childhood.

Inguinal hernias and hydroceles
During its descent into the scrotum the testis is accompanied by a pouch of peritoneum, the processus vaginalis. The processus begins to close at birth and is normally completely obliterated during the first year. Both inquinal hernias and

Inguinal hernia and hydrocele

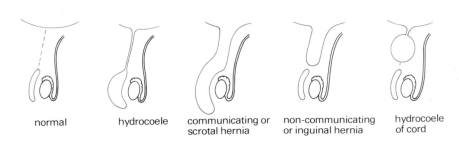

normal   hydrocoele   communicating or   non-communicating   hydrocoele
                                     scrotal hernia   or inguinal hernia   of cord

hydroceles are due to persistent patency of the processus vaginalis. Where the processus remains very narrow, it fills with peritoneal fluid and the infant or child presents with a hydrocele. If a hydrocele is present at birth it is worth waiting four months or so because spontaneous closure of the patent processus may occur. Beyond this age, closure is unlikely and ligation of the processus at the deep ring is indicated. Urgent operation is indicated if an older child suddenly develops a hydrocele, without a history of trauma, since this is sometimes the presenting feature of testicular tumour. Hydroceles may develop considerable tension since the processus often has uni-directional flap valves within it; operation should not be unduly delayed because testicular atrophy may result.

Where the processus remains wide in part or all of its course, an inguinal or inguino-scrotal hernia results. If the processus is wide enough to allow bowel to enter, spontaneous resolution can never occur and operation is essential. The younger the child the more urgent the operative procedure: in a neonate one should operate within two to three days; in a one- to three-month old baby, within one to two weeks, and in all the other children within a month. Irreducibility is very common in young babies and it not only puts them at risk of bowel ischaemia but also, more commonly, of testicular ischaemia.

The child with a hernia may present with a history of a swelling which comes and goes; and in this case, the only evidence of the presence of a hernial sac may be the thickening of the spermatic cord on the affected side. Almost as commonly, however, the swelling appears suddenly and is apparently irreducible, thus requiring emergency admission. If the history is short (that is, less than 12 hours), there is no reddening of the skin over the hernia and the child is well, Gallows traction is applied to the lower limbs and an intramuscular dose of diamorphine is given. In 99 per cent of children, after an hour or so of undisturbed sleep the hernia will either have reduced spontaneously or it will be easily reducible by manipulation. Following such an episode, the child should be kept in hospital, and herniotomy (ligation of the hernial sac at the deep ring) performed after two to three days when the oedema has subsided. If the hernia does not reduce with conservative means or if the bowel within the hernial sac is clearly strangulated, emergency operation is essential. This can be one of the most difficult operations in a neonate or young infant. All infants noted to have a hernia should be referred to a surgeon immediately for elective surgery.

THE PREPUCE

The prepuce is closely adherent to the glans penis during the first year of life and any attempt at retraction must be avoided until spontaneous separation occurs. This is usually in the second year but may be delayed until four years of age. Ammoniacal dermatitis of the prepuce is common, and often confused with balanitis. Because of this, circumcision should never be performed until a child is out of nappies.

Phimosis
Phimosis refers to stenosis of the preputial orifice. It may be congenital but more often results from recurrent balanitis or traumatic retraction of the foreskin. It

leads to ballooning and a poor stream during urination, as well as further attacks of balanitis. Treatment is by circumcision.

Paraphimosis

This can only occur in a child with a moderate phimosis, a preputial aperture slightly less than the size of the coronal sulcus. Following forcible retraction the foreskin is trapped in the retracted position. Treatment is by reduction under anaesthesia, with or without a dorsal slit, followed six weeks later by circumcision.

Hypospadias

The urethra opening on to the ventral aspect of the penis, at a point proximal to a normal site, is one of the commonest congenital abnormalities of the male genitalia, occurring in 1 in 350. The severity varies from a glandular orifice to scrotal and perineal types. There may also be a ventral curvature or chordee of the penis distal to the abnormal urethral meatus which becomes more conspicuous during erection. Failure of fusion of the ventral part of the foreskin results in a redundant dorsal hood. Surgical repair is indicated if the boy is incapable of a socially acceptable urinary stream while standing, or where the deformity may interfere with normal sexual intercourse. It is absolutely essential to conserve the foreskin so that it may be used in these corrective procedures.

BIBLIOGRAPHY

Black D A K 1972 Renal disease, 3rd edn. Blackwell, Oxford
Chantler C 1976 Management and prognosis of renal disease in childhood. In: Hull D (ed) Recent advances in paediatrics — 5. Churchill Livingstone, Edinburgh, p 259–304
James J A 1976 Renal disease in childhood, 3rd edn. Mosby, St Louis
Johnston J H 1969 Posterior urethral valves. In; Rickham P P, Johnston J H (eds) Neonatal surgery, 1st edn. Butterworth, London, p 532–542
Rubin M I, Barratt T M 1975 Pediatric nephrology. Williams & Wilkins, Baltimore
Smellie J M, Normand I C S 1975 Bacteriuria, reflux and renal scarring. Archives of Diseases of Childhood 50: p 581–585
Winterborn M H 1977 The management of urinary infections in children. British Journal of Hospital Medicine 17: p 453–461

12
Blood

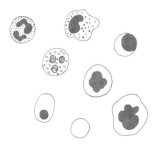

The interpretation of haemoglobin concentrations and white blood counts during infancy and childhood demands some knowledge of the physiological adjustments occurring during this period. The polycythaemia present at birth is followed by a progressive fall in haemoglobin concentration, reaching its minimum at two to three months. This fall is paralleled by relative erythroid hypoplasia in the marrow; however the haemoglobin concentration of healthy infants seldom falls below 10 g/100 ml.

During the fourth and fifth months, iron deficiency contributes to the anaemia and may be corrected by oral iron supplements. Folate deficiency may also occur particularly in infants born before term. Premature infants are also liable to develop anaemia during the first four months of life simply because the blood volume, in line with body size, increases rapidly at a time when the bone marrow is relatively hypoplastic.

Age-related changes in haemoglobin concentration

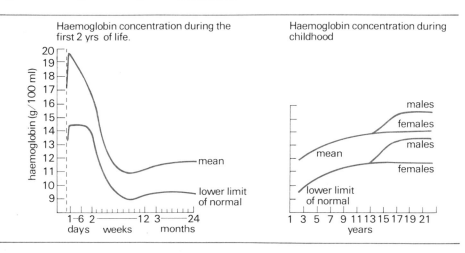

Age-related changes in white cell count

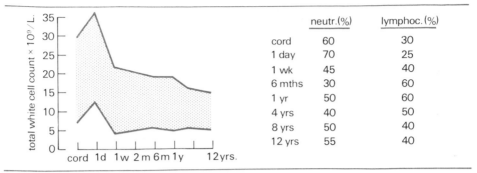

	neutr.(%)	lymphoc.(%)
cord	60	30
1 day	70	25
1 wk	45	40
6 mths	30	60
1 yr	50	60
4 yrs	40	50
8 yrs	50	40
12 yrs	55	40

The white cell count, which is high at birth, rapidly falls to normal adult levels. During the first four years of life lymphocytes predominate rather than neutrophils.

IRON DEFICIENCY ANAEMIA

Anaemia in children may be suggested by tiredness, lethargy or pallor, but it is often only discovered during investigation for other conditions, particularly infection and poor weight gain. Overt gastrointestinal bleeding is rare in childhood. Although it is important to exclude serious underlying problems, the majority of childhood anaemia is due to dietary iron deficiency.

Three-quarters of the total body iron of a newborn infant is found in circulating haemoglobin. In the full-term infant this reserve is adequate to meet requirements for the first four to six months but probably lasts only six weeks in the

Causes of anaemia

	Neonatal	Infancy	Childhood
Haemorrhage	Feto-Maternal Twin-to-twin Placental Subaponeurotic Cephalhaematoma	Hiatus hernia	Hiatus hernia Meckel's diverticulum Epistaxis
Haemolytic	Rhesus incompatibility ABO incompatibility Spherocytosis G6PD deficiency	Acquired Sickle cell Thalassaemia Spherocytosis	Acquired Sickle cell Thalassaemia Spherocytosis
Infection	Intra-uterine (CMV, rubella) Septicaemia Urinary tract	Urinary tract	Chronic infection Chronic disease
Bleeding disorders	Haemorrhagic disease of the newborn	Haemophilia Christmas disease	Haemophilia Christmas disease
Deficiency		Physiological Prematurity Iron Folate Bone marrow depression	Iron Folate Bone marrow depression

Iron balance in infancy

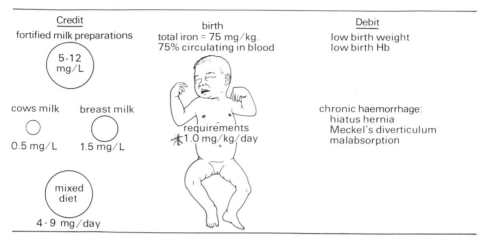

premature. The dietary requirements of a normal infant for elemental iron are 1 mg/kg/day. Although breast milk has a relatively low iron content, it is probably unnecessary to give iron supplements, particularly if mixed feeding is introduced at four to six months. It might even be contraindicated because recent research has demonstrated that the iron binding globulin of breast milk, lactoferrin, has bacteriological properties and that this effect is reduced if the protein becomes iron saturated.

In any community between 10 and 60 per cent of children may be iron deficient, depending on dietary and social habits. The higher figures occur in children of immigrant populations or those who live in impoverished inner city areas. A hypochromic microcytic blood film is usually sufficient evidence to justify a trial of oral iron therapy. The history may provide clues to alternative diagnoses, for example pica suggests lead poisoning, and recurrent vomiting raises the possibility of reflux oesophagitis. Children who fail to respond to an adequate course of iron warrant more detailed investigation including serum iron and iron binding capacity, radiological studies of the gastrointestinal tract, and renal and thyroid function tests. Intestinal malabsorption may present with iron deficient anaemia, and there may be associated folate deficiency. There is some evidence that severe

Serum iron and iron binding capacity in the investigation of anaemia

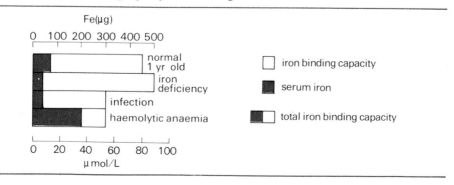

iron deficiency may itself impair the integrity and function of the intestinal mucosa, so that iron replacement may have to be administered parenterally. Iron treatment should be continued for three months to replenish iron stores as well as correct haemoglobin concentrations.

Iron preparations

Ferrous gluconate (Ferlucon) elixir	250 mg/5 ml dose contains 30 mg of elemental iron
Ferrous fumerate (Fersamal) syrup	140 mg/5 ml dose contains 45 mg of elemental iron
Ferrous sulphate (BPC) mixture	60 mg/5 ml dose contains 12 mg of elemental iron
Ferrous gluconate tablets	300 mg contains 36 mg of elemental iron
Ferrous sulphate tablets	200 mg contains 60 mg of elemental iron

APLASTIC ANAEMIA

A pancytopenia necessitates marrow examination which may show either reduced cellularity without infiltration, aplastic anaemia, or invasion by malignant cells. Aplastic anaemia may be inherited or acquired.

Fanconi's anaemia

An autosomal recessive condition, Fanconi's anaemia is the most common of the inherited types, and presents in boys at four to seven years of age and in girls between six and ten years of age. Bruising and purpura are the usual presenting complaints with anaemia appearing more insidiously. Associated features include abnormal pigmentation, short stature, skeletal and renal malformations and there may be chromosomal breakages. The condition is progressive but the deterioration may be delayed with androgens and corticosteroids. Most children with Fanconi's anaemia die within a few years of diagnosis and some develop acute leukaemia. Bone marrow transplantation from a compatible sibling or donor offers the main hope of therapy in the future.

Acquired aplastic anaemia

This may occur at any age. Although some cases follow the ingestion of certain drugs such as chloramphenicol, the majority have no obvious provoking factor. Aplastic anaemia may occur following hepatitis B infection. If the bone marrow is moderately cellular at diagnosis there is a greater chance that spontaneous remission may occur. The majority have severe pancytopenia, respond poorly to corticosteroids and androgens, and die of infection within a year. Again compatible bone marrow transplantation offers some hope for the future. Transplantation is more successful in those patients who have had the least blood transfusions and it is important therefore to explore the availability of suitable donors early in the course of the illness.

HAEMOLYTIC ANAEMIAS

Haemolytic anaemias may be congenital or acquired. Some of the acquired group produce problems in the first days of life and are due to maternal antibodies haemolysing the infant's cells.

The pathogenesis of haemolytic anaemias

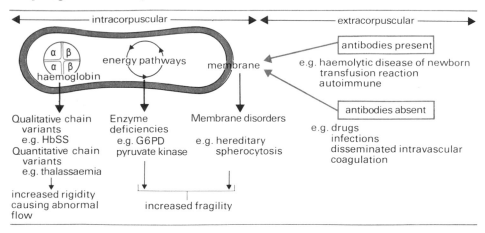

Hereditary haemolytic anaemias

The majority of haemolytic anaemias encountered in infancy and childhood are due to disorders of the red cells. They are characterised by anaemia, an increased reticulocyte count, an unconjugated hyperbilirubinaemia and skeletal changes secondary to compensatory marrow hyperplasia.

Hereditary spherocytosis is an autosomal dominant condition in which the red cell membrane is abnormally permeable to sodium. The resulting spherocytes are not diagnostic of hereditary spherocytosis as they are found in a wide variety of haemolytic anaemias. The disorder may present as neonatal jaundice and has been confused with ABO incompatibility. In later childhood it produces anaemia, chronic malaise and splenomegaly. The continuous high rate of bilirubin excretion leads to pigmented gall stones so that, eventually, gall bladder disease is common. The haemoglobin concentration generally runs in the range of 9 to 11 g/100 ml, but may drop during an infection because of an increased rate of haemolysis and also because there may be an associated hypoplastic crisis. Jaundice may also become conspicuous in these episodes. The diagnosis is confirmed by demonstrating the increased osmotic fragility. Splenectomy is indicated in all symptomatic cases but is usually delayed until after the age of four years because of the risk of overwhelming septicaemia in young splenectomised children. Continuous prophylactic antibiotics are recommended to prevent this hazard. Following splenectomy the red cell survival is returned to normal although spherocytosis persists.

Hereditary elliptocytosis is another autosomal dominant condition affecting membrane permeability but the majority of patients are asymptomatic.

The osmotic fragility test in the diagnosis of hereditary spherocytosis. Metabolic pathways of the red blood cell

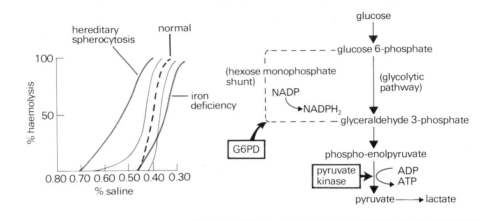

Hereditary red cell enzyme deficiencies

Two important pathways are essential for the normal function of the mature red cell. The hexose-monophosphate pathway provides a supply of reduced nicotinamide adenine-dinucleotide which is essential for protection against oxidative damage. The glycolytic or Emden-Meyerhof pathway provides the majority of energy for the cell. Deficiency of many of the enzymes in these two pathways has been described but the most important deficiencies are those of glucose-6-phosphate dehydrogenase (G6PD) and pyruvate kinase.

Glucose-6-phosphate dehydrogenase deficiency. There are many variants of this enzyme, each having a different geographical distribution. The form seen in black Americans results in haemolysis when the person is exposed to antimalarial and other drugs. The Mediterranean and oriental variants often present in the newborn period with jaundice due to excess haemolysis and they

An abbreviated list of drugs to be avoided by patients with glucose-6-phosphate dehydrogenase deficiency. A typical drug induced crisis in such a patient

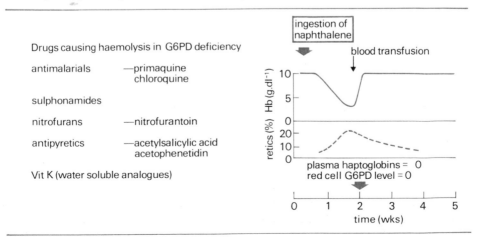

may require an exchange transfusion. These conditions are also 'drug sensitive'. Ingestion of Fava beans is a well recognised hazard in affected Mediterranean peoples. Patients with glucose-6-phosphate dehydrogenase deficiency should be given a list of drugs to avoid. The condition is inherited by the sex-linked mode.

Pyruvate kinase deficiency is considerably less common and affects mainly North European populations. It causes neonatal jaundice, anaemia and splenomegaly. Splenectomy is occasionally of benefit.

Disorders of haemoglobin synthesis

These fall into two main categories: those in which there is an aminoacid substitution in the globin portion of the molecule, the haemoglobinopathies; and those in which there is relative failure of globin chain synthesis, the thalassaemia syndromes. It is unusual for these conditions to present in the newborn period when fetal haemoglobin is the predominant haemoglobin type.

The developmental changes in the haemoglobins of intra- and extrauterine life

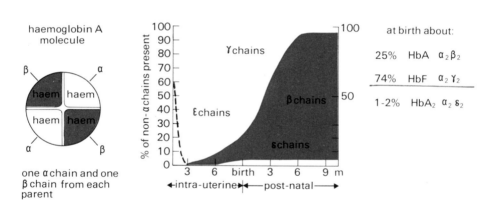

Normal and abnormal haemoglobins in later childhood

normal			abnormal		
different polypeptide chains in various haemoglobins			HbS	α_2 β_2^s	sickle cell disease
% after age 3 yrs			HbAS	α_2 β β^s	sickle cell trait
HbA	α_2	β_2 (98-99%)			
HbF	α_2	γ_2 (0-2%)	Hb Barts	γ_4	thalassaemia
HbA$_2$	α_2	δ_2 (1-3%)	HbH	β_4	

Sickle cell anaemia is by far the most common of the haemoglobinopathies; 15 per cent of all negroes carry the gene that causes valine to replace glutamine in the sixth position of the beta chain. The homozygous condition is referred to as sickle cell anaemia or disease, and the heterozygote as sickle cell trait. The disease is a serious condition with a number of important complications in addition to the chronic anaemia. Painful swelling of the hands and feet is a common early presentation. The splenomegaly of the younger child becomes less prominent as repeated infarctions produce an 'autosplenectomy'. Crises are usually precipitated by infection and may be complicated by dehydration, poor tissue perfusion, hypoxia and acidosis. The anaemia is sometimes exacerbated by temporary marrow failure and folate deficiency. Treatment is largely symptomatic with antibiotics, warmth and adequate fluids. In developed countries the prognosis for a normal life is moderately good. The heterozygote is asymptomatic except under conditions of low oxygen tension as might occur at high altitude or under general anaesthesia.

Features of sickle cell disease

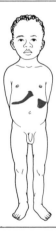

Crises	Clinical features
painful	pallor; icterus
haemolytic	
aplastic	haemic murmur; hepatomegaly
hepatic	splenomegaly (after 8 yrs of age only 10%)
megaloblastic	
	chronic leg ulcers
Acute infarction:	renal involvement:
abdominal	haematuria
pulmonary	defective urine concentration
neurological	
hands and feet syndrome	infections:
aseptic necrosis—femoral	pneumococcal septicaemia
and humeral heads	salmonella osteomyelitis

Thalassaemia syndromes are most common among Asian and Mediterranean races, and are subdivided into alpha and beta thalassaemia depending on the chain affected by the synthetic failure. Beta thalassaemia is the more common, the homozygous state resulting in a severe haemolytic anaemia with hypochromic microcytic cells. The compensatory bone marrow hyperplasia produces a characteristic overgrowth of the facial and skull bones, as well as fragile limb bones. Although death may be delayed by repeated transfusion, the problems of chronic iron overload result in progressive organ failure. Desferrioxamine and other iron chelating agents have been used in an attempt to reduce the positive iron balance but as yet with little significant advantage. Recently improved results have been reported using continuous subcutaneous infusions of desferrioxamine. Techniques for haemoglobin identification in the mid-term fetus may permit antenatal diagnosis and selective abortion. The heterozygous beta thalassaemia produces a mild anaemia which may be confused with iron deficiency. Haemoglobin electrophoresis permits identification of these abnormal haemoglobin types.

Features of thalassaemia major

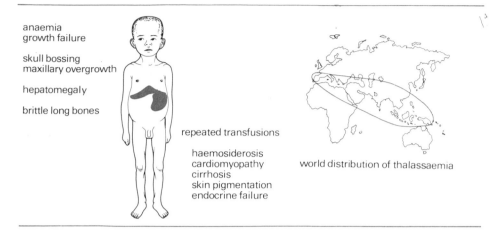

anaemia
growth failure

skull bossing
maxillary overgrowth

hepatomegaly

brittle long bones

repeated transfusions

haemosiderosis
cardiomyopathy
cirrhosis
skin pigmentation
endocrine failure

world distribution of thalassaemia

BLEEDING DISORDERS

A variety of disorders may lead to excessive bleeding in childhood. A past history
may be important in distinguishing congenital from acquired problems. Previous
surgery, including dental extractions, without undue bleeding provides good
evidence against an inherited disorder. Tonsillectomy is notorious for putting a
considerable strain on coagulation systems and may uncover mild haemophilia. A
family history is often helpful in diagnosing sex-linked recessive disorders such as
haemophilia or Christmas disease, but may be absent in up to a third of new cases.
A dominant pattern of inheritance is characteristic of Von Willebrand's disease
and hereditary telangiectasia. The character of the bleeding problem together
with four basic tests of coagulation should make it possible to decide from which
group of disorders a patient is suffering. These tests also serve as screening
procedures in cases of suspected child abuse or before liver or jejunal biopsy.

Classification of bleeding disorders

Presentation		Mechanism	Diagnosis
injury provoked skin and mucosal bleeding		defective blood vessels	hereditary haemorrhagic telangectasia allergic or post-infectious vasculitis Vit C deficiency—scurvy
		thrombocytopenia	idiopathic thrombocytopenia chronic immune thrombocytopenia
		platelet function defect	drug induced thrombocytopenia thrombasthenia
spontaneous and injury provoked		coagulation disorder	haemophilia A B Von Willebrand's Vit K deficiency liver disease
deep haematomas haemarthrosis haematuria			

Key investigations in the evaluation of a bleeding disorder

---

1. Full blood count including platelet count (normal 150–400 × 10⁹/l; bleeding occurs when below $40 \times 10^9/l$).
2. Ivy's bleeding time (normal less than six minutes). An abnormal result with normal platelet count is suggestive of a qualitative platelet abnormality.
3. Prothrombin time. A test of the extrinsic pathway: Factors II (prothrombin), V, VII and X together with fibrinogen. (Normal = control ± 20%).
4. Partial thromboplastin time. A test of the intrinsic pathway: Factors, V, VIII, X, XI, XII and XIII together with prothrombin and fibrinogen. (Normal = control ± 20%).

Normal results in these four tests exclude all deficiencies other than factor XIII, (fibrin stabilising factor) deficiency.

Inherited deficiencies of each of the coagulation factors have been described; they are all rare with the exceptions of haemophilia A and B, and von Willebrand's disease.

Haemophilia

Haemophilia A occurs in approximately 1 in 14 000 males and is six times more common than haemophilia B, otherwise known as Christmas disease. Haemophilia A is due to the synthesis of abnormal factor VIII with resulting reduced biological activity. It is transmitted as a sex-linked recessive, and carrier females are asymptomatic but may be detected because of an excess of immunoreactive factor VIII over that which is biologically active. The severity of haemophilia is linked to the degree of deficiency of factor VIII; concentrations of factor VIII less than 1 per cent of normal causes severe problems, 1 to 5 per cent causes moderate problems, and 5 to 20 per cent only mild symptoms. Spontaneous bleeding into joints and muscles with resulting orthopaedic problems is the main hazard.

It is essential to treat all bleeding incidents promptly by replacing the missing factor. Until relatively recently, this necessitated the use of fresh frozen plasma, but currently the availability of cryoprecipitate concentrates and purified dried

Coagulation pathways. Characteristic laboratory results in idiopathic thrombocytopenia (ITP), Von Willebrand's disease, haemophilia, and Vitamin K deficiency

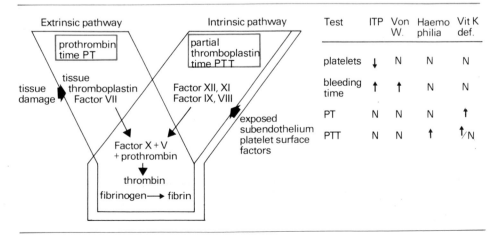

Test	ITP	Von W.	Haemo philia	Vit K def.
platelets	↓	N	N	N
bleeding time	↑	↑	N	N
PT	N	N	N	↑
PTT	N	N	↑	↑/N

human factor VIII have enabled the use of small volumes and therefore simplified treatment. Many families have now been trained to treat bleeding episodes at home. In general, the aim of replacement is to increase the factor VIII level to a biologically effective concentration of 10 to 20 per cent. Activity up to 50 per cent of normal may be necessary to combat severe trauma or surgery. Physiotherapy has a vital role in maintaining the strength of muscles which might otherwise become weakened during periods of immobilisation and therefore increase joint susceptibility to further damage.

Von Willebrand's disease

Von Willebrand's disease is an autosomal dominant disorder characterised by prolonged bleeding time, low factor VIII and reduced platelet adhesiveness. Treatment is as for haemophilia. Aspirin should not be given.

Thrombocytopenia

Idiopathic thrombocytopenic purpura is the most common of the thrombocytopenias and is thought to have an immunological basis as it often follows one to two weeks after a viral infection. There is a clear relationship with rubella. Platelet bound IgG antibodies are detectable in a significant proportion of cases. Problems usually develop when the platelet counts fall below $40 \times 10^9/l$, and in the severe cases the count may be below $5 \times 10^9/l$. The common presenting features are petechiae and superficial bruising but mucosal bleeding may also occur. Rarely haemorrhage occurs into the brain or viscera. As the differential diagnosis includes acute leukaemia and aplastic anaemia, it is justifiable to perform a marrow examination immediately to demonstrate the normal or increased number of megakaryocytes which are characteristic of idiopathic thrombocytopenia.

In children, 85 per cent have an acute self-limiting course and the majority have recovered spontaneously by six months. In those who have only mild symptoms no treatment is necessary, but where there is a risk of severe generalised bleeding or bleeding into a solid organ, a short course of corticosteroids may help by producing a temporary elevation of the platelet count. Long courses of corticosteroids should be avoided and refractory cases should be considered for splenectomy; if this fails immunosuppression with azathioprine may be successful.

Drug-induced thrombocytopenia is unusual in childhood but is becoming increasingly recognised following the use of cotrimoxazole. Thrombocytopenia may occur in the neonatal period as a complication of rhesus disease, intra uterine infection or due to maternal drug ingestion. It may also occur transiently in the infant of a mother with idiopathic thrombocytopenia. There is also a group of rare hereditary thrombocytopenias.

Haemorrhagic disease of the newborn

This coagulation disturbance arises from vitamin K deficiency and the resulting impairment of hepatic production of factors II, VII, IX and X. It characteristically develops between the second and fourth days of life and presents with gastrointestinal bleeding. Breast fed infants, premature infants and those exposed to perinatal asphyxia are most at risk. The occasional tragedy due to this readily preventable condition merits the prophylactic use of vitamin K_1 in all newborn infants shortly after birth (intramuscular dose 0.5 to 1 mg).

Disseminated intravascular coagulation (DIC)

Severe disturbances such as septicaemia, shock and acidosis may promote simultaneous activation of both the coagulant and the fibrinolytic pathways, with a resulting consumption of platelets, fibrinogen, factors V and VIII but without the formation of insoluble fibrin. Soluble complexes of fibrin monomers circulate as fibrin degradation products and their detection is a further indication of consumptive coagulopathy. DIC should be suspected in a gravely ill child with both shock and generalised bleeding. Every attempt should be made to determine and treat the underlying cause. In the neonatal period this may be asphyxia, profound hypothermia, infection or severe rhesus disease. In infancy it may complicate hypertonic dehydration and produce renal vein thrombosis, manifest by oliguria, haematuria and bilateral renal masses.

The haemolytic uraemic syndrome

This is a disease of infants in which a prodromal gastrointestinal or respiratory illness is followed by acute renal failure, microangiopathic haemolytic anaemia with numerous burr cells and thrombocytopenia. It has been most frequently recognised in South America.

Meningococcal septicaemia

Meningococcal septicaemia is classically associated with progressive purpura but may progress to a consumptive coagulopathy. Similar features can develop in septicaemia due to other bacterial, viral and rickettsial infection. Therapy must always be directed at the underlying cause but these gravely ill children need close haematological supervision in case there is a place for cautious heparinisation. Intervention with anticoagulants is still of questionable merit.

BIBLIOGRAPHY

Biggs R 1978 The treatment of haemophilia A and B and von Willebrand's disease. Blackwell, Oxford
Oski F A, Naiman J L 1966 Hematologic problems in the newborn. Saunders, Philadelphia
Weatherall D J, Clegg J B 1972 The thalassaemia syndromes, 2nd edn. Blackwell, Oxford
Willoughby M L N 1977 Paediatric haematology. Churchill Livingstone, Edinburgh

13
Malignancy

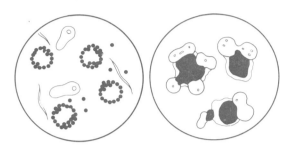

Malignancies are now second only to accidents in the mortality tables of children aged 1 to 15 years. Childhood malignancies fall into two main categories: those which are found more commonly and almost exclusively in children; and those which are manifestations of tumours found in all age groups. The former group which includes nephroblastomas, neuroblastomas and retinoblastomas evolves from malignant transformation of developing tissues. Genetic influences are probably greater than environmental factors and the spectrum of susceptible organs is quite different to that seen in adults where bronchus, gastrointestinal tract and breast predominate. It has long been recognised that complete cure is possible in nephroblastoma, and the carefully monitored introduction of more aggressive modes of therapy has demonstrated that an increasing number of malignancies are amenable to cure. This progress is the result of better understanding of the natural history of tumours and the introduction of expert multidisciplinary management schedules. These schedules while bringing rewards, also impose a great burden on the child and family.

LEUKAEMIA

Leukaemia is the most common malignant disease in childhood, occurring in

Epidemiology of childhood leukaemia

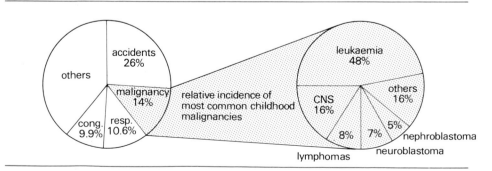

Age distribution of acute leukaemia

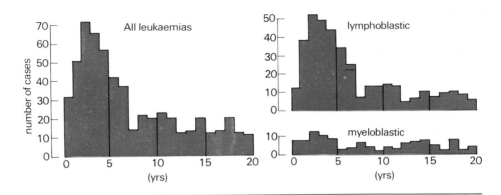

about 1 in 30 000 children under the age of 14 years. Acute lymphoblastic leukaemia accounts for 86 per cent, acute myeloblastic leukaemia for 13 per cent and chronic myeloid leukaemia for 1 per cent. Acute leukaemias are characterised by the presence of blast cells in the peripheral blood, as distinct from chronic leukaemias where excessive numbers of normal looking leucocytes are present.

The aetiological basis of leukaemia remains a mystery. A familial incidence is very rare and there is no definite evidence of viral involvement. Leukaemia is a relatively common cause of death in children with Down's syndrome, as the incidence is 10 to 18 times that in normal children.

Clinical manifestations

A minority, 15 per cent, of children with acute leukaemia present rapidly over a few days; the majority, 85 per cent, develop symptoms more insidiously over weeks and months. Common initial complaints include pallor, fever, recurrent infections, malaise and abnormal bruising. Childhood leukaemia is notorious for its varied presentations, and it must be considered in the diagnosis of any unusual illness especially if accompanied by hepatosplenomegaly, lymphadenopathy or bone tenderness.

Clinical features of acute leukaemia

fatigue and pallor	80%		hepatomegaly	60%
anorexia	45%		splenomegaly	70%
fever	55%		abdominal pain	20%
skin or mucosal bleeding	30%		lymphadenopathy	25%
Infections:			bone pain	25%
sore throats	20%			
other	20%			

Clinical suspicion must not be conveyed to parents until laboratory investigation has provided complete confirmation. Doctors and nurses must also be sensitive to the sometimes irrational fears of leukaemia that arise when parents have failed to grasp the meaning of relatively innocent diagnoses such as iron deficiency anaemia and infectious mononucleosis. Idiopathic thrombocytopenia may alarm doctors until the characteristic bone marrow appearance has been revealed!

Careful examination of peripheral blood and a bone marrow aspirate is generally sufficient to confirm or refute the diagnosis of acute leukaemia. Blast cells are usually apparent and account for between 1 per cent and nearly 100 per cent of the white cell count. The total white cell count is typically in the range 20 to $50 \times 10^9/l$ but can be lower than $10 \times 10^9/l$, subleukaemic leukaemia, or in excess of $100 \times 10^9/l$. Peripheral blood blast cells may be undetectable in the subleukaemic variety. A normochromic normocytic anaemia and a thrombocytopenia are invariable. Bone marrow examination is essential to the diagnosis, and provides an important parameter by which to judge subsequent remission. Recently more refined studies of lymphoblastic cells show that the term acute lymphoblastic leukaemia refers to a heterogenous group of cell lines derived from T, B, 'null' or 'common' cells. The T cell leukaemias appear to have a particularly bad prognosis.

Management

As soon as the diagnosis has been made with certainty both parents are seen together so that the nature of the disease, its treatment and prognosis may be discussed in detail. This initial talk has usually to be repeated because of the distress of the first conversation. While the ultimate aim is one of curing the disease, this has to be balanced against the ability of the child and family to tolerate all components of management.

In the U.K. specific treatment plan has evolved as the result of controlled studies under the auspices of the Medical Research Council. Chemotherapy lasts two to three years and aims at as complete eradication of malignant cells as is possible. This eradication must be directed not only at the bone marrow but also at the central nervous system, and current programmes include cranial irradiation and intrathecal methotrexate. In judging the effectiveness of therapy it is a useful

Treatment of acute leukaemia

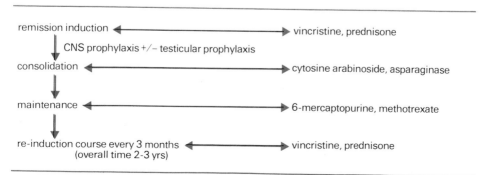

The tumour cell mass

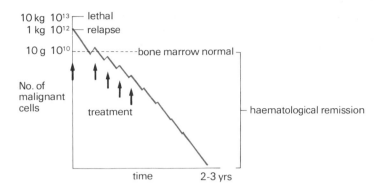

concept to consider the total leukaemia cell load, which may be 10^{11} to 10^{12} cells, or more than a kilogram of malignancy at the time of diagnosis. Each course of treatment is thought to produce a 'two log kill', equivalent to reducing the tumour mass from 1 kg to 10 g. Apparent remission with a normal marrow examination is compatible with the persistence of 10 g of malignant cells in the body. This model of total tumour mass is also applicable to disseminated solid tumours. Chemotherapeutic agents are selected on the basis of selective toxicity towards tumour cells, speed of effect, and according to their impact on the phases of cellular divison.

Cytotoxic agents and the dividing cell

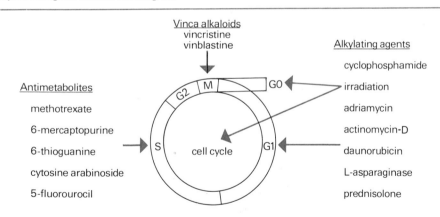

G1-resting phase; S-synthesis of DNA; G2-premitotic phase; M-mitosis and division; G0-latent phase

Immunosuppressed children are susceptible to infection and up to 15 per cent die from this cause without any evidence of marrow relapse. Chickenpox and measles are particular hazards, but high titre zoster immune globulin protects against the former and pooled gammaglobulin usually has an adequate titre against measles.

Leukaemia: complications of the disease and its treatment

	Infections —
bleeding	chickenpox, pertussis
hair loss	measles
bone marrow depression	gram negative septicaemia
fevers	pneumocystis
bone involvement	cytomegalovirus
testicular involvement	fungal infections
CNS involvement	
meninges	
eyes	

Clinical features of meningeal leukaemia

Signs and symptoms	%
vomiting	80
headache	69
papilloedema	69
weight gain	29
palsies	16
visual disturbance	7
fits	7
nausea without vomiting	4
ataxia	4
vertigo	2

Current treatment regimes have resulted in the survival of 30 to 50 per cent of children for more than four years and it is hoped that survival for this length of time indicates cure. The question of stopping potentially toxic therapy after a sufficiently prolonged remission is important as unnecessary immunosuppression has a mortality risk of its own.

Survival rates in acute leukaemia

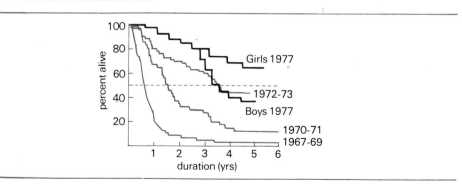

NEPHROBLASTOMA (WILMS' TUMOUR)

A nephroblastoma originates from embryonal kidney and is made up of tissues in various stages of differentiation. The incidence is approximately 1 in 10 000 live

Nephroblastoma: clinical features and investigation

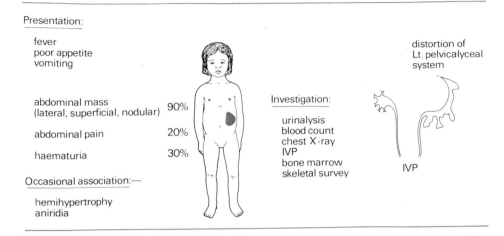

Presentation:

fever
poor appetite
vomiting

abdominal mass   90%
(lateral, superficial, nodular)

abdominal pain   20%

haematuria   30%

Occasional association:—

hemihypertrophy
aniridia

Investigation:

urinalysis
blood count
chest X-ray
IVP
bone marrow
skeletal survey

distortion of
Lt. pelvicalyceal
system

IVP

births (i.e. 70 new cases each year in the United Kingdom). 60 per cent present before the age of three years, and it is marginally more common in boys than girls. The left kidney is affected more frequently than the right, and 10 per cent of tumours are bilateral.

The resulting abdominal mass is usually asymptomatic and often comes to light through accidental palpation. It is important to investigate all cases of haematuria with this diagnosis in mind. The IVP is sometimes, but not always, diagnostic of nephroblastoma, showing the intrarenal origin of the tumour and the resulting distortion of the pelvicalyceal system. It is also necessary to determine whether the contralateral kidney is normal. 40 per cent of tumours have metastasised by the time of diagnosis but secondaries amenable to surgery or irradiation do not necessarily prevent complete cure. Nephrectomy is no longer regarded as an emergency but should be performed promptly. The involved kidney together with ureter, lymph nodes and adjacent infiltrated tissues is removed and formal staging is decided upon. Chemotherapy with vincristine is commenced at the time of surgery. Actinomycin and adriamycin have been introduced into programmes for metastasised tumour. Radiotherapy is directed towards the renal bed and metastases but care is taken to protect the spine and opposite kidney.

Treatment of nephroblastoma

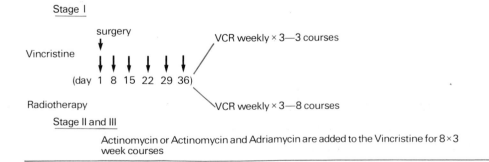

Stage I

surgery

Vincristine

(day 1 8 15 22 29 36)

VCR weekly × 3—3 courses

VCR weekly × 3—8 courses

Radiotherapy

Stage II and III

Actinomycin or Actinomycin and Adriamycin are added to the Vincristine for 8 × 3 week courses

The prognosis depends on the initial stage of the tumour. Tumours limited to the kidney and completely resected (Stage I) are associated with a five-year survival rate of at least 80 per cent. Stage IV tumours with haematogenous metastases have less than a 10 per cent five year survival rate. In general terms, survival free of disease at two years is equivalent to a cure.

NEUROBLASTOMA

A neuroblastoma originates from tissues of neural crest origin namely the adrenal medulla and sympathetic nervous system. Although they are usually highly malignant, there is an interesting spectrum of disease and histological examination of infant deaths show that localised, '*in situ*' tumours may occur 14 to 40 times as frequently as those which are symptomatic. There is also a gradation between the rapidly proliferating neuroblastoma and the benign ganglioneuroma. Cases have been reported in which neuroblastomas have spontaneously matured into ganglioneuromas.

These tumours occur most commonly in the first four years of life with an incidence of approximately 1 in 8000 live births, so that there are about 80 new cases each year in the United Kingdom.

The clinical manifestations are varied depending on the site of the primary tumour and the extent of metastases. The latter are commonly responsible for the symptoms. 65 to 75 per cent of cases are abdominal, most arising in the adrenal medulla but some in the retroperitoneal sympathetic ganglia. The remainder arise in sympathetic ganglia in the neck, thorax and pelvis, and the extra-abdominal sites appear to have a better prognosis.

Those tumours which are abdominal in origin usually produce a mass which crosses the mid-line and which may be difficult to distinguish from the liver. The liver may well be involved in metastases. It is therefore important to exclude primary liver pathology such as a hepatoblastoma. Features useful in confirming the presence of a neuroblastoma include the diffuse, speckled calcification sometimes seen on a plain abdominal X-ray, and elevated levels of catecholamine

Neuroblastoma: clinical features and investigation

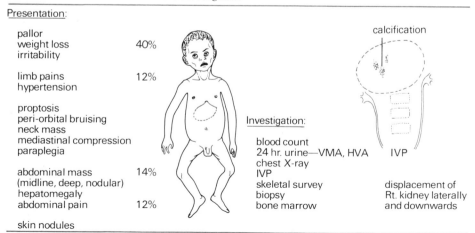

Presentation:

pallor	
weight loss	40%
irritability	
limb pains	12%
hypertension	
proptosis	
peri-orbital bruising	
neck mass	
mediastinal compression	
paraplegia	
abdominal mass	14%
(midline, deep, nodular)	
hepatomegaly	
abdominal pain	12%
skin nodules	

calcification

Investigation:

blood count
24 hr. urine—VMA, HVA   IVP
chest X-ray
IVP
skeletal survey   displacement of
biopsy   Rt. kidney laterally
bone marrow   and downwards

degradation products in the urine. Raised levels of homovanyllic acid (HVA) and especially vanillylmandelic acid (VMA) are present in over 90 per cent of affected children. The high frequency of metastases makes a careful systemic review and skeletal survey important. Bone metastases are more common than pulmonary.

Surgery is directed towards complete resection where possible but not at the expense of causing severe mutilation. Postoperative irradiation is invariably indicated but in immediate proximity to the spine and kidneys it introduces problems of subsequent scoliosis and radiation nephritis. A case for chemotherapy has not been fully established but combined vincristine and cyclophosphamide are frequently used.

Unfortunately the prognosis for children with this tumour has not shown any significant improvement over the last 20 years. The prognosis is influenced by the site of the tumour and by the age of the child. The figures are more favourable in children under the age of two years and an interesting group of infants show spontaneous recovery in spite of metastases to subcutaneous tissue, liver and bone marrow. Recent research suggests an immunological mechanism for this regression and raises the possibility of new therapeutic approaches for the future.

HISTIOCYTOSIS X

Histiocytosis X is the term used to describe a spectrum of disease in which there is an abnormal proliferation of histiocytes. There is some debate as to whether this represents a single disease entity and whether it is inflammatory or neoplastic in origin. Current opinion favours a malignant pathology and by convention it is divided into three main categories. It is a rare disease in the United Kingdom, about 40 new cases presenting each year.

Eosinophilic granuloma of bone

This is the most benign end of the spectrum and consists of isolated lesions of bone occurring most commonly in the skull, ribs, clavicles and vertebrae. They present with pain, swelling, a lump and occasionally spinal cord signs. The typical radiographic appearance is of a well demarcated lytic lesion but a full skeletal survey and a biopsy are necessary to confirm the diagnosis. Accessible lesions are treated by currettage at the time of biopsy and only 5 per cent become multifocal. Inaccessible lesions may be treated with radiotherapy.

Hand-Schuller-Christian disease

This is a more disseminated variety commonly presenting as a persistent ear discharge but there may also be a seborrhoeic-like rash, bone lesions of the skull and mastoid, exophthalmos, diabetes insipidus and hepatosplenomegaly.

Letterer-Siwe disease

Letterer-Siwe Disease is at the most severe end of the spectrum and behaves as a highly malignant and generalised disorder. It typically presents in infancy as failure to thrive, fever, a haemorrhagic seborrhoeic rash, lymphadenopathy and hepatosplenomegaly. There may be pancytopenia and the ESR is elevated. The diagnosis is largely based on clinical appearance but should be confirmed by biopsy of either the enlarged glands or the skin rash.

Both the Hand-Schuller-Christian and Letterer-Siwe diseases require treatment with combined chemotherapy using chlorambucil, vinblastine, methotrexate and cyclophosphamide. The prognosis depends upon the extent of the disease and whether involved organs show impaired function.

OTHER MALIGNANCIES

Rhabdomyosarcoma

This is a rare but highly malignant tumour, originating from smooth muscle fibres and occurring most frequently in the first two years of life. It may present as a swelling around the orbit or nasopharynx, in the bladder, vagina or uterus and occasionally in the limbs. It can be responsible for a haemorrhagic vaginal discharge. Treatment requires radical surgery, radiotherapy and chemotherapy with vincristine, actinomycin and cyclophosphamide.

Non-Hodgkin's lymphoma

This highly malignant disorder used to be termed lymphosarcoma but the recent realisation that they consist of T cells has shown that they are closely allied to T cell leukaemias. The usual sites of presentation are the gastrointestinal tract producing intestinal obstruction or intussusception, the anterior mediastinum with superior venocaval obstruction, and in the peripheral lymph nodes. The prognosis is very poor as apparently well localised tumours may metastasise. Current management regimes combine surgery, radiotherapy and multiple chemotherapy.

Hodgkin's disease

This is rare in children but there is some evidence that genetic factors play a part in its aetiology, there being a significant association with certain HLA types. It is also four times more common in boys than girls. The presenting features include lymphadenopathy, with or without systemic symptoms such as fever, sweating and weight loss. The staging and treatment programmes which have proved so successful in adult practice are being increasingly applied in the childhood disease but splenectomy is less commonly practised because of the risk of septicaemia. Radiotherapy is most effective for localised disease and chemotherapy with the MOPP combination (Mustine, Oncovin, Procarbazine and Prednisone) is used in disseminated cases.

Retinoblastoma

This is a very rare but important tumour of the eye with frequency of approximately one in 30 000 live births. There is a strong familial incidence particularly if the condition is bilateral. The spread is either into the orbit or along the optic nerve, and intracranial extensions are the usual cause of death. The diagnosis must be suspected whenever a white pupillary reflex replaces the normal red one and must be rapidly followed by an adequate ophthalmological examination. Treatment may involve enucleation of the eye together with radiotherapy and chemotherapy.

BIBLIOGRAPHY

Jones P G, Campbell P E 1976 Tumours of infancy and childhood. Blackwell, Oxford.
Lascari A D 1973 Leukemia in childhood. Thomas, Springfield.
Malpas J S 1976 The effect of treatment on lymphomas and childhood solid tumours. Journal of
    the Royal College of Physicians 10: 183-193.
Malpas J S 1977 Leukaemia in children. British Journal of Hospital Medicine 17: 444.
Williams I G 1972 Tumours of childhood. Heinemann, London.

14
Growth

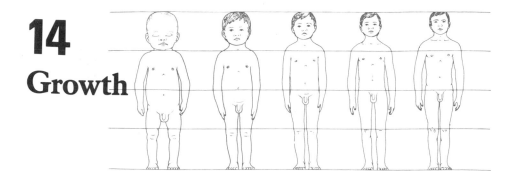

Accurate measurements of height, weight and head circumference plotted on record charts provide an invaluable illustration of growth and development. Growth reflects not only general health but also the nutritional and emotional environment of a child, and disordered growth may be the only obvious manifestation of disease or deprivation.

HEAD GROWTH

At birth the head circumference, 32 to 37 cm, is three-quarters of its adult value, 52 to 57 cm, and the majority of post-natal growth occurs in infancy. The anterior fontanelle which normally measures approximately 2.5 by 2.5 cm at birth, may no longer be palpable by six months but often remains patent until 18 months.

Microcephaly is commonly associated with brain hypoplasia.

Head circumference chart (after Nellhaus)

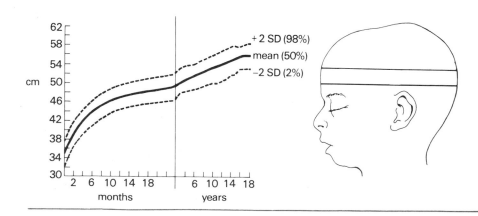

Macrocephaly refers to an enlarged skull cavity without increased intracranial pressure. The brain is also enlarged due to glial overgrowth and mental handicap is common.

Hydrocephalus must be considered when serial head circumference measurements deviate away from a normal growth curve and where there are signs of raised intracranial pressure. This condition more than any other emphasises the need for accurate measurement and careful plotting on an appropriate chart.

Asymmetrical skulls and craniosynostosis

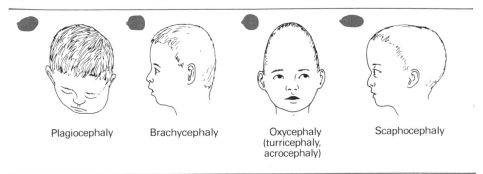

| Plagiocephaly | Brachycephaly | Oxycephaly (turricephaly, acrocephaly) | Scaphocephaly |

Asymmetrical skulls are caused by inequality of growth rates at the coronal, sagittal and lambdoid sutures. The inequality may be an innocent postural effect as is commonly the case in mild plagiocephaly or may be due to premature fusion of the sutures, craniosynostosis.

Premature craniosynostosis occurs as an isolated congenital deformity, as a component of certain inherited syndromes, and secondary to metabolic disorders such as hypophosphatasia and idiopathic hypercalcaemia. It has also been reported after excessive thyroxine replacement therapy. Localised forms of craniosynostosis produce characteristic skull shapes and in some there are potentially damaging pressure effects upon the brain, eyes, and cranial nerves. Infants suspected of having this condition require prompt referral to a neuro-surgical centre experienced in assessing and treating these problems. Craniectomy or reconstruction of the sutures is usually performed in the first few months of life, and may have to be followed by cosmetic procedures.

HEIGHT AND WEIGHT

Height increase or velocity is rapid in infancy and then progressively slows until the pubertal growth spurt. Birth length is doubled by approximately four years and trebled by 13 years. Puberty causes a brief acceleration of the height velocity from a mean of 5 to 6 cm per year to a brief peak of approximately 10 cm per year. Linear growth ceases when the long bone epiphyses fuse, an event closely related to sexual maturity and adrenal androgen release.

Body weight is the most sensitive index of nutritional status and general health. On average half the adult weight is reached by 9 to 11 years.

Growth charts (after Tanner and Whitehouse)

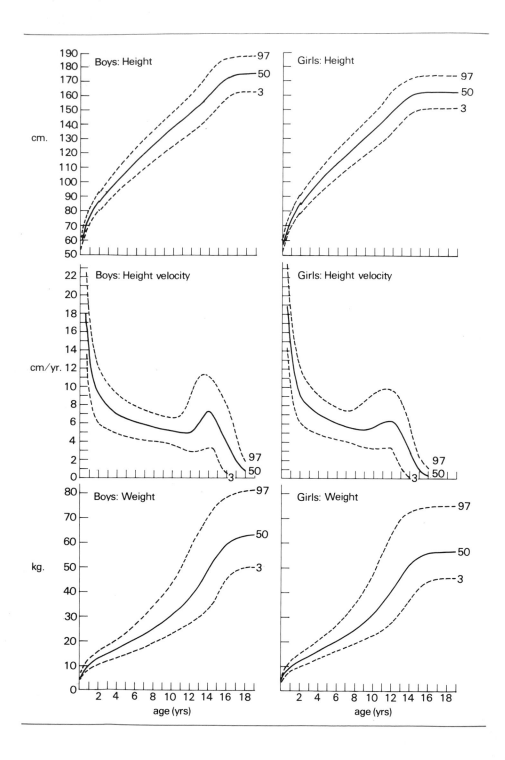

SHORT STATURE

Short stature, defined as a height below the third centile, occurs in many healthy children but each case should be carefully evaluated and particular attention must be paid to those who are severely short with a height less than minus three standard deviations, those whose parental heights suggest that they should be above the third centile, and those in whom serial measurements show progressive deviation from the normal. The investigation of these children must take into account the multiple genetic and environmental factors which influence growth.

Genetic and environmental causes of short stature

Familial short stature. Adult height is subject to polygenic inheritance and has therefore a normal distribution. In assessing a problem of short stature it is useful to plot the parents' height centiles on the child's growth chart. The theoretical correlation between the child's eventual height and the mid-parental value is 0.71. It must be remembered that parental short stature may have resulted from inherited disease, for example skeletal dysplasia, or from still relevant environmental influences.

Familial growth delay. A separate group of genes regulates the tempo of growth and there may be a familial pattern of delayed puberty with retarded skeletal maturation but eventually normal adult height. This variant is commoner in boys and can cause considerable distress in adolescent years. Recognition of the problem and sympathetic explanation provides a considerable boost to their morale and it is rarely justified to artificially accelerate puberty with exogenous androgen treatment.

Low birth weight conditions. The majority of pre-term and small-for-gestational age infants achieve normal adult size. A minority have permanently restricted growth. They are a heterogenous group consisting of infants exposed to external influences such as congenital infection or maternal drugs, or having intrinsic disorders, for example chromosomal anomalies. A number of syndromes include low birth weight and subsequent growth restriction. Russell-Silver syndrome combines these features with a triangular facies, small mandible and body asymmetry.

Causes of short stature (after Lacey and Parkin)

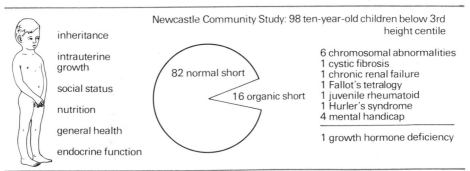

Newcastle Community Study: 98 ten-year-old children below 3rd height centile

inheritance

intrauterine growth

social status

nutrition

general health

endocrine function

82 normal short

16 organic short

6 chromosomal abnormalities
1 cystic fibrosis
1 chronic renal failure
1 Fallot's tetralogy
1 juvenile rheumatoid
1 Hurler's syndrome
4 mental handicap

1 growth hormone deficiency

Social deprivation. Short statue is most prevalent in the lower social classes and reflects the superimposition of a disordered environment on genetic potential. It is not easy to define the latter as successive generations have usually been exposed to the same adverse factors. Growth hormone release is depressed in emotionally deprived children but rapidly reverts to normal when they are provided with love and reasonable care. These disturbed children may also show bizarre, compulsive eating behaviour, to the extent that they develop distended abdomens and bouts of vomiting.

Nutritional starvation produces a different response with exaggerated growth hormone secretion but a block at the hepatic level where there is diminished synthesis of the somatomedins, growth factors which mediate in the peripheral anabolic effects of growth hormone.

Systemic causes

Those sufficient to restrict growth are usually severe and can be diagnosed by careful history and examination. Exceptions are chronic renal disease and malabsorption. Coeliac disease is a particular problem in that it may mimic hypopituitarism producing subnormal height velocity, delayed bone age and suppressed growth hormone responses. A jejunal biopsy may therefore be necessary in doubtful cases.

Endocrine causes of short stature

Growth hormone deficiency. This is relatively uncommon but has provided a major stimulus to basic research in this field, and its therapy has resulted in the establishment of specialised growth clinics. In the majority of affected children it is an isolated deficiency and an underlying fault cannot be defined. 10 to 15 per cent have a familial basis. Multiple pituitary hormone failure suggests secondary hypopituitarism produced by inflammatory, traumatic or neoplastic disorders in the suprasellar region.

Growth hormone deficiency must be confirmed by serial accurate height measurements and by a subnormal response to provocation tests such as insulin induced hypoglycaemia or arginine infusion. Limited supplies of human growth hormone are available for the treatment of proven cases and it has no place in the management of other varieties of growth failure.

Craniopharyngioma. This is a rare but important condition to exclude whenever there is a possibility of secondary hypopituitarism. The tumour is composed of expanding cystic remnants of Rathke's pouch, a dorsal protrusion of the embryonic stomatodoeum, and its strategic location results in life threatening pressure effects. Headache and defective vision are more common initial complaints than short stature, but visual field assessment and a lateral skull X-ray are essential in the assessment of short children.

Juvenile hypothyroidism results in progressive growth failure and is characterised by severe retardation of skeletal development. It is readily confirmed by performing thyroid function tests and responds well to thyroxine replacement.

Pressure effects and clinical features of craniopharyngioma

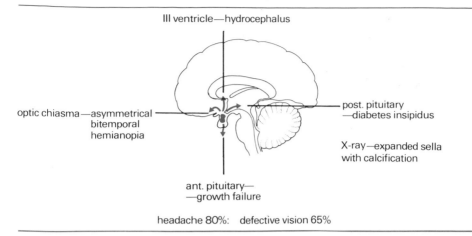

III ventricle—hydrocephalus

optic chiasma—asymmetrical
bitemporal
hemianopia

post. pituitary
—diabetes insipidus

X-ray—expanded sella
with calcification

ant. pituitary—
—growth failure

headache 80%: defective vision 65%

Adrenal insufficiency, hypoparathyroidism and pubertal disorders account for a small number of children with short stature. Corticosteroid therapy at a dosage in excess of prednisone 5 mg per day or its equivalent interferes with linear growth. Alternate day single dose corticosteroid regimes permit more normal growth.

Investigation of short stature

In the majority of children the history will reveal a genetic or social basis for their problem and detailed investigation is therefore inappropriate. Those lacking such an explanation, having definitely abnormal growth, or having additional signs or symptoms require accurate measurement or anthropometry. In addition to an accurate measurement of height, which provides the basis for longitudinal growth assessment, there must be some comparison of trunk versus leg length to allow recognition of disproportionate short stature. Pubertal staging, optic fundi and visual field assessment are essential parts of the physical examination. Laboratory investigations are guided by the clinical findings but in general are limited to total blood count, plasma electrolytes, creatinine, calcium, phosphorus, alkaline phosphatase and thyroid function. Turner's syndrome is not rare and hence there is a case for chromosomal analysis in short girls. Random measurements of basal growth hormone levels are misleading and a more formal provocation is required. A commonly used out-patient procedure is the exercise test in which the serum growth hormone level is measured 20 minutes after finishing 10 minutes of strenuous exercise. Radiographs of the left wrist and hand for bone age determination and a skull X-ray for pituitary fossa examination complete the initial assessment.

It is unnecessary to subject children to more formal assessment of growth hormone secretion, such as insulin-induced hypoglycaemia, until they have had at least six months of longitudinal growth assessment. Exact height measurement at three monthly intervals enables the height velocity to be determined. A subnormal velocity confirms the case for further detailed investigation. The combination of serial height measurements and bone age determinations is not

Longitudinal growth assessment

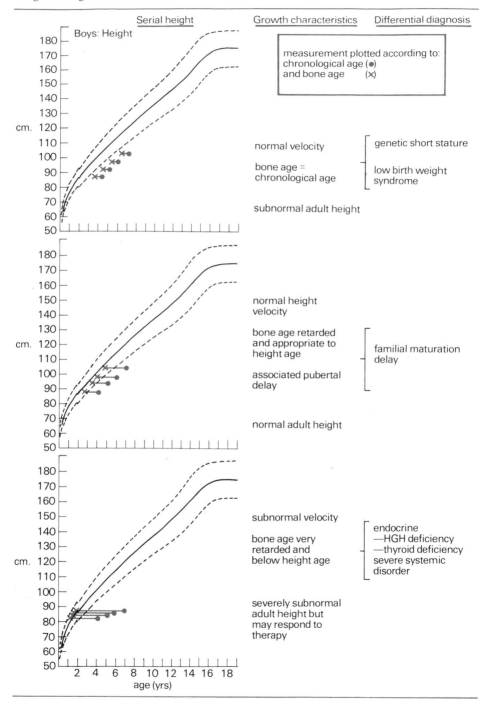

only a useful tool in the diagnosis of short stature, but provides a parameter by which therapy may be judged.

Disproportionate short stature

Calculation of the ratio of upper and lower body segment lengths will reveal cases of disproportionate short stature. Skeletal disorders account for the majority of this group and may be classified into those where abnormality originates in the skeleton, or has a systemic metabolic basis, for example mucopolysaccharidoses. They may also be divided into those with short limbs or short trunks, the latter usually having kyphoscoliosis. Exact diagnosis, confirmed by radiological and metabolic studies, is essential for genetic counselling.

Achondroplasia

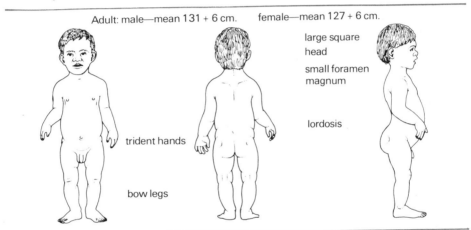

Adult: male—mean 131 + 6 cm.　female—mean 127 + 6 cm.

large square head

small foramen magnum

lordosis

trident hands

bow legs

EXCESSIVE HEIGHT

The great majority of tall children come from tall families and accept their stature as normal. An unusually tall child may have an underlying disorder but these are usually readily excluded. Occasionally, girls apparently destined to have an adult height above 5 feet 10 inches (178 cm) are brought for advice and possible medical intervention. Prediction of final height is not easy as it is influenced by the time of menarche and the rate of skeletal maturation as well as by the linear grow rate in childhood. Tables are available for predicting adult height but they are liable to errors of approximately 5 cm either way. Exogenous oestrogen therapy has been

Pathological causes of excessive height

Endocrine disorders	Other disorders
Pituitary — eosinophilic adenoma Thyrotoxicosis Precocious puberty (early stages)	Cerebral gigantism (Soto's syndrome) Marfan's syndrome Homocystinuria

used to promote accelerated skeletal maturation and a premature cessation of linear growth in girls but the benefits are often marginal, and there is concern about the risks of interfering with the humoral mechanism of puberty and of increasing the incidence of reproductive tract neoplasia. The orthopaedic approach to this problem, epiphyseal stapling, retains its place in a very small group of children with asymmetrical growth. Irradiation of the growing epiphyses has rightly been abandoned because of the high risk of inducing osteosarcomata.

BIBLIOGRAPHY

Beighton P 1978 Inherited disorders of the skeleton. Churchill Livingstone, Edinburgh.
Lacey K A, Parkin J M 1974 Causes of short stature. A community study of children in Newcastle-upon-Tyne. Lancet I: 42-45.
Marshall W A 1977 Human growth and its disorders. Academic Press, London.
Nellhaus G 1968 Head circumference from birth to eighteen years. Pediatrics 41: 106-114.
Sinclair D 1973 Human growth after birth, 2nd edn. Oxford University Press, Oxford.
Smith D W 1977 Growth and its disorders. Saunders, Philadelphia.
Tanner J M, Whitehouse R H, Takaishi M 1965 Standards from birth to maturity for height, weight, height velocity and weight velocity; British children. Archives of Diseases of Childhood 41: 613-635.

15
Endocrine

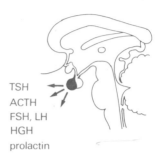

TSH
ACTH
FSH, LH
HGH
prolactin

Although the fetus is totally dependent on a maternally regulated environment, fetal endocrine systems differentiate and commence autonomous activity in the first trimester. The placenta is relatively impermeable to peptide hormones so that most fetal hypothalamic-pituitary-endocrine gland circuits evolve independently of any direct interference from maternal hormone levels. The adrenal cortex is an exception in that the placenta actively participates in steroid metabolism and this is reflected in the major transition from fetal to adult cortex activity with birth.

Trophic hormones are first detectable in the anterior pituitary between five and eight weeks' gestation, and serum levels of thyroid stimulating hormone (TSH) and the gonadotrophins (LH and FSH) reach adult levels by 16 to 20 weeks. This early surge of trophic hormone activity may relate to endocrine gland development prior to the establishment of sensitive feedback mechanisms.

The endocrine factors which control human fetal growth have yet to be defined. Anencephalic infants with absent growth hormone have relatively little reduction in body weight although there are delays in skeletal and lung maturation. The mean birth weight of hypothyroid infants is greater than normal. These apparent anomalies may be resolved by greater knowledge of the role in fetal growth of the new generation of growth promoting peptide hormones, somatomedins, epidermal growth factor, fibroblast growth factor and nerve growth factor.

Delivery and the demands of an independent existence result in major endocrine adjustments. In the case of TSH and thyroid hormone release the change is abrupt, but for other systems such as the gut and pancreas the transition occurs progressively with the introduction of oral feeds.

PUBERTY

Puberty is a series of physical and physiological changes which convert the child to an adult capable of reproduction. The physical events include a growth spurt, alteration of body proportion and the development of sexual organs and secondary sexual characteristics. There is great variability in the onset and order

The normal age range of puberty (after Marshall and Tanner)

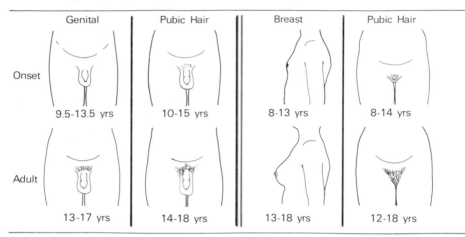

of these events. 95 per cent of girls commence puberty between 9 and 13 years with breast formation (80 per cent) or pubic hair growth (20 per cent) as a first event. Menarche occurs at a mean age of 13.5 years and is closely correlated with skeletal maturity so that it is suspicious to find a girl still amenorrhoeic with a bone age of over 15 years. Boys have a later puberty with onset for 95 per cent being between 9.5 and 13.5 years, the first sign being enlargement of the testes, rapidly followed by growth of the penis and pubic hair. It is not unusual to find infantile genitalia in a boy aged 15 years if there is delayed skeletal maturation. A standardised scheme for recording genital, breast and pubic hair maturation has been described by Tanner.

Physiology of puberty
The newborn infant is capable of releasing high levels of the gonadotrophins, testosterone and oestradiol but this transient hormonal activity is subsequently inhibited by a very sensitive gonadohypothalamic feedback mechanism. Puberty follows the elevation of the threshold for this feedback inhibition but the mechanisms responsible for this readjustment are not known. The pineal gland may be partly responsible for hypothalamic suppression of gonadotrophin release as tumours which destroy this gland or its connections sometimes result in precocious puberty. Longitudinal studies of normal children show a rise of FSH levels at the onset of puberty and a later rise of LH which is paralleled by testosterone and oestradiol. Adrenal androgen output is correlated with pubic hair growth, skeletal maturation and possibly the age of menarche. The link between the hypothalamic pituitary axis and adrenal sex hormones is a mystery.

Precocious puberty
Precocious puberty is termed 'true' or intracranial when it is controlled by the hypothalamic-pituitary axis, and 'false' when an extracranial or exogenous source of hormone is responsible.
    Early puberty is relatively common in girls and there may be a family history. Detailed assessment is unnecessary unless puberty commences before the age of

Causes of precocious puberty

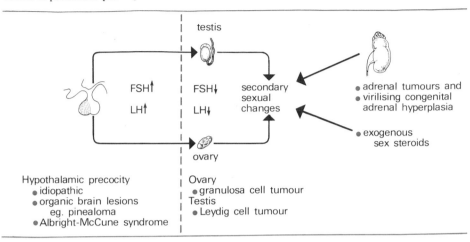

Hypothalamic precocity
 • idiopathic
 • organic brain lesions
     eg. pinealoma
 • Albright-McCune syndrome

Ovary
 • granulosa cell tumour
Testis
 • Leydig cell tumour

six years or menses before eight years, or if puberty pursues an abnormal sequence of events with virilisation or is accompanied by other problems such as neurological symptoms, hypertension or abnormal growth. Of girls commencing puberty early, 90 per cent have no demonstrable abnormality. Precocious puberty in boys (defined as having an onset earlier than nine years) is more frequently pathological (60 per cent of cases) and requires careful evaluation.

The Albright-McCune syndrome consists of unilateral pigmentation, cystic bone lesions and precocious puberty. It is commoner in girls and the basic endocrine derangement is still unresolved.

Premature thelarche is an isolated transient phase of breast development in girls and is not uncommon during infancy and childhood. There are no other signs of puberty and recognition of this innocent occurrence should obviate further investigation.

Premature pubarche refers to isolated development of pubic and axillary hair and is again more common in girls. There may be slight advance in the bone age and marginal increase in urine oxosteroid levels but other signs of sexual development are absent.

Gynaecomastia in adolescent boys is common and may be uni- or bilateral. It is usually transient and does not indicate underlying endocrine problems unless there is other evidence of testicular failure.

Delayed puberty

Delayed puberty may indicate a gonadal failure with elevated gonadotrophin levels, or a disorder of the hypothalamic-pituitary axis in which case they are reduced. Ovarian dysgenesis is a component of Turner's syndrome, XO karyotype, but it can also occur independently. In males, gonadal dysgenesis occurs in Klinefelter's syndrome, XXY karyotype. Gonadal failure may also follow irradiation or exposure to cytotoxic therapy.

The testicular feminisation syndrome is suggested by amenorrhoea and absent pubic hair in a girl with normal breast development. In this familial disorder genetic males with testes develop as phenotypic females because of end-organ resistance to testosterone.

Haematocolpos. Increasing abdominal distention and monthly discomfort without bleeding calls for examination of the vulva, as an imperforate hymen may produce retention of menstrual products.

Normal sexual differentiation

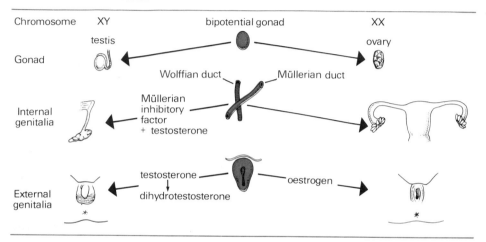

DISORDERS OF SEXUAL DIFFERENTIATION

Parents expect the sexual identity of their offspring to be immediately obvious. Ambiguity of the external genitalia at the time of birth causes great distress and sensitive explanation is vital. Complete diagnostic evaluation requires special expertise as it has to consider the long term functional role of the individual as well as the precise gender. A genetic male with functioning testes but feminised external genitalia is better reared as a girl.

The majority of intersex problems represent female or male pseudo-hermaphroditism rather than true hermaphroditism. The recognition of virilising

A classification of ambiguous genitalia

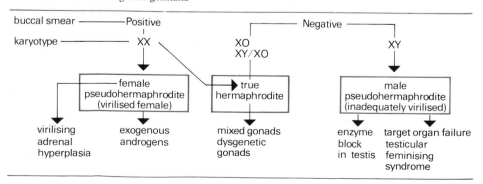

congenital adrenal hyperplasia must be a priority in order to avert a salt-losing crisis. The exact nature of other types may necessitate laparotomy and gonad biopsy. After assigning the appropriate gender, management may involve reconstructive surgery, hormonal substitution and possibly removal of gonads. The latter is particularly indicated in gonadal dysgenesis because of the risk of neoplastic transformation. Reconstructive surgery to the external genitalia should be completed before 18 months of age if possible because of the psychological implications.

ADRENAL GLANDS

During intrauterine development the adrenal cortex is considerably enlarged due to a thick inner fetal zone. This zone, which accounts for 80 per cent of the cortex at full term, involutes rapidly after birth leaving the outer adult zone to synthesise essential mineralocorticoids and glucocorticoids. The fetal cortex acts in a mutually dependent relationship with the placenta to synthesise oestriol and dihydroepiandrosterone. The measurement of these steroids in the maternal serum or urine provides an index of feto-placental health. The increasing development of the adult zone at term may be a factor in initiating the onset of labour; anencephalic infants with secondary adrenal hypoplasia, but without polyhydramnios tend to have prolonged gestation.

Congenital adrenal hyperplasia

This group of inherited, autosomal recessive disorders is caused by the absence of essential enzymes in the pathway of cortisol and aldosterone synthesis. The resulting interruption of the adrenohypothalamic feedback stimulates excessive corticotrophin (ACTH) release and overactivity of the biosynthetic steps prior to the block, with an accumulation of androgenic steroids. The commonest variety is 21-hydroxylase deficiency, 1 in 5000 to 1 in 50 000 live births. Affected female infants are virilised at birth with clitoral hypertrophy and variable fusion of the labia minora. The most masculinised girls may be confused for males with

Congenital adrenal hyperplasia

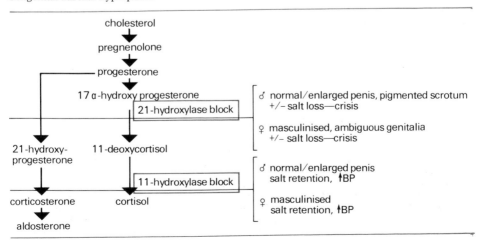

hypospadias and cryptorchidism. Prompt recognition of this problem is less easy in males and they may not be diagnosed prior to an adrenal crisis in the second week of life. The crisis, often preceded by vomiting and poor weight gain, is biochemically characterised by low serum sodium and high potassium. Grossly elevated serum ACTH and 17-hydroxyprogesterone levels suggest the 21-hydroxylase deficiency. This may be confirmed by elevated concentrations of urinary pregnanetriol and 17-oxosteroids. A salt-losing crisis demands urgent therapy with intravenous saline, glucose and hydrocortisone. Long-term management must aim to suppress the hyperplastic adrenal glands and provide replacement hydrocortisone and a salt-retaining steriod, fludrocortisone. The correct replacement is that which permits normal linear growth and maintains serum 17-hydroxyprogesterone and the urinary steroids within acceptable limits. Surgical correction of the masculinised female perineum is commenced in the first year. Adult men and women are capable of normal fertility but should remain on hydrocortisone and fludrocortisone. Among the rarer forms of congenital adrenal hyperplasia, 11-beta-hydroxylase deficiency results in virilisation and salt retention with hypertension. Affected children may present with excessive growth, but the advanced bone age considerably limits their final adult stature.

Cushing's syndrome

This rare disorder is due to sustained high cortisol levels of either exogenous or endogenous origin. The commonest endogenous cause in children is an adenoma or carcinoma of the adrenal cortex. It should be considered when acne and masculinisation accompany the usual signs of cortisol excess. Distinction must be made between these potentially malignant unilateral tumours and the rarer problem of bilateral adrenal hyperplasia due to pituitary microadenomata. An IVP will probably show kidney displacement in the former. ACTH levels are suppressed by the tumour and elevated urinary steroid metabolites fail to diminish during a dexamethasone load. Adrenal tumours require unilateral adrenalectomy and additional radiotherapy if there is histological evidence of capsule invasion. In acquired bilateral adrenal hyperplasia, management is either

Cushing's syndrome

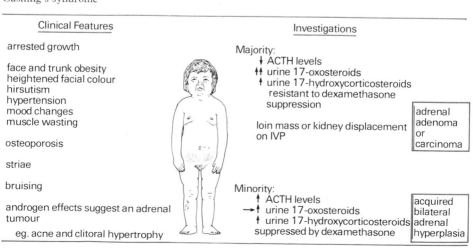

Clinical Features	Investigations	
arrested growth	Majority:	
	↓ ACTH levels	
face and trunk obesity	↑↑ urine 17-oxosteroids	
heightened facial colour	↑ urine 17-hydroxycorticosteroids	
hirsutism	resistant to dexamethasone	
hypertension	suppression	
mood changes		adrenal
muscle wasting		adenoma
	loin mass or kidney displacement	or
osteoporosis	on IVP	carcinoma
striae		
bruising	Minority:	
	↑ ACTH levels	acquired
androgen effects suggest an adrenal	→↑ urine 17-oxosteroids	bilateral
tumour	↑ urine 17-hydroxycorticosteroids	adrenal
eg. acne and clitoral hypertrophy	suppressed by dexamethasone	hyperplasia

directed against the pituitary adenomata using high voltage radiation and trans-
sphenoidal microsurgery, or relies on bilateral total adrenalectomy.

Adrenal cortical failure (Addison's disease)
This uncommon disorder has an autoimmune basis and may occur in association
with diabetes mellitus, thyroiditis and hypoparathyroidism. Children either
present with an insidious onset of weakness, weight loss and increased pigmentation or become acutely ill following a brief episode of diarrhoea and vomiting.
An adrenal crisis demands urgent therapy with intravenous glucose and saline
together with hydrocortisone. Long term replacement consists of hydrocortisone
(25 to 30 mg/m² surface area/day) and fludrocortisone 0.1 to 0.2 mg daily. With all
patients on corticosteroid replacement therapy, the child must be provided with a
steroid warning card and the parents advised of the necessity of increasing the
dosage during times of illness.

THYROID

The thyroid originates from a ventral extension of the endoderm foregut which
migrates caudad to lie at the level of the upper trachea. Developmental failures
may be classified as hypoplasia or maldescent. Hypoplasia varies from absence of
detectable thyroid and early severe hypothyroidism, to lesser degrees which
remain asymptomatic until later childhood. An ectopic gland may account for a
lingual mass or produce a thyroglossal cyst. A sinus may occur along the line of
descent.

Physiology
The fetal thyroid contains colloid and iodoproteins by ten weeks gestation; plasma
TSH is detectable at this stage and there is evidence for early activity of the
pituitary-thyroid axis. The fetal thyroid preferentially releases 'reverse T3', a
molecule which differs from tri-iodothyronine by the location of a single iodine
atom. Reverse T3 is thought to be inactive and its place in physiology has not been

Ectopic sites of the thyroid gland. Neonatal thyroid function

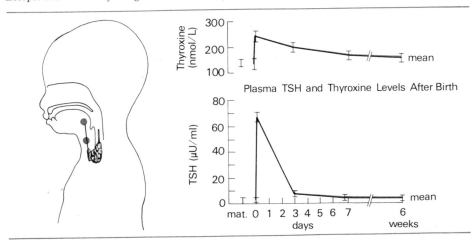

Plasma TSH and Thyroxine Levels After Birth

established. There is minimal transplacental passage of maternal thyroxine to the fetus.

Following birth there is a surge of TSH release later paralleled by increased thyroxine (T4) and tri-iodothyronine (T3). TSH levels return to the normal adult range by one week but T4 and especially T3 show a slower decline to adult values. The definition of normal neonatal thyroid function is essential for the development of screening programmes to detect congenital hypothyroidism.

Hypothyroidism

Congenital hypothyroidism is relatively common, 1 in 6000 live births. Central nervous system development appears critically dependent on thyroxine from late pregnancy through the first months of infancy. In some infants brain development may be irreversibly damaged before birth, in others brain damage may be avoided by early detection and adequate treatment. It is important that affected infants are identified as soon as possible after birth.

Congenital hypothyroidism

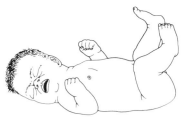

coarse facies	umbilical hernia
dry skin	constipation
hoarse cry	prolonged jaundice
hypotonia	

Goitrous hypothyroidism. A hypothyroid infant with a goitre has probably been exposed to maternal goitrogens such as antithyroid drugs, iodine containing preparations, phenylbutazone or PAS. The goitre may cause life threatening tracheal compression. Inborn errors of thyroxine biosynthesis account for familial goitrous hypothyroidism but these conditions seldom present in the newborn.

Juvenile hypothyroidism. Hypothyroidism occurring in later childhood presents with growth failure and abnormal skeletal delay. As thyroxine levels are adequate in the early critical phase of brain development there is no intellectual impairment.

L. thyroxine sodium is the standard therapy for hypothyroidism. Infants require a relatively higher dose, 5 μg per kg per day, diminishing to 2 to 3 μg per kg in later childhood. The dose is monitored by checking height and bone age increments as well as biochemical parameters. Therapy must be life long.

Hyperthyroidism

Neonatal hyperthyroidism is an uncommon disorder but must be anticipated in all infants of mothers with a history of thyrotoxicosis. Maternal thyroid stimulating immunoglobulins may traverse the placenta to overstimulate the fetal thyroid producing irritability, fever, diarrhoea and poor weight gain. Although transient the condition is potentially fatal and may require antithyroid therapy or propranolol.

Juvenile hyperthyroidism is uncommon but the features are similar to those seen in adults with the addition of excessive growth and occasional abnormal choreiform movements. The diagnosis is confirmed by elevated plasma thyroxine levels. Medical management using carbimazole is the treatment of choice. An initial two year course may result in spontaneous remission in 25 to 75 per cent of cases, and a further course should be completed before considering surgical management. Radioactive iodine is to be avoided in childhood.

Autoimmune thyroiditis
Goitres due to autoimmune thyroiditis are less rare than previously considered. The majority are asymptomatic but there may be signs of mild hyperthyroidism or progressive hypothyroidism. A positive thyroid antibody test confirms the diagnosis. Therapy with replacement thyroxine is indicated for significantly enlarged goitres or biochemical hypothyroidism. Goitrogen consumption and familial goitrous hypothyroidism enters the differential diagnosis.

Isolated thyroid nodules
These must be carefully investigated by isotope scans and biopsy to exclude carcinoma.

PARATHYROID GLANDS

Hypoparathyroidism
Transient hypoparathyroidism is a common neonatal event and the resulting hypocalcaemia may cause convulsions or apnoeic episodes. Permanent hypoparathyroidism is rare and has to be distinguished from conditions in which there is organ unresponsiveness to circulating parathyroid hormone, the pseudohypoparathyroidism syndromes.

True hypoparathyroidism is confirmed by demonstrating increased urinary phosphate or cyclic AMP excretion during an infusion of parathyroid hormone.

Pseudohypoparathyroidism syndromes are refractory to parathyroid administration and the children may show the other features; short stature, round facies, short metacarpals, ectopic calcification and mental retardation.

Classification of hypoparathyroidism

Transient neonatal	Prematurity, cerebral injury Maternal diabetes Maternal hyperparathyroidism
Permanent life-long	Isolated hypoplasia Di George syndrome. Thymus aplasia, defective immunity, candidiasis, cardiac lesions Autoimmune — associated diabetes mellitus, Addison's disease, chronic hepatitis, etc. Post-thyroidectomy
Pseudohypoparathyroidism syndromes	

Pseudopseudohypoparathyroidism is part of the group of X-linked disorders in which the typical physical abnormalities are not accompanied by biochemical derangement.

Treatment of hypoparathyroidism. Acute symptomatic hypocalcaemia requires urgent correction with intravenous calcium, 0.1 mmol elemental calcium per kg bodyweight per hour. 10 per cent calcium gluconate should be diluted to 2 per cent for use and the infusion must be carefully monitored.

Permanent hypoparathyroidism and pseudohypoparathyroidism are treated with supraphysiological doses of vitamin D or related compounds which act by promoting intestinal calcium absorption and by mobilising bone calcium. The dose of vitamin D is adjusted to maintain the plasma calcium level in the low normal range (2.15 to 2.40 mmol/l). Chronic overdosage carries the risk of nephrocalcinosis and renal failure.

Features of hypoparathyroidism

Acute Hypocalcaemia	Chronic Hypocalcaemia
Convulsions	Convulsions
	calcification of basal ganglia
neuromuscular excitability	headache, vomiting (raised intracranial pressure)
Chvostek sign	photophobia
Trousseau sign	cataracts
carpopedal spasm	poor dentition
	chronic diarrhoea
	Investigation: serum calcium ↓ serum phosphorus ↑ alk. phos.—normal

DIABETES

Diabetes mellitus is the disorder which results from insulin deficiency. In most juvenile diabetics, this is due to irreversible islet beta cell damage. Diabetes is rare in infancy but the incidence rises to approximately 1 in 1200 among schoolchildren. Children account for only 4 to 6 per cent of the total diabetic population but the life-long complications of the disease emphasise their importance.

Aetiology

The failure of the islet beta cells in diabetes is poorly understood but appears to be the end result of both environmental and genetic factors. Genetic influence is less important in juvenile than in maturity onset diabetes; less than 50 per cent of identical twins of young diabetics develop the disorder compared with 100 per cent in maturity onset diabetics, and only 10 per cent of affected children have a diabetic parent or sibling. The histocompatibility types HLA-B8 and HLA-BW15 are found more commonly in juvenile diabetes than in the control population or in maturity onset cases, and it is likely that the gene conferring susceptibility to diabetes is linked to these HLA loci. Environmental influences are suggested by autumn and winter peaks, case clustering and an association with viral infections such as mumps and coxsackie B4.

A unifying hypothesis proposes that viral beta cell damage in genetically susceptible individuals triggers a sequence of autoimmune destructive processes. Islet cell antibodies commonly appear during the initial phase after the onset of symptoms.

Clinical features

The symptoms are characteristic and the diagnosis is seldom in doubt if glycosuria and ketonuria are detected. Young diabetics always require prompt diagnosis and therapy, but the correct diagnosis may be confused by a coincidental febrile illness and the hyperventilation mistakenly interpreted as being due to pneumonia. Diabetes may be confirmed by a single blood glucose estimation and glucose tolerance tests are rarely necessary. Early diagnosis saves lives and allows an organised introduction to the principles of diabetic management; often as an out-patient. Ketoacidosis obviously necessitates urgent admission.

Features and duration of symptoms in childhood diabetes

Clinical Features

Early:	Late:		
polyuria	vomiting	**Duration of symptoms before diagnosis**	
(secondary nocturnal	abdominal pain		
enuresis)	hyperventilation		
thirst	(metabolic acidosis)	0-2 wks	20%
lethargy	shock		
weight loss	coma	2-6 wks	52%
anorexia			
(increased appetite		6 wks plus	28%
unusual)			
constipation			

Diabetic ketoacidosis

The basic principles of treatment consist of insulin therapy, fluid and electrolyte replacement and the correction of provoking factors. Low dose insulin regimes are favoured as these provide for more predictable control of blood sugar and largely avoid hypoglycaemia and hypokalaemia. Although metabolic acidosis may be prominent it is unnecessary to administer sodium bicarbonate unless there is severe circulatory failure.

Long term management

It is not possible to return diabetics to a physiologically normal state with current methods of insulin administration. Management must be a compromise aimed at the following objectives; a happy child leading a full life and equipped for a normal adult role; normal growth; education and motivation to maintain the best possible diabetic control. Current clinical and experimental studies support the belief that optimal control reduces the long term risk of microvascular disease. In practice good control means freedom from symptoms and minimal glycosuria but occasional mild hypoglycaemia is acceptable. The essentials of management are diet, appropriate insulin and education in the techniques and understanding of diabetes.

Diet. A regulated carbohydrate intake is essential for adequate control. Carbohydrate is adjusted to approximately 40 per cent of the total caloric intake and is based on readily recognisable 10 gram portions which are divided among three main and three snack meals. An average ten year old boy requires 2000 calories per day and a carbohydrate intake of 200 grams per day divided into 20×10 gram portions, distributed as 4, 2, 5, 2, 5, 2.

Insulin. Most children can be controlled on combinations of short and medium duration insulins. Purified or monocomponent porcine insulins are replacing less pure preparations.

Young children may have satisfactory control on a single morning injection but it is wise to introduce a twice daily regime in the prepubertal child. There can only be very approximately guides to insulin requirements but children seldom require more than 1 unit per kg per day of the pure porcine insulins. Injections are the focal point of the diabetic day and correct technique must be stressed. This can only be learned by demonstration. A standard insulin syringe (BS 1619, 20 units

A scheme for the management of diabetic ketoacidosis

1.	Initial management Assess circulatory status Weigh Insert I.V. line and send samples to laboratory Stop oral intake and insert nasogastric tube Attach ECG monitor
2.	Identify provoking factors, e.g. infection
3.	Fluid, electrolyte and insulin management Calculate total fluid requirement (deficit + maintenance + losses) Replace $\frac{1}{3}$ 0–4 hr $\frac{1}{3}$ 4–12 hr $\frac{1}{3}$ 12–24 hr

Treat shock i.v. N saline or plasma	i.v. soluble insulin initial dose 0.25 u/kg continue 0.10 u/kg/hr
Extracellular replacement: i.v. N saline + KCl until blood glucose <14 mmol/l	using infusion pump until blood glucose <14 mmol/l
Intracellular replacement: i.v. 0.2 N saline in 5% dextrose and KCl	reduce insulin to 0.05 u/kg/hr (adjust according to blood glucose)
Graded re-introduction of oral fluids 2-hourly milk/sugar drinks	start 8-hourly soluble insulin 0.5–2.0 u/kg/day
Regular diet	establish on medium-acting insulin

A selection of insulin preparations

Type		Origin	pH	Approximate time of action (hr)		
				Onset	Peak	Duration
Short-acting	Soluble	Ox	3	0–1	3–6	10
	Actrapid MC	Pig	7	0–1	2–5	7
	Leo Neutral	Pig	7	0–1	1–4	8
Medium-acting	Isophane	Ox	7	1–2	6–14	24
	Semitard MC	Pig	7	1–2	4–9	16
	Leo Retard	Pig	7	1–2	4–12	24
Long-acting	Monotard MC	Pig	7	2–3	6–14	36

per ml) is used with 26-gauge disposable needles which can be reused if, like the syringe, they are stored in industrial spirit. Injection problems include pain due to too shallow needle insertion, fat hypertrophy due to inadequate spacing of injections, and fat atrophy which may be linked to poor technique but may also have an immune basis. The latter seldom occurs with the new pure insulins.

Urine tests. Glycosuria is a crude parameter of control but is currently the only practical approach. The clinitest method is widely used but the tablets are caustic and potentially dangerous if eaten. Tests are performed on the second voided sample before main meals and the family should learn how to make appropriate insulin adjustments. Acetest tablets may be reserved for periods of poor control such as during coincidental illness.

Problems in diabetic control
Poor control and so-called brittle diabetes with recurrent ketoacidosis and hypoglycaemia may arise from several causes.

Hypoglycaemia. Parents have a great fear of insulin reactions and this naturally leads to caution in attaining freedom from glycosuria especially in evening tests. In older children reactions are usually easily preventable by ready access to glucose tablets or adjustment of diet and insulin doses.

The Somogyi phenomenon refers to reactive hyperglycaemia, glycosuria, and ketonuria after hypoglycaemic episodes which are often transient, nocturnal and escape detection. Excessive insulin dosage is a common cause.

Poor growth. Children with early onset diabetes tend to have reduced adult height but improved control minimises this shortening. Chronically bad control may produce dwarfism, hepatomegaly and facial obesity, the Mauriac syndrome.

Behaviour. Parents require advice on how to cope with injection trauma, dietary delinquency, fake urine tests and pseudo-hypoglycaemia. Urine tests must not be regarded as times of judgement. Adolescents may become introspective and depressed about the future so that poor control and carelessness may be a symptom of their distress.

Factors which influence diabetic control

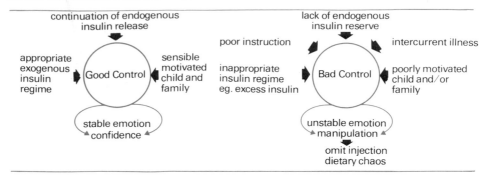

Long term complications

The microvascular disease responsible for retinopathy and nephropathy is related to duration of diabetes and seldom occurs within ten years of onset. After 20 years 80 per cent have some retinal changes but only a minority develop significant visual impairment. Sub-capsular snowstorm cataracts are occasionally seen in childhood.

Chronic renal failure accounts for half of all deaths in patients who develop diabetes before the age of 20. Proteinuria is the first sign of renal disease and the mean duration of diabetes before its onset is 15 years. Once detected the average life expectancy is five years but some survive considerably longer. Diabetic renal damage is a consequence of the metabolic derangements of the disease, and its avoidance is a stimulus to attaining more physiologically normal blood sugars in young diabetics.

HYPOGLYCAEMIA

Hypoglycaemia is rare after the newborn period but must be considered in the assessment of non-febrile seizures, particularly those occurring early in the morning and after prolonged fasts. A blood glucose of less than 2.2 mmol/l is diagnostic and the urine should also be tested for ketones, a helpful step in distinguishing the two main categories of disorders which cause recurrent hypoglycaemia: substrate deficiency and hyperinsulinism. In children where there is no obvious explanation, a carefully monitored period of starvation with serial determinations of plasma glucose, insulin, cortisol, growth hormone, betahydroxybutyrate and lactic acid is the most useful investigation.

Substrate deficiency

Ketotic hypoglycaemia is the commonest cause of hypoglycaemia after the first year. Affected children are usually small, slim and most susceptible to attacks during coincidental illness. Nocturnal fits associated with vomiting and unconsciousness develop and ketonuria is prominent. Monitored starvation results in a more pronounced hypoglycaemia and ketonaemia than normal, but insulin levels are very low. Limited gluconeogenic reserves probably account for this disorder.

Causes of hypoglycaemia in infancy and childhood

Substrate deficiency (ketones usually present)	*Hyperinsulinism* (ketones absent)
1. ketotic hypoglycaemia	1. pancreatic
2. hepatic enzyme deficiencies	nesidioblastosis
glycogen storage diseases	insulinoma
galactosaemia	2. mesenchymal tumours
hereditary fructose intolerance	3. prediabetes mellitus
3. exogenous hepatotoxins and poisons	
Reye's syndrome	
alcohol, aspirin	
unripe Akee fruit	
4. endogenous hepatotoxins	
tyrosinosis	
maple syrup urine disease	
5. endocrine deficiencies	
pituitary, adrenal	

Hypoglycaemia can be avoided by regular bedtime snacks and additional glucose drinks during illness. The problem resolves spontaneously in later childhood.

Hyperinsulinism

Nesidioblastosis is a rare problem of young infants in which developmental disorganisation of the islet cells and inappropriate insulin release results in refractory hypoglycaemia. The latter may be partially controlled using continuous infusions of glucose, and diazoxide. The most successful long-term therapy is a 75 to 80 per cent resection of the pancreas.

Insulinomas account for most cases of hyperinsulinism in older infants and children, and again extensive resection of the pancreas is indicated.

BIBLIOGRAPHY

Cornblath M, Schwartz R 1976 Disorders of carbohydrate metabolism in infancy, 2nd edn. Saunders, Philadelphia
Craig O 1977 Childhood diabetes and its management. Butterworth, London
Gardner L I 1969 Endocrine and genetic diseases of childhood. Saunders, Philadelphia
Hamilton W 1972 Clinical pediatric endocrinology. Butterworth, London
Walshe P 1979 Screening for neonatal hypothyroidism. British Journal of Hospital Medicine 21: 28–36

16
Skin

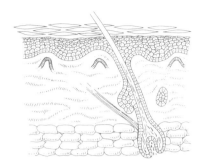

Man consists mainly of water and it is his skin which stops him from drying out. In addition, the skin protects the body from physical, chemical and biological insult. The superficial layer of the epidermis, stratum corneum, with its compact horny cells provides an effective barrier to the passage of substances in either direction. The dermis, with its high collagen content, gives skin its ability to stretch and mould. Its numerous blood vessels and sweat glands are important in the control of body temperature.

The epidermis develops in the third week of fetal life, and is initially composed of two layers, an outer periderm and an inner basal layer. The periderm is equipped with absorptive microvilli and actively transfers substances between amniotic fluid and fetal tissues. It is normally shed long before term, but occasionally it persists as a horny cocoon, creating the so-called 'collodion baby'. The basal or germinative layer gives rise to the definitive multi-layered epidermis, and this differentiation is largely complete when keratinisation establishes the stratum corneum in the sixth month of fetal life. An extremely premature infant has thin, poorly keratinised epidermis, and is therefore vulnerable to excessive skin water losses after birth.

The sebaceous glands are active from mid gestation, and their secretion, together with the residue of the periderm, accounts for the vernix caseosa. The vernix provides a greasy coating to the newborn skin and may have bacteriocidal properties. Term infants are able to sweat within two to five days after birth, but there may be a delay of two to three weeks in the premature. Sebum and sweat retention are common in the newborn:

Milia
These are minute sebaceous material cysts which give rise to yellowish-white specks over the nose and face. Although they may be very conspicuous in the first days of life, they disappear spontaneously by three to four weeks.

Miliaria

This is possibly the most frequent skin eruption in the first weeks of life, and reflects sweat gland immaturity and the tendency to overheat babies. It arises as crops of papules or papulo-vesicles over the face, trunk and napkin area. It generally resolves rapidly with appropriate clothing and ventilation, but may occasionally become secondarily infected.

RASHES OF EARLY INFANCY

Infantile seborrhoeic dermatitis

Seborrhoeic dermatitis is a distinctive erythematous and scaly, non-eczematous eruption of unknown cause. It usually starts during the second or third month of life as cradle cap or napkin dermatitis which spreads rapidly, sometimes giving psoriasis-like lesions over much of the body. The child is never ill and is not

Seborrhoeic dermatitis

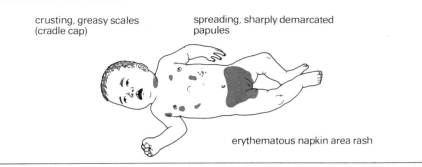

crusting, greasy scales (cradle cap)

spreading, sharply demarcated papules

erythematous napkin area rash

distressed by it. In its mildest form, just one or two lesions may be present in the flexures giving rise to an erroneous diagnosis of atopic eczema. Very mild corticosteroid and antiseptic combinations such as 1 per cent hydrocortisone and 3 per cent clioquinol will usually clear it.

Napkin rashes

Rashes in the napkin area are very common and not always indicative of poor

Napkin area rashes

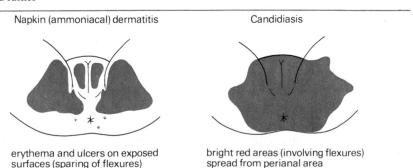

Napkin (ammoniacal) dermatitis

Candidiasis

erythema and ulcers on exposed surfaces (sparing of flexures)

bright red areas (involving flexures) spread from perianal area

mothering. The main causes are napkin dermatitis, candidiasis and seborrhoeic dermatitis.

Napkin dermatitis is caused by prolonged contact with wet napkins. Bacterial conversion of the urine to ammonia creates an alkaline irritant. Simple measures are usually effective; frequent napkin changes, careful washing at each change and the application of a protective cream such as zinc and castor oil ointment. The napkin should be rinsed thoroughly after washing and used with disposable napkin liners.

Candidiasis is commonly superimposed on a napkin rash and warrants treatment with nystatin ointment.

ATOPIC ECZEMA

Atopic eczema affects 3 per cent of children and usually has its onset between two and eighteen months of age. There is often a family history of other atopic disorders, hay fever or asthma. Itching is very prominent and scratching frequently results in secondary infection. It has a fluctuating course with approximately 50 per cent resolving by eighteen months and few continue to have a problem beyond childhood. Although skin prick tests for specific allergens are often positive, they provide little guide to clinical management as multiple factors are usually involved. There is some preliminary evidence that breast feeding and total avoidance of cow's milk protein in the first few months of life may reduce the incidence of atopic problems in genetically susceptible infants.

Management
Atopic eczema is a very taxing illness for child and family. Disturbed nights, irritability and the often alarming appearance add to the burden. The parents have an active role in management and need careful sympathetic instruction.

Atopic eczema

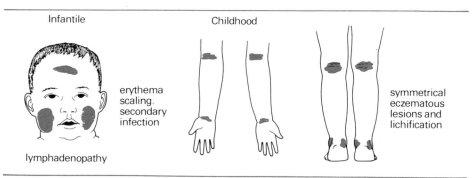

The skin is often dry because of an associated ichthyosis; the avoidance of all soap and the use of emulsifying ointment in its place helps to correct this. Corticosteroid ointments applied once or twice daily benefit the affected areas but should be used sparingly and the potency kept to the minimum necessary to control the disease. One percent hydrocortisone cream or ointment, or betamethasone cream diluted to 1 in 10 with cetomacrogol cream, are usually adequate for all but the most stubborn patches. Secondary infection may be treated with a topical antibiotic, for example chlortetracycline or neomycin combined with a corticosteroid. If the child is pyrexial, or deeper spread of infection occurs, a systemic antibiotic should be given. The control of scratching and the provision of undisturbed nights are valuable assets. Antihistamines, for example trimeprazine tartrate or promethazine, used as night sedation are well tolerated and valuable if given as a short course during exacerbations. Other useful measures include using cotton underclothes rather than wool, avoiding heat and light bandaging of the limbs at night. The hands must never be tied to prevent scratching. Children must *not* be vaccinated against smallpox or come into contact with a recently vaccinated person. They are at risk of developing widespread and potentially fatal vaccinia. There is no contraindication to immunisation against diphtheria, whooping cough, tetanus and poliomyelitis, but these should be given when the eczema is in a less acute phase. Primary infection with herpes simplex virus may give a very severe reaction known as Kaposi's varicelliform eruption.

INFECTIONS AND INFESTATIONS

Bacterial

Impetigo is a highly contagious superficial skin infection which passes rapidly through a vesicular phase and usually presents with typical golden brown crusts. Topical therapy with the application of 3 per cent chlortetracycline cream is adequate for limited infections. More extensive lesions require a systemic antibiotic, for example erythromycin. Refractory or atypical cases raise the possibility of an underlying cause such as scabies, scalp pediculosis or an immune deficiency.

Bacterial skin infection

Scalded skin syndrome   Impetigo

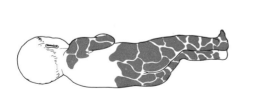 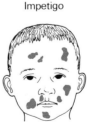

golden crusts

staphylococcus

streptococcus

Bullous impetigo of the newborn may have serious complications , for example osteomyelitis and pneumonia, and the mortality is high. Systemic antibiotics are required, for example flucloxacillin.

Toxic epidermal necrolysis (Lyell's disease, Ritter's disease or staphylococcal scalded skin syndrome) results from epidermal cleavage due to toxins of staphylococcus phage type 71. Typically, young infants and children develop acute inflammation and soreness which evolves into a generalised exfoliation, the scalded skin syndrome. Even ordinary handling can result in skin loss and extreme care is necessary in the nursing of these children.

Viral

Primary herpes simplex infection is usually asymptomatic but it can produce a gingivostomatitis in young children. It presents with fever, irritability, and difficulty in swallowing. The latter is caused by extensive shallow ulcers of the buccal, gingival and pharyngeal mucosae. Occasionally there may be a vulvovaginitis or a keratoconjunctivitis.

Herpetic encephalitis is a rare but grave complication. Gingivostomatitis requires careful nursing to ensure an adequate fluid intake. Idoxuridine paint may accelerate healing if it can be successfully applied to the ulcerated mucosa.

Herpes zoster is not uncommon in children and usually settles without leaving post herpetic neuralgia. Povidone-iodine paint will reduce infectivity and the likelihood of secondary infection.

Viral warts affect most children at some time during childhood. They are harmless and self limiting, and treatment is only indicated if there is discomfort. This is most likely on the pressure bearing areas of the soles. The application of a salicylic acid based wart paint is usually all that is required.

Molluscum contagiosum is more likely to affect covered areas of the body. The individual lesions can be cleared by pricking the centre with a sharpened stick dipped in liquid phenol.

Fungal infection

Fungal infections due to the usual human dermatophytes are uncommon in childhood; a diagnosis of athlete's foot is nearly always wrong. Susceptibility to animal ringworm, especially *Microsporum canis* from cats and dogs, is quite high and scalp involvement is unique to children.

Fungal skin infection

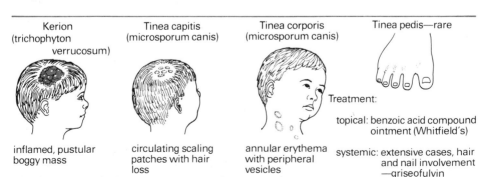

Kerion (trichophyton verrucosum)	Tinea capitis (microsporum canis)	Tinea corporis (microsporum canis)	Tinea pedis—rare
inflamed, pustular boggy mass	circulating scaling patches with hair loss	annular erythema with peripheral vesicles	Treatment: topical: benzoic acid compound ointment (Whitfield's) systemic: extensive cases, hair and nail involvement —griseofulvin

Infestations

Scabies is due to a mite which is spread by close family contact and invades the horny layer of the skin where it lays its eggs. The burrows are generally over hands, wrists, elbows, feet and genitalia but can occur on the face of babies. Infestation provokes an intense itch and a secondary erythematous papular rash. The mite may be identified using a low power lens and a needle. The whole family should be treated by a single application of benzyl benzoate emulsion to all the skin surfaces below the neck. A less irritating alternative is 1 per cent gamma benzene hexachloride.

Skin infestation

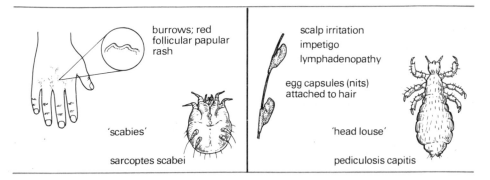

Pediculosis capitis

Pediculosis capitis or head lice infestation is common in our schools. It may present as a persistent itch with secondary dermatitis or be found on routine hair examination. The oval nits are easily seen firmly adhering to the hair shaft. The mature lice are less often visible. The application of 0.5 per cent malathion solution is effective against the lice and nits.

CONGENITAL SKIN LESIONS

Birth marks

Strawberry naevus (superficial cavernous angioma). A third of these elevated lesions occur on the face and become conspicuous and grow rapidly in the first month of life. In spite of parental pressure, management must be conservative with the reassuring knowledge that spontaneous disappearance occurs by the age of five or six years.

Capillary naevus (port wine stain). This defect in dermal blood vessels can occur anywhere but is commonest on the upper half of the body. There is no tendency to fade or spread. Usually it is an isolated cosmetic problem, but occasionally there may be meningeal involvement as well, for example in the Sturge-Weber syndrome.

Pigmented naevi. These naevi are rarely evident at birth and start to appear at the age of two years. In childhood they are usually flat or only slightly elevated. Histologically they show junctional activity but malignancy is extremely rare.

With maturation the majority lose their junctional elements and become intradermal and completely benign. Extensive macular pale brown 'cafe au lait' spots are a feature of neurofibromatosis.

Ichthyosis
The most frequent form is an autosomal dominant condition characterised by dry finely scaling skin. It may coincide with and complicate atopic dermatitis. Restoration of skin moisture with an emollient cream is the basis of treatment.

Congenital anhidrotic ectodermal dysplasia
This is a rare, sex-linked, recessive condition producing loss of sweat glands, dental hypoplasia, and sparse hair, eyebrows and eyelashes. These children are intolerant of heat.

Epidermolysis bullosa
This condition is a pathological susceptibility to blistering and there are a number of genetic varieties. The severity ranges from blistering with unusual trauma to serious life threatening scarring and deformity, despite careful handling.

Incontinentia pigmenti
This rare condition is almost exclusively restricted to females and is usually obvious at birth. Groups of vesicles evolve through warty papules to bizarre patterns of pigmentation. There is associated eosinophilia, dental and eye abnormalities.

Xeroderma pigmentosum
This autosomal recessive condition is manifest by dry photosensitive skin liable to freckling, keratoses and malignant transformation.

Acrodermatitis enteropathica
This produces progressive mucocutaneous ulceration and is associated with bowel pathology. It responds to treatment with zinc.

OTHER COMMON SKIN DISORDERS

Psoriasis
This commonly presents as an acute guttate rash following an upper respiratory tract infection. An eruption of small discrete red scaling lesions may develop rapidly and cover much of the body. Resolution usually occurs after two months or so, but the existence of the psoriatic tendency has been indicated and the more typical plaques on elbows, knees and scalp may develop at any time. Treatment should be kept to a minimum compatible with asymptomatic control. The application of coal tar and salicylic acid ointment after bathing is a useful measure.

Pityriasis rosea
This is an acute self limiting eruption giving rise to erythematous scaling macules

with a central distribution. It may superficially resemble guttate psoriasis but is distinguished by a herald patch, which appears three or four days before the main eruption, and by the frequent presence of itching and fine scaling. A mild corticosteroid ointment may help resolution.

Granuloma annulare
These skin lesions consist of asymptomatic dermal nodules usually on the fingers or toes. It is a harmless condition but resolution may be slow, taking years rather than months.

Alopecia areata
These areas of localised hair loss on the scalp have a characteristic margin of exclamation mark hairs. The alopecia is usually self-limiting and possibly related to periods of school or other stress. Rare cases progress to alopecia totalis. It should be distinguished from habitual hair pulling, trichotillomania, and ringworm of the scalp in which there is an obvious inflammatory element.

Acne
Acne occasionally occurs in a child less than eighteen months old and reflects physiological adjustments in the responsiveness of sebaceous glands to postnatal hormone changes. Its occurrence later in childhood, but before the onset of puberty, requires further investigation in case of underlying adrenal pathology. It is, of course, very common in adolescence but the problem should not be discounted because it may dominate life and give rise to self-imposed isolation. It is linked to the onset of sebaceous gland activity and the production of free fatty acids in follicles which are blocked, with resulting comedones or blackheads, inflammation and pustules. Treatment is directed at removing the keratin plugs, for example with benzoyl peroxide, and suppression of lipolytic bacteria with long term low dose antibiotics, usually tetracycline 250 mg twice daily.

Erythema nodosum
These tender erythematous nodules occur most frequently over the pretibial region. They appear in crops and may be associated with fever and arthralgia. An underlying problem may be streptococcal infection, tuberculosis, *Mycoplasma pneumoniae*, food or drug sensitivity. In the majority no underlying condition will be found.

BIBLIOGRAPHY

Solomon L M, Esterly N B 1973 Neonatal dermatology. Saunders, Philadelphia.
Solomon L M, Esterly N B, Loeffel E D 1978 Adolescent dermatology. Saunders, Philadelphia.

17
Bone and Joint

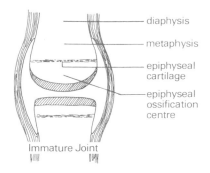

diaphysis

metaphysis

epiphyseal cartilage

epiphyseal ossification centre

Immature Joint

Bone tissue can be detected in the eight-week fetus. It arises from precursor mesenchymal cells which either evolve into osteoblasts and osteocytes capable of primary ossification, or into chondroblasts and chondrocytes which give rise to an initial cartilagenous model. Tissue oxygen concentration, mechanical stress and hormonal agents are some of the factors known to dictate the type of bone development. In the limbs there are also complex interactions between skeletal formation and the ectodermal covering. Mineralisation which is essential to bone structure depends on the transplacental passage of calcium, phosphorus and vitamin D or its metabolites. This mineral transfer is maximal in later gestation and the calcium content of the fetus is doubled in the last month. The calcium deficit created by premature delivery increases the requirement for vitamin D in the postnatal period. Following delivery, the skeleton continues its growth, both in length and weight. It also undergoes considerable remodelling, particularly in the first two years when the rate is 10 times that which occurs in adult life. Maturation is accompanied by progressive endochondral ossification with the appearance of epiphyseal centres and the disappearance of the growth cartilages. This maturation is subject to genetic and environmental controls and may be quantified to provide the bone age, a valuable parameter in assessing growth and its disorders.

ARTHRITIS

A swollen, painful joint requires prompt evaluation as it may be the first sign of severe systemic illness. Young children present with fever, limp or pseudo-paralysis rather than specific joint symptoms. The problem may be localised to a single joint, in which case pyogenic infection must be excluded, or involve several joints, a polyarthritis.

Polyarthritis in childhood

Infection	Bacterial — pyogenic, tuberculosis
	Viral — rubella, mumps, infectious
	mononucleosis.
Post-infectious	Rheumatic fever
Allergic	Henoch Schönlein purpura, other allergies
Collagen vascular disease	Rheumatoid arthritis, systemic lupus
	erythematosis, dermatomyositis
Haematological disease	Leukaemia, haemophilia, sickle cell disease
Gastrointestinal tract	Ulcerative colitis, Crohn's disease
disorders	
Trauma and synovitis	

Pyogenic arthritis

In pyogenic arthritis the joint is usually hot, swollen and acutely tender and more than one joint may be involved. Movement of the affected joint is restricted and very painful. The joint must be aspirated and the fluid examined by microscopy and culture, and also blood samples taken for culture at the same time. Osteomyelitis adjacent to a joint may produce a sympathetic effusion but the tenderness will be on the bony metaphysis rather than over the joint. The commonest infecting organism is *Staphylococcus pyogenes*, and flucloxacillin given intravenously is the treatment of choice. Surgical drainage is frequently required if diagnosis is delayed beyond 48 to 72 hours from the onset of symptoms. During the acute phase of the illness the joint is splinted, but later physiotherapy and mobilisation is essential to prevent joint flexion from developing into a permanent deformity.

Rheumatic fever
See Chapter 9.

Features of rheumatic fever

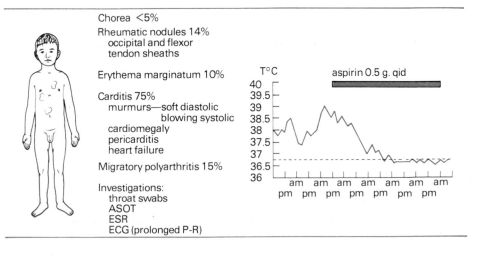

Chorea <5%
Rheumatic nodules 14%
  occipital and flexor
  tendon sheaths

Erythema marginatum 10%

Carditis 75%
  murmurs—soft diastolic
              blowing systolic
  cardiomegaly
  pericarditis
  heart failure

Migratory polyarthritis 15%

Investigations:
  throat swabs
  ASOT
  ESR
  ECG (prolonged P-R)

T°C   aspirin 0.5 g. qid
40
39.5
39
38.5
38
37.5
37
36.5
36
  am am am am am am am
  pm pm pm pm pm pm pm

Tuberculous arthritis

Tuberculous arthritis is now very rare in Europe but occasionally presents in the spine and the larger synovial joints.

Viral arthritis

Viral arthritis may be confused with rheumatic fever or juvenile chronic polyarthritis.

Henoch Schönlein purpura

This is a diffuse, self-limiting allergic vasculitis. It is common in young children but the precipitating factors have not been fully identified. The clinical picture is readily recognisable; the majority resolving quickly and requiring only analgesics. A minority have more severe gastrointestinal manifestations and may warrant a brief course of corticosteroid therapy. The renal lesion is discussed elsewhere.

Features of Henoch Schönlein purpura   *1/3 preceded by URTI.*

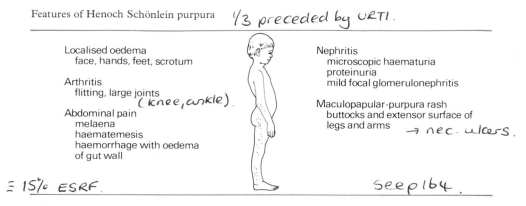

Localised oedema
   face, hands, feet, scrotum

Arthritis
   flitting, large joints
      (knee, ankle).

Abdominal pain
   melaena
   haematemesis
   haemorrhage with oedema
   of gut wall

≡ 15% ESRF.

Nephritis
   microscopic haematuria
   proteinuria
   mild focal glomerulonephritis

Maculopapular-purpura rash
   buttocks and extensor surface of
   legs and arms   *→ nec. ulcers.*

see p 164.

Allergic polyarthritis

A transient allergic reaction consisting of an urticarial rash and synovitis is not uncommon. It may follow mild upper respiratory tract infections, drug or dietary allergen exposure.

Juvenile chronic polyarthritis (Still's disease)

There are three major sub-groups of rheumatoid disease in childhood: a systemic variety, 20 per cent; polyarthritis, 50 per cent; and oligoarthritis in which joint involvement is limited to one to four joints, 30 per cent. The peak incidence is in the one- to five-year age group with a smaller peak at puberty. The diagnosis is largely clinical as affected children seldom have a positive rheumatoid factor test.

Systemic juvenile chronic polyarthritis may not have prominent joint symptoms and should be considered when there is difficulty in establishing the cause of a remitting fever, hepatosplenomegaly and abdominal pain. Acute lymphatic leukaemia and metastatic neuroblastoma may produce a similar clinical picture and a marrow examination may therefore be necessary.

Polyarticular juvenile chronic polyarthritis presents with painful swelling and stiffness of both large and small joints. It has a symmetrical distribution and characteristically involves the temporo-mandibular joints and the cervical

Features of systemic juvenile chronic polyarthritis, Still's disease

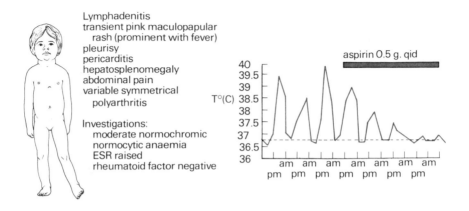

spine as well as limb joints. Systemic signs are minimal, usually weight loss and mild anaemia. The arthropathy of psoriasis or large bowel inflammation, Crohn's disease and ulcerative colitis, can produce a similar picture.

Oligoarticular juvenile chronic polyarthritis is a chronic large joint disorder often associated with chronic iridocyclitis and a positive anti-nuclear factor test. Some older girls do have a positive IgM rheumatoid factor and have a disease equivalent to the adult pattern. Adolescent boys with the HLA B27 type are liable to juvenile ankylosing spondylitis.

Management. The priorities in therapy are to reduce joint inflammation and to avoid deformity. Aspirin, (80 to 90 mg/kg/day) is the most effective drug. It may have to be supplemented by one of the non-steroid anti-inflammatory agents, for example indomethacin or ibruprofen. Chronic disease may require gold injections, penicillamine or chloroquine but these drugs introduce a significant risk of toxicity problems. Corticosteroids are avoided except in the control of severe systemic illness and iridocyclitis.

Exercise, hydrotherapy and night splints are part of a carefully tailored programme which is essential to maximise long-term joint mobility. In 70 to 80

Knee and hand involvement in juvenile chronic polyarthritis. A fifteen-year follow-up of 100 children (after Calabro).

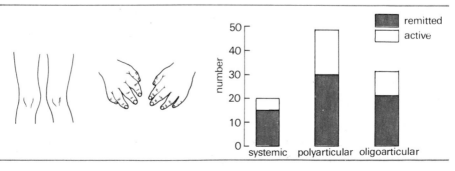

per cent of cases a useful independent life is possible and the active inflammatory component of the disease eventually remits spontaneously.

OSTEOMYELITIS

Osteomyelitis is usually haematogenous in origin and affects the metaphyses of long bones. The epiphyseal plate of growing bones normally prevents spread into the adjacent joint space. *Staphylococcus pyogenes* accounts for 90 per cent, with *Haemophilus influenzae* and *Streptococcus pyogenes* as less common isolates. Children with sickle cell disease are susceptible to salmonella infections and the site is frequently atypical.

The anatomy of osteomyelitis and its distribution in 93 children, 89 with a single site and four with double sites — in parenthesis (after Mollan and Piggot)

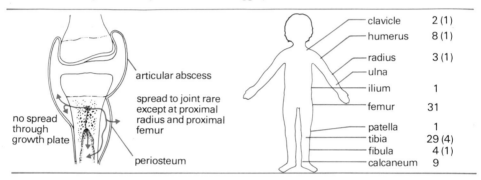

clavicle	2 (1)
humerus	8 (1)
radius	3 (1)
ulna	
ilium	1
femur	31
patella	1
tibia	29 (4)
fibula	4 (1)
calcaneum	9

Clinical features. The infected limb is painful and immobile. Swelling and occasionally redness may be seen if diagnosis is delayed. Examination of all inexplicably febrile children must include careful palpation of the limbs looking for areas of local swelling and tenderness. The adjacent joint may contain a sterile or sympathetic effusion. Repeated blood culture is the most satisfactory method of determining the responsible organism and therefore establishing its antibiotic sensitivity. X-rays are not of diagnostic help in the first 10 to 14 days. The first radiological signs are subperiosteal new bone formation and spotty rarefaction. Radioisotopic bone scan will show abnormality at a much earlier stage but is seldom necessary.

Management. Prompt, effective antibiotic therapy is essential for a successful outcome. Neglected cases are liable to develop irreversible bone necrosis, draining sinuses and limb deformity. Appropriate antibiotic regimes include high dosage intravenous flucloxacillin and/or fucidin for one to two weeks followed by oral therapy until there is clinical response and radiological evidence of healing. Lack of response in the first 48 hours of therapy is an indication for surgical exploration and drainage.

Infantile cortical hyperostosis (Caffey's disease)
This is a rare but characteristic disorder of infants manifest by irritability, fever, and non-suppurative tender painful swelling of bone. It usually effects one or

more of the following; mandible, clavicle, ulna, humerus and ribs, shows abnormal subperiosteal new bone formation but no bone necro

NORMAL POSTURAL VARIATIONS

These are common problems which arouse much parental anxiety. Reassurance is usually more appropriate than expensive shoe modifications or unnecessary physiotherapy.

In-toe gait. This may originate in the foot (metatarsus varus), in the tibia (tibial torsion), or in the femora (persistent anteversion of the femoral neck). These conditions are symmetrical, pain free and are accompanied by normal mobility. They generally resolve in three to four years.

Out-toe gait is also common in the first two years of life and may be unilateral. It always corrects spontaneously.

Causes of in-toe gait

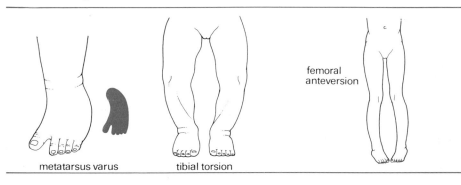

metatarsus varus   tibial torsion   femoral anteversion

Genu varum (bow legs). Outward curving of the tibia often associated with tibial torsion, is not uncommon and corrects with growth. Severe examples should raise the suspicion of Blount's disease, a rare developmental anomaly of the proximal tibial epiphyses.

Genu valgum (knock-knees) is frequent in the 2- to $4\frac{1}{2}$-year age-group and is usually innocent if symmetrical and independent of any other abnormality. Severe and progressive cases raise the possibility of rickets which is most frequently seen among Asian immigrant children. Rickets may be confirmed by the X-ray appearance of the typical frayed epiphyseal changes and by an elevated serum alkaline phosphatase.

Flat feet. The medial arch of the foot develops within two to three years of walking. It is largely obliterated by a fat pad in younger children. Persistent flat feet may be familial or reflect joint laxity. It is insignificant if the foot is pain free, mobile and develops an arch when standing on tiptoe. Neurological problems and pathological joint laxity are occasional underlying causes. Severe convex flat foot

Knock knees and flat feet

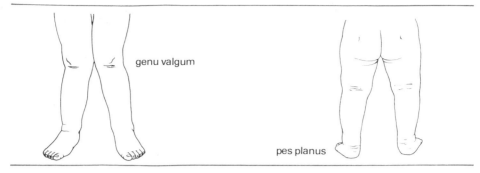

genu valgum

pes planus

is occasionally due to congenital vertical talus, in which condition early surgical treatment can avoid crippling deformity in later life.

SCOLIOSIS

Scoliosis refers to spinal curvature in the coronal plane and is best detected by asking the child to bend over at the waist with the arms hanging freely.

Innocent postural scoliosis is corrected by full flexion and does not evolve into the structural form.

Structural scoliosis is fixed and accompanied by rotation of the vertebral bodies which in the thoracic spine produces thoracic cage deformity, the classical 'rib hump'. The main curvature may be compensated for by secondary curvatures so that the head is aligned with the pelvis. Scoliosis is commonly asymptomatic but can develop into a disagreeable cosmetic problem.

80 to 85 per cent of structural scoliosis is of the idiopathic variety occurring mainly in girls during the rapid adolescent growth period, 10 to 14 years. Infantile (0 to 2 years), and juvenile (3 to 9 years) forms also occur. Family studies indicate a genetic basis. A small proportion are produced by congenital vertebral anomalies, hemivertebrae, neurofibromatosis or osteogenesis imperfecta. Neuromuscular disorders such as muscular dystrophy and Marfan's disease may result in secondary scoliosis.

Structural scoliosis, its anatomy and clinical detection

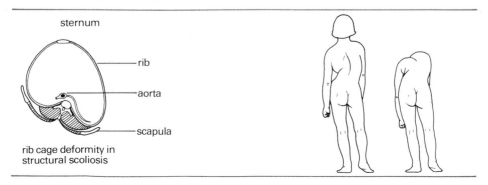

sternum

rib

aorta

scapula

rib cage deformity in structural scoliosis

Physiotherapy has no place in preventing the evolution of structural scoliosis. The Milwaukee brace worn for 23 hours a day provides a distraction force between head and pelvis as well as pressure on the posterior displaced ribs. It halts progression in 70 per cent of cases. Surgical correction and fusion is reserved for patients with pulmonary or spinal cord complications, unstable spines or progressive deformity. The deformity rarely deteriorates after skeletal maturity although it may worsen during pregnancy and in old age.

HIP DISORDERS

Congenital dislocation of the hip

Early detection is essential as it permits a relatively simple course of treatment with the likelihood of an excellent outcome. Delayed diagnosis and advanced secondary changes in the hip and adjacent tissues complicates the problem so that the management is prolonged and the outcome often less than totally satisfactory.

The basic fault remains to be determined but there are definite genetic influences. Familial joint laxity is a factor and girls are more susceptible than boys (6:1). There is a striking geographical variation with the incidence in north-west Europe being 1.5 true dislocations per 1000 births, as opposed to the Bantu race where the condition is almost unknown. Unilateral cases are more common than bilateral (2:1). Infants born by breech presentation and with extended hips are especially susceptible. Down's

Screening tests. These techniques must be learnt by practical instruction from an expert. The infant should be content and relaxed, and is placed on his back on a firm flat surface. The hips are flexed at a right angle and the knees are also held flexed. Starting with the knees together the hips are slowly abducted through a complete 90° arc. A dislocated hip slips back into the acetabulum during abduction, producing a palpable clunk. Restricted abduction is also a suspicious finding. Minor clicks may originate from the knee, especially if it is not kept immobile, but there should be little confusion with the genuine 'clunk'. Doubtful cases must be examined by an experienced doctor and many of the early clicks disappear after the first week of life.

Careful screening of all newborn infants will detect a hip clunk in between 1:80 and 1:120. It would appear therefore that of all infants detected as having joint

Ortolani test for congenital dislocation of hip

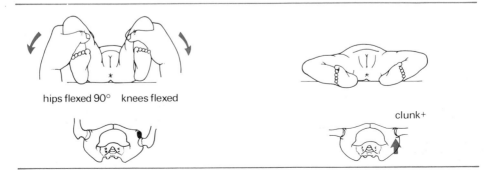

hips flexed 90°   knees flexed

clunk+

Congenital dislocation of hip, radiology and management

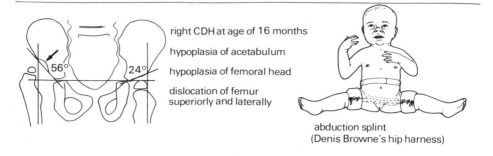

right CDH at age of 16 months

hypoplasia of acetabulum

hypoplasia of femoral head

dislocation of femur
superiorly and laterally

abduction splint
(Denis Browne's hip harness)

laxity at birth, less than 10 per cent eventually prove to have true dislocation. The infant whose hips are still suspect in the second and third weeks, are usually fitted with an abduction appliance such as the Von Rosen splint. Hips which are more equivocal are reviewed subsequently and have an X-ray examination of the hip at about four months to ensure that the femoral head is normally located. The splint is retained until the acetabulum shows signs of developing satisfactorily and the head is sufficiently ossified to confirm its congruity within it. The time period is variable, extending from two to four months.

It is unfortunately true that dislocated hips are still missed in spite of the widespread introduction of screening procedures. Suspicion is raised by a child with a shortened leg, or with a gait in which the affected foot is placed flat on the ground while the opposite knee is flexed. It does not generally delay the onset of walking but may well cause frequent falls. Bilateral cases have a symmetrical gait and tend to present even later if missed in the neonatal period. Attempted reduction of the hip involves initial traction followed by more prolonged splintage or in the event of failure, operative intervention. The latter may involve open reduction, femoral osteotomy and acetabular reconstruction.

Transient synovitis

This is the most common cause of hip pain or limp in children. It is a unilateral, self-limiting condition of ill-defined aetiology although many follow a mild upper respiratory tract infection. Boys in the age group 2 to 12 years (average six years) are most susceptible. It usually has a sudden onset with limp, and pain of variable severity. Abduction, full extension and internal rotation are restricted and there may be tenderness over the anterior aspect of the hip. There is usually no leucocytosis, and the ESR is normal or only mildly elevated. X-rays are normal. The diagnosis can only be made after observation and exclusion of Perthe's disease, septic arthritis or adjacent osteomyelitis, tuberculous arthritis, rheumatoid disease, a slipped femoral epiphyses, or an osteoid osteoma.

Transient synovitis seldom lasts for more than a few days or weeks and treatment consists of simple analgesics and bed rest often with simple skin traction. Approximately 6 per cent of cases considered to have transient synovitis subsequently develop features of Perthe's disease, and long-term studies have suggested an increased incidence of degenerative changes in the affected joint.

Perthe's disease

This results from episodes of segmental avascular necrosis of the femoral head. The necrotic bone is gradually replaced by new bone, but recovery can be complicated by residual deformity of the femoral head. It is most common in the four to eight-year age group and the ratio of boys to girls is 5:1. The underlying cause has not been established but it is suspected that the femoral head disorder is part of a more generalised growth disturbance in which skeletal development is retarded.

Limp, with or without pain, is the presenting complaint and hip mobility, especially abduction and internal rotation, is limited. The hip X-ray reflects the natural history of the bone necrosis; initial increase in density followed by fragmentation and reossification. The identification of the femoral head at risk of deformity is central to management; the head at risk is usually treated by 'containment' in the acetabulum either by femoral osteotomy or bracing. The healing phase during which the head requires protection lasts two to four years.

Slipped capital femoral epiphyses

In this condition there is a gradual displacement of the femoral head downwards and posteriorly. It results from a high shear force during the adolescent growth spurt (girls at age 10 to 14 years and boys at 12 to 16 years) and is bilateral in 25 per cent of patients. Obese children with delayed skeletal and sexual maturity are especially susceptible. Pain in the region of the hip, thigh or knee accompanied by a limp are the typical features. The early radiological appearances are easily overlooked and a lateral projection is essential to detect epiphyseal slipping. A suggestive history warrants repeat X-rays after four to six weeks if the initial examination is negative. Treatment is by manipulation or internal fixation.

KNEE DISORDERS

The knee is a common source of complaint among adolescents. In assessing the cause of knee pain, the hip must also be examined as hip pain is often referred to the knee.

Osgood Schlatter disease is a painful tenderness of the tibial tuberosity at the site of insertion of the patellar tendon, traction apophysitis. It is aggravated by quadriceps contraction, and temporary restriction of vigorous exercise is sufficient therapy in most cases.

Chondromalacia patellae indicates softening of the articular cartilage of the patellae usually as the result of indirect trauma, for example unaccustomed games activity. The retropatellar pain is worse on rising from prolonged sitting or on stairs, and is accompanied by crepitus. Avoidance of repetitive knee bending and physical recreation is usually adequate advice. Occasional cases have patellar misalignment worthy of surgery.

⚬ immobilize or
⚬ paring.
⚬ patellectomy

Talipes

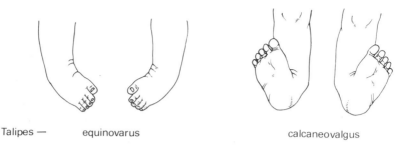

Talipes —   equinovarus   calcaneovalgus

TALIPES (CLUBFOOT)

Talipes equinovarus

The fixed clubfoot is one of the most complex deformities facing orthopaedic surgeons as it represents disruption of complicated interrelationships between bone, ligament and muscle. The incidence is 1.2 per 1000 live births, rising by 20-fold where there is an affected first degree relative. Males are more at risk with a ratio of 3:1, and 50 per cent of cases are bilateral. All cases must be examined carefully to exclude an underlying neurological problem.

Treatment is largely determined by the rigidity of the deformity and by the secondary changes. In the earliest stages, gradual manipulative correction is combined with strapping. Over a period of six to eight weeks this results in correction of approximately 60 per cent of cases. If the hind foot remains in an equinus position operation is required to release the responsible soft tissue shortening. Manipulation and strapping is continued until the foot will evert and dorsiflex beyond the neutral position. In the final stages, Denis Browne's boottee splints, in which open-ended boots are attached to a crossbar, are worn at night. The whole course of treatment may continue until at least five years of age. Failure to achieve early true correction may result in the need for corrective bone surgery later in childhood.

Talipes calcaneovalgus

In this deformity the foot is dorsiflexed and everted but the underlying structural abnormality is less profound and the foot is more amenable to simple manipulation.

GENETIC BONE AND JOINT DISORDERS

Marfan's disease (autosomal dominant)

This disease consists of arachnodactyly, hypermobile joints, ocular abnormalities, and a high arched palate. There are commonly associated deformities of the spine and chest. The prognosis is determined by associated cardiovascular problems such as dilated aortic root, dissecting aortic aneurism and billowing mitral valve incompetence.

Cleido-cranial dysostosis (autosomal dominant)
The features include absence of part of all of the clavicle, and delayed ossification of the skull with persistent open skull sutures. Affected children also tend to be short.

Osteogenesis imperfecta (autosomal dominant, occasionally recessive)
In this condition there is an underlying failure in collagen metabolism resulting in multiple fractures of fragile bones, lax joints and thin skin. Blue sclerae, scoliosis, hypoplastic teeth and progressive deafness are also features. The congenital form may be of such severity that the fetus dies in utero or shortly after birth. The later onset variety is compatible with a reasonable prognosis and may present in adolescence as 'osteoporosis'.

Osteopetrosis or marble bone disease (autosomal recessive or autosomal dominant)
The recessive form is more severe causing bone marrow failure and early death. The dominant or less severe form presents in childhood as facial paralysis, bone fractures and osteomyelitis.

BONE CYSTS AND TUMOURS

Features suggestive of a bone tumour include pain, swelling or a limp. Fortunately the majority of underlying lesions are benign; atypical osteomyelitis, incomplete fracture of normal bone, a simple cyst or an osteoid osteoma.

Simple bone cysts
Simple bone cysts are most frequent in the diaphysis and present acutely as painful pathological fractures or as a chronic ache. The X-ray appearances are usually typical.

Osteoid osteoma
This may present with intermittent and often nocturnal pain, classically responding to aspirin. X-rays show extensive periosteal thickening with a focus of dense new bone surrounding a centrally placed radiolucent nidus. Typical cases may be treated conservatively but where there is doubt or failure to respond to simple analgesia, biopsy and excision of a central nidus provides almost instant relief of pain.

Ewing's tumour and osteosarcoma
These are the two most common malignant primary bone tumours in childhood. The former has to be distinguished from neuroblastoma which commonly metastasises to bone. Radiology can normally distinguish Ewing's tumour, which produces characteristic periosteal new bone formation, from osteosarcoma where there is more prominent bone destruction and infiltration. The introduction of combined local radiotherapy, or ablative surgery with chemotherapy, has brought a note of optimism to these previously dismal conditions. Osteosarcoma is less responsive to chemotherapy but recent programmes combining high dosage

methotrexate, folinic acid 'rescue', adriamycin and early radical amputation demonstrates remarkably improved results up to the present time.

BIBLIOGRAPHY

Asher C 1975 Postural variations in childhood. Butterworth, London.
Blockey, N J 1976 Children's orthopaedics — practical problems. Butterworth, London.
Calabro J J 1976 Clinical features of Still's disease. In: Jayson M I V (ed) Still's disease, Academic Press, London.
Fixsen J A 1977 Borderline orthopaedic abnormalities in children. Hospital Update 3: 185-191.
Lloyd-Roberts G C 1971 Orthopaedics in infancy and childhood. Butterworth, London.
Mollan R A B, Piggot J 1977 Acute osteomyelitis in children. Journal of Bone and Joint Surgery 59B: 2.

18
Brain, Nerve, Muscle

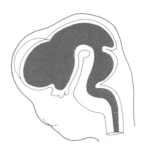

All who are concerned with the safe passage of children from conception to adulthood, have as a prime goal the preservation of normal brain development. Potential hazards have effects which are largely determined by the degree of differentiation of the nervous system. In the first trimester genetic and environmental influences may disrupt embryogenesis and produce malformations which either abort or reach term as gross anomalies, for example anencephaly and spina bifida. In later fetal life and during infancy insults are more likely to produce focal, irreversible pathology in differentiated tissue, lesions which may well be the basis of cerebral palsy.

In addition to interference with structural differentiation, the brain is also susceptible to problems during its various growth spurts. In the human fetus maximal neuronal proliferation occurs in the mid-trimester and is relatively protected from maternal malnutrition and placental dysfunction, but is vulnerable to viral infection, radiation, drugs and excessive alcohol. Glial multiplication and myelination occurs over a more extended period from the third antenatal trimester through the first two years of life and is therefore exposed to the effects of intra- and extra-uterine malnutrition, perinatal asphyxia and inborn errors of metabolism. We are only on the threshold of understanding how these hazards may influence the subtler components of growth, dendritic proliferation and synaptic connectivity.

INTRA-CRANIAL INFECTION

Acute infection of the meninges may be viral, aseptic meningitis, or bacterial, acute purulent meningitis, in origin. Meningitis may also be due to tuberculosis and rarer pathogens such as fungi and protozoa. Leukaemic cell infiltration can cause a sterile meningitis.

Acute purulent meningitis
Purulent meningitis is relatively common in childhood especially in pre-school

Bacterial meningitis: clinical features and common causative organisms

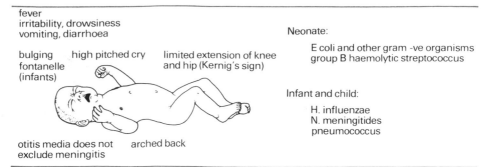

fever
irritability, drowsiness
vomiting, diarrhoea

Neonate:

E coli and other gram -ve organisms
group B haemolytic streptococcus

bulging   high pitched cry
fontanelle
(infants)

limited extension of knee
and hip (Kernig's sign)

Infant and child:

H. influenzae
N. meningitides
pneumococcus

otitis media does not
exclude meningitis

arched back

years, 35 percent of childhood cases occurring in the first year and 80 per cent in the first five years of life. It is essential to make an early diagnosis as delay results in death, over 100 per year in U.K., and a high incidence of neurological complications.

The characteristic features of meningeal irritation, neck stiffness and Kernig's sign are often absent in children under 18 months of age. Neonates and young infants are more likely to present with a fever, poor feeding, vomiting and drowsiness. In many in this age group a convulsion is the first sign of illness. An infant who has a fever with convulsion almost invariably warrants a lumbar puncture. A partially treated meningitis may be the reason why a child with an otitis media or other upper respiratory tract infection fails to respond to an antibiotic and becomes increasingly drowsy. On the other hand children with an upper respiratory tract infection, cervical lymphadenitis or pneumonia may show meningismus, that is they have the signs of meningeal irritation in the absence of intracranial disease.

Treatment. For children older than three months an intravenous high dosage ampicillin regime, 300 to 400 mg/kg/day, is appropriate until the microorganism and its antibiotic sensitivities have been identified. *Haemophilus influenzae* is normally sensitive to ampicillin but requires this high dosage to be maintained for at least 10 days. Chloroamphenicol is the drug of choice for resistant strains. *Neisseria meningitidis* and *Diplococcus pneumoniae* are sensitive to parenteral benzylpenicillin, 250 000 units/kg/day.

Lumbar puncture

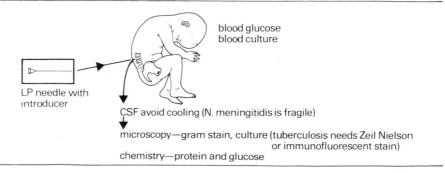

blood glucose
blood culture

LP needle with
introducer

CSF avoid cooling (N. meningitidis is fragile)

microscopy—gram stain, culture (tuberculosis needs Zeil Nielson
                              or immunofluorescent stain)
chemistry—protein and glucose

Cerebrospinal fluid findings in meningitis

	Normal*	Acute purulent meningitis	Aseptic (viral) meningitis	Tuberculous meningitis
appearance	clear	cloudy	usually clear	opalescent
cells/mm³	0–5 lymphocytes	10–100 000 polymorphs	15–2000 lymphocytes	250–500 lymphocytes
glucose mmol/l	2.8–4.4 (CSF>60% blood)	low (CSF<60% blood)	normal (CSF>60% blood)	very low (CSF<60% blood)
protein g/l	0.15–0.35	0.5–5.0	0.2–1.25	0.45–5.00

*in the postnatal period normal CSF contains a higher cell and protein content.

Children with meningococcal infections often have a widespread purpuric rash and are liable to develop septicaemic shock. Purpura in a febrile child suggests major infection and must always be regarded seriously, for treatment should be commenced as soon as possible. Other children in the family are also vulnerable and should be provided with prophylaxis, sulphadiazine, 100 mg/kg/day for five * days. Nasal carriage of *N. meningitidis* is relatively common but difficult to eradicate. *Rifampicin 48 hrs per close contacts* *

Neonatal meningitis is a serious illness with a high mortality and the majority of survivors have neurological sequelae. Therapy must be directed towards the ventriculitis which is often associated. Systemic therapy with either ampicillin and gentamicin, or chloramphenicol may have to be supplemented by intrathecal and possibly intraventricular antibiotic administration.

Complications. Meningitis is often complicated by convulsions and there is an argument for the prophylactic use of phenytoin. Inappropriate anti-diuretic hormone release often accompanies intra-cranial problems and can lead to hyponatraemia which may be prevented by careful restriction of intravenous and oral fluids. Subdural effusions are probably frequent but the majority are small and insignificant. Occasionally, an enlarging head circumference and bulging fontanelle suggests a larger accumulation. This may be visualised by transilluminating the skull, and confirmed by performing a subdural tap when a fluid containing a high protein content can be aspirated. A rapidly increasing head circumference may also be a consequence of an obstructive hydrocephalus. Ten to 20 per cent of all children surviving meningitis have long term neurological abnormality; convulsions, deafness, or spasticity.

Recurrent meningitis raises the possibility of a congenital mid-line sinus, or a post-traumatic dural defect providing communication with an air sinus. An immune deficiency should also be considered.

Viral meningitis

Viral meningitis is commoner than it is realised. It may be accompanied by a macular rash or preceded by upper respiratory tract or gastrointestinal complaints. The symptoms of viral meningitis are usually less abrupt and milder than with acute purulent meningitis. Cerebrospinal fluid examination and culture is obviously essential to make the distinction. Serial viral titres, nasopharyngeal and rectal swabs may identify the virus.

Tuberculous meningitis

Tuberculous meningitis must be considered in every case of aseptic meningitis or encephalitis. It follows the rupture of a tubercle (Rich's focus) into the cerebrospinal fluid and evolves as the resulting inflammatory reaction and arteritis develops. The cerebrospinal fluid examination is not always diagnostic in early cases. A tuberculin skin test is positive in 75 per cent and a chest X-ray shows a suggestive lesion in 80 per cent. Treatment is dealt with in the section dealing with tuberculosis.

Brain abscess

This is a relatively rare condition, there is usually a predisposing cause. Although it is essential to consider lumbar puncture in every child at risk of having intracranial infection, this procedure should be deferred if there are features of raised intracranial pressure. A neurosurgical opinion must be sought.

Brain abscess: aetiology, clinical features and treatment

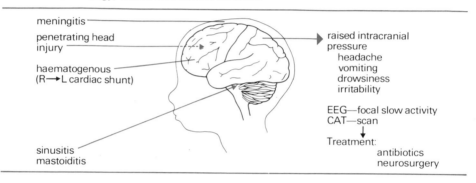

Encephalitis

Encephalitis produces fever, disturbed consciousness, convulsions and focal neurological signs. The majority of cases are viral and there may also be features of meningitis or spinal cord involvement (meningoencephalitis and encephalomyelitis). Viral invasion of nervous tissue may result in immediate inflammation and destruction, mainly of grey matter, or may provoke a delayed immunologically mediated demyelination of white matter.

An encephalitis-like illness without fever or aseptic meningitis raises the possibility of a 'toxic' or metabolic encephalopathy. Lead poisoning and drug ingestion must always be considered.

Herpes simplex encephalitis is the most common sporadic severe encephalitis. Only 10 to 15 per cent have associated herpetic gingivostomatitis or skin lesions. Focal seizures and neurological signs are frequent and may suggest a temporal lobe space occupying lesion. The mortality rate is 70 per cent and neurological sequelae are frequent in the survivors. The cerebrospinal fluid contains a variably elevated white cell count and may be blood stained. Electroencephalography and computerised axial tomography helps to distinguish this encephalitis from a cerebral abscess or tumour. The development of potentially successful anti-viral therapy, adenosine arabinoside, has emphasised

Viral meningoencephalitis

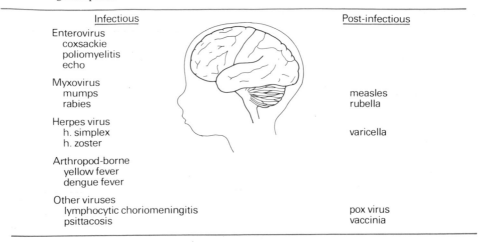

Infectious	Post-infectious

Enterovirus
  coxsackie
  poliomyelitis
  echo	

Myxovirus
  mumps
  rabies
	measles
	rubella

Herpes virus
  h. simplex
  h. zoster
	varicella

Arthropod-borne
  yellow fever
  dengue fever	

Other viruses
  lymphocytic choriomeningitis
  psittacosis
	pox virus
	vaccinia

the need for prompt identification of the virus. At present brain biopsy with electron-microscopy is alone in fulfilling this requirement.

Post-infectious encephalitis
The more common varieties have the following frequencies; measles 1 in 1000; live measles vaccine 1 in 1 000 000; varicella 1 in 1000; rubella 1 in 5000, vaccinia 1 in 100 000.

Measles encephalitis commences with irritability, drowsiness and multiple seizures two to four days after the appearance of the rash. The EEG shows a severe diffuse abnormality. The course varies from complete recovery in a few days to death in status epilepticus or grossly impaired recovery. There is no specific treatment.

Varicella causes a relatively benign encephalitis, often an acute self-limiting cerebellar ataxia.

Subacute sclerosing panencephalitis (SSPE) is a prototype of human slow virus infection which is now recognised as a late complication of measles. The disease may progress over a period of years or death can occur as soon as six weeks after onset. The persistence of virus in the brain may be due to a defective immune response when measles is acquired at an early age. It enters the differential diagnosis of degenerative brain disorders.

Reye's syndrome refers to the association of acute encephalopathy with diffuse fatty infiltration of the liver. Viral infections, particularly influenza B and varicella, have been linked to certain epidemics but the aetiology of this often fatal condition is largely a mystery.

EPILEPSY AND CONVULSIONS

The definition of terms is important when discussing epilepsy and other causes of transient loss of consciousness in children. The diagnosis of epilepsy has major medical and social implications. Unfortunately it is common for the diagnosis to be made in error and for inappropriate drug regimes to be initiated.

Epilepsy implies a primary disorder of the brain producing recurrent electrical disturbances and resulting in epileptic attacks. It can only be diagnosed if there has been more than one epileptic attack. A child who has only had one convulsion cannot be said to have epilepsy because he may never have another.

A convulsion is a non-specific term and refers to all major motor attacks both epileptic and non-epileptic. The terms fit and seizure are also used in this context.

Clinical types of epilepsy

Major motor or grand-mal epilepsy is by far the most common type and consists of loss of consciousness, falling, an initial transient stiffness or tonic phase which may be associated with cyanosis, and then generalised rhythmic jerking, the clonic phase. The attack is usually over in a few minutes and is followed by a period of post-ictal drowsiness. If the clonic phase is prolonged beyond 20 minutes the child is said to be in status epilepticus. This is a medical emergency as it may lead to death from asphyxia or exhaustion.

Focal motor epilepsy consists of twitching or jerking of one side of the face, one arm or one leg. Consciousness is usually retained or only slightly impaired and the child does not usually fall. Sometimes jerking can be seen to spread across one side of the face or along a limb; this is called a 'Jacksonian march'. A focal motor attack may proceed to a major motor attack with loss of consciousness, falling and generalised convulsions. Focal motor epilepsy often falls into the secondary or symptomatic category.

Psychomotor or temporal lobe epilepsy is often difficult to diagnose in children because the child finds it hard to describe the complex sensory phenomena. Any stereotyped episodic behaviour such as lip smacking or well organised motor phenomena associated with momentary loss of awareness may represent temporal lobe epilepsy.

The differential diagnosis of convulsions

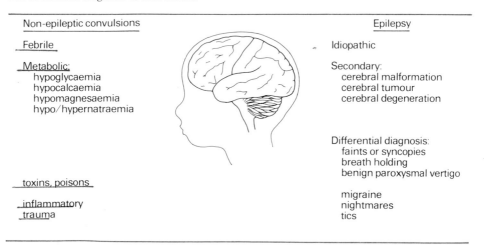

Non-epileptic convulsions	Epilepsy
Febrile	Idiopathic

Metabolic:
   hypoglycaemia
   hypocalcaemia
   hypomagnesaemia
   hypo/hypernatraemia
	Secondary:
	   cerebral malformation
	   cerebral tumour
	   cerebral degeneration

	Differential diagnosis:
	   faints or syncopies
	   breath holding
	   benign paroxysmal vertigo

toxins, poisons	migraine
inflammatory trauma	nightmares tics

Myoclonic epilepsy is characterised by single or repetitive contractions of muscles or groups of muscles. Myoclonic seizures are usually due to underlying brain damage, for example the result of perinatal hypoxia. A variant of this form of epilepsy, akinetic attacks, results in sudden loss of body tone and a fall to the ground.

Infantile spasms represent a rare form of epilepsy seen only in young children. It usually commences between three and eight months of age. The majority show typical flexion, jack-knife or salaam spasms, which may occur as often as several hundred times a day. The spasm involves sudden flexion of the trunk at the neck, trunk and limbs and lasts one to three seconds. It may be preceded by a cry. Although treatment may control the spasms, it does not affect the associated mental deterioration, and many children are left severely handicapped.

Petit-mal attacks consists of episodes of impaired consciousness without falling or involuntary movements. The child stops whatever he is doing and looks vacant for 5 to 20 seconds and then continues as if nothing had happened. Characteristically petit-mal attacks can be induced by hyperventilation. They are not seen under the age of two years, have their peak incidence between five and nine years, and seldom persists into adult life. Petit mal epilepsy with diagnostic three cycle per second spike-wave discharges on EEG is a relatively rare condition. Petit mal-like attacks without this specific EEG finding are much more common.

Some children with epilepsy cannot easily be classified into any of the above categories.

All children with suspected epilepsy should be fully assessed. A careful and detailed history from someone who has witnessed the attacks is of the utmost importance. General examination with special emphasis on developmental and neurological aspects is also required. A skull X-ray and fasting blood sugar and calcium estimations are often indicated. An EEG may help to decide if doubtful attacks are epileptic or not, and may give some help in deciding the kind of epilepsy present. Caution is necessary as a normal EEG is seen in a number of children with attacks highly suggestive of epilepsy, and conversely abnormal discharges may occasionally be seen in EEGs from children who have never had an attack of any kind.

A child with infantile spasms usually has a very severe EEG abnormality termed hypsarrhythmia. Some children have photosensitive epilepsy induced for example by a flickering television screen, and this may be confirmed by the EEG. Focal motor and psychomotor attacks are associated with cortical spike foci. There is no single EEG pattern which characterises major motor convulsions and many kinds of EEG abnormality may be seen.

Management. Children with epilepsy require regular drug therapy in an attempt to prevent further convulsions. Experience has shown that certain categories of epilepsy respond best to particular groups of anticonvulsants.

Drug therapy in epilepsy

Type of epilepsy	Drug of first choice	Other drugs
Grand mal epilepsy	Phenytoin	Sodium valproate Carbamazepine
Focal epilepsy	Carbamazepine	Phenytoin
Temporal lobe epilepsy	Carbamazepine	Phenytoin
Petit mal epilepsy	Ethosuximide	Sodium valproate
Myoclonic epilepsy	Clonazepam	Sodium valproate Ketogenic diet
Infantile spasms	ACTH or corticosteroids	Clonazepam Ketogenic diet
Status epilepticus	Diazepam i.v.	Paraldehyde i.m.

Optimal drug dosage and susceptibility to side-effects vary from individual to individual, and serum anticonvulsant levels are valuable in assessing therapy. The regime should be kept as simple as possible and it is seldom necessary to use more than two drugs.

A diagnosis of epilepsy raises considerable fears not only in the family but among school teachers and social contacts. Children with epilepsy do not require much limitation of their activities. For obvious reasons they are advised not to cycle in traffic but they may swim provided there is a responsible adult in attendance. The great majority of children with epilepsy attend ordinary schools and are average scholars. More than 60 per cent of children diagnosed as having epilepsy seem to 'grow out' of their seizure tendency during childhood and anticonvulsant therapy can be discontinued if they have been free of convulsions for two to three years. A very small minority of children continue to have frequent epileptic attacks despite anticonvulsant therapy. The overall prognosis for childhood epilepsy is good with modern management.

Anticonvulsants: dosage and side-effects

	Side-effects	
Drug	Common	Rare
Phenytoin 4–8 mg/kg/day	cerebellar ataxia** gum hyperplasia hirsutism, rashes	rickets toxic encephalopathy facial coarsening
Carbamazepine 10–20 mg/kg/day	rash* fatigue* dizzyness*	bone marrow depression hepatic toxicity
Sodium valproate 20–40 mg/kg/day	drowsiness* nausea*	thrombocytopenia (high dosage) hair loss*
Phenobarbitone 3–6 mg/kg/day	irritability** overactivity**	rickets
Ethosuximide 20–40 mg/kg/day	nausea* rashes	bone marrow depression
Clonazepam 0.05–0.2 mg/kg/day	drowsiness** salivation**	

* Transient if drug continued
** May settle with slight dose reduction

Treatment of status epilepticus. It is unfortunate that many children await arrival at a casualty department before any attempt is made to stop status epilepticus. Every family doctor should be prepared to terminate these attacks as promptly as possible. The child should first be placed in a position which assures patency of the airway. Diazepam given intravenously, 0.2 to 0.3 mg per kg, is the drug of choice as it acts almost immediately. There is a risk of provoking apnoea if it is injected too quickly or if an excessive dose is administered. It is ineffective if given intramuscularly, but can be given rectally. Paraldehyde given intramuscularly, 0.15 ml per kg, is a satisfactory alternative. A plastic syringe is safe as long as the injection is used promptly. Intramuscular phenobarbitone is too slow-acting to be useful.

Febrile convulsions

Febrile convulsions are very common and affect some 4 per cent of all children, most often in the second year of life. The usual history is that the child is noticed to be unwell and hot and then has a major motor seizure lasting a few minutes. There is often a family history of febrile convulsions. On examination the child has a high temperature, and frequently evidence of upper respiratory tract infection. More serious conditions such as meningitis or urinary tract infections must always be excluded. The attacks are considered to be benign if they last less than 10 minutes and there are no persisting neurological signs. The prognosis for benign febrile convulsions is good, although recurrences are common. The risk of recurrence may be minimised by advising the parents to use tepid sponging and antipyretics whenever the child becomes febrile.

Prolonged febrile convulsions are a cause for concern for there is evidence that they may result in cerebral scarring particularly in the temporal lobe region. It is not possible to forecast whether a recurrent attack is going to be benign or prolonged and potentially damaging. For this reason it is generally recommended that a child who has had an atypical or recurrent convulsion should commence prophylactic anticonvulsant therapy. There is still doubt as to the most effective way of providing this prophylaxis. Regular phenobarbitone (4 to 5 mg/kg) as a single night time dose has had some success but unfortunately it causes significant behavioural problems in some children. Sodium valproate may prove to be a useful alternative.

Febrile convulsions: age incidence and recurrence rate

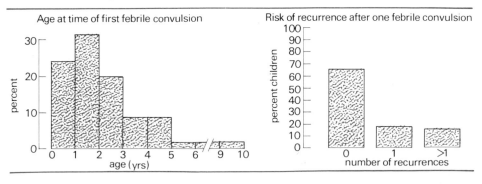

Other causes of transient loss of consciousness

Breath holding attacks are common in toddlers. The history that the attacks had been precipitated by physical or psychological hurt and that the child recovered immediately, helps to distinguish them from epilepsy. Drug treatment is not necessary and the attacks cease spontaneously.

Syncope or fainting is not uncommon among older children. Careful history reveals likely predisposing factors such as immobility or fear, and rapid recovery without any post-ictal phase.

Benign paroxysmal vertigo may present as sudden attacks of falling, swaying or dizziness but consciousness is not lost. Impaired vestibular function is revealed by caloric tests. No treatment is indicated as these attacks are brief and disappear spontaneously.

Migraine, day dreams, night terrors, hysteria and masturbation also enter the differential diagnosis.

Tics or habit spasms are irregular contractions of muscle groups, for example blinking and jerking or facial grimacing. They can be controlled voluntarily but feelings of tension increase until the movement has to be repeated. They are often a reflection of underlying emotional disturbance and should not be confused with focal epilepsy.

NEUROMUSCULAR DISORDERS

Muscle and lower motor neurone disorders present as floppiness, delayed motor milestones, abnormal gait, clumsiness or progressive muscle weakness.

Muscle disorders

The muscular dystrophies are characterised by progressive degeneration of certain groups of skeletal muscles and are frequently hereditary. A number of different forms have been distinguished on clinical and genetic grounds. Muscular dystrophy is the commonest cause of muscle disease in childhood.

Duchenne's muscular dystrophy is the commonest and most serious type of muscular dystrophy, 30 per 100 000 live born males. Inheritance is as a sex-linked recessive but mutations are frequent and said to be responsible for 30 per cent of isolated cases. The female carriers are usually asymptomatic. Symptoms appear in the first five years of life and consist of frequent falls, a lordotic waddling gait and difficulty climbing stairs. Prominence of the calf muscles is an early feature and is called 'pseudo-hypertrophy' because the muscles although enlarged are weak. Due to weakness of the gluteal muscles, boys with this condition 'climb up' their legs when they rise from the lying position (Gower's sign). The diagnosis of Duchenne's dystrophy is made by finding a serum creatinine phosphokinase 30 to 200 times higher than normal, myopathic changes on electromyography, and characteristic muscle biopsy features.

Most of these boys are unable to walk by the age of 8 to 11 years and are confined to a wheelchair. They develop scoliosis and an equinus deformity of the feet due to

Duchenne's muscular dystrophy: early and late clinical features, and the muscle biopsy appearance

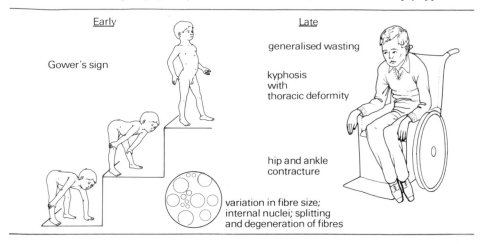

muscular weakness and imbalance. The pseudo-hypertrophy is replaced by muscle wasting. Respiratory infections precipitate death by age 15 to 25. Intellectual development is usually normal but there is a slightly increased frequency of mild mental handicap.

Genetic counselling is important in Duchenne's dystrophy, and female carriers may be detected by finding a moderately raised serum creatinine phosphokinase. Where women are carriers, the prospective parents may elect to have all male pregnancies terminated because of the 1 in 2 risk to the fetus. A method for confirming disease in the unborn fetus is being developed.

Becker's muscular dystrophy is a milder form of sex-linked recessive muscular dystrophy.

Facioscapulohumeral muscular dystrophy has an autosomal dominant pattern of inheritance and presents in late childhood or early adolescence. There may be a marked variation in the severity of the disease within affected families. Shoulder girdle weakness is an early feature followed by facial involvement and inability to close the eyes tightly. Winging of the scapulae is another feature. This condition has a very slow progression and may be compatible with a normal life span.

Limb girdle dystrophy also presents in later childhood or early adult life. The pelvic girdle muscles are most affected. It has autosomal recessive inheritance.

Myotonic dystrophy was previously considered to be a disease of adult life but it is now realised that onset in childhood is not uncommon. It differs from the other muscular dystrophies, not only in the presence of myotonia, but also because of the widespread involvement of other tissues. Both males and females are affected and the inheritance is of an autosomal dominant. The muscle weakness characteristically involves the facial and neck muscles producing a myopathic facies, ptosis, an open mouth and a sagging jaw. Myotonia is seen as delayed opening of the eyes after closure or difficulty in relaxing the grasp. Distal limb weakness may also be present. Other features include cardiac involvement, cataracts, testicular atrophy and adrenal dysfunction.

In the congenital form infants have feeding and respiratory difficulties. Many die in the newborn period but those who survive show considerable recovery. The majority are, however, educationally subnormal. It is interesting that in every congenital case the mother is the affected parent.

Congenital myopathies are a complex group of disorders which can only be characterised after detailed examination of muscle obtained at biopsy, for example central core disease and nemaline myopathy.

Metabolic myopathies. Type II glycogen storage disease, acid maltase deficiency, is an autosomal recessive condition in which muscle weakness is a major feature. In the infantile form (Pompe's disease) infants present with cardiac failure, hepatomegaly and gross hypotonia. The majority die before 18 months.

Neuromuscular junction disorders
Myasthenia gravis is now recognised as being an autoimmune disorder. It is more common in girls. The onset is usually gradual with ptosis, strabismus, difficulty in chewing, loss of facial expression and arm weakness being common manifestations. The weakness may be very variable and is characteristically induced by fatigue. The diagnosis is confirmed by showing prompt improvement after an intravenous injection of edrophonium. The treatment of myasthenia involves the use of long-acting anticholinesterase drugs such as neostigmine or pyridostigmine. Thymectomy also has a place. Infants born to mothers with myasthenia gravis are susceptible to a transient form of the illness.

Neuromuscular disorders

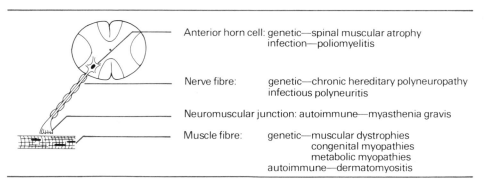

Anterior horn cell: genetic—spinal muscular atrophy
infection—poliomyelitis

Nerve fibre: genetic—chronic hereditary polyneuropathy
infectious polyneuritis

Neuromuscular junction: autoimmune—myasthenia gravis

Muscle fibre: genetic—muscular dystrophies
congenital myopathies
metabolic myopathies
autoimmune—dermatomyositis

Nerve fibre disorders (neuropathies)
Infectious polyneuritis (Guillain-Barré syndrome) presents as a rapidly evolving flaccid paralysis and is commonly preceded by symptoms suggestive of viral infection. It usually involves both distal and proximal muscles and may affect the respiratory muscles. Facial weakness is common. The cerebrospinal fluid often shows a considerable elevation of protein but no cellular response. The weakness progresses over a matter of days and then remains stationary for some

weeks before entering a slow recovery phase. There is no specific treatment but respiratory complications must be avoided. It is essential to distinguish spinal cord problems which may need surgical evaluation from acute infectious polyneuritis.

Anterior horn cell disorders

Acute Werdnig-Hoffman disease (spinal muscular atrophy Type I) is the early infantile form, has an autosomal recessive inheritance, and an incidence of 1 in 20 000 births. Mothers may notice a lack of fetal movements and the infants can be floppy and weak at birth. Symptoms are always present within the first few months of life. In spite of the extreme muscle weakness, the infants are alert and watchful. Muscle fasciculation, especially in the tongue, is a feature. The diagnosis is made by electromyography and muscle biopsy. The condition is progressive and usually leads to death from respiratory failure before 18 months of age.

There are milder forms of spinal muscular atrophy with later onset, for example the Kugelberg-Welander form.

Acute Werdnig Hoffman disease: clinical features and muscle biopsy appearance

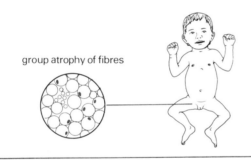

group atrophy of fibres

alert facial expression
  fasciculation of tongue

deformed chest
  see-saw respiration

frog position
  absent reflexes

Floppy infant syndrome

Paralytic and non-paralytic causes of floppiness in infants

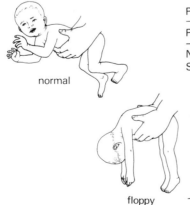

normal

floppy

Paralytic and non-paralytic causes of floppiness in infants

Paralytic	Non-paralytic

Neuromuscular disorders
Spinal cord lesions
  e.g. birth trauma
	Brain disorders
	  e.g. cerebral palsy
	    degenerative CNS disease
	    Prader-Willi syndrome
	Chromosomal disorders
	  e.g. Down's syndrome
	Systemic disorders
	  e.g. malnutrition
	    congenital heart disease
	    hypothyroidism
	Connective tissue disorders
	  e.g. osteogenesis imperfecta
	Benign hypotonia

The term floppy infant is reserved for babies who have marked hypotonia. A useful test is to hold the baby in ventral suspension.

Benign hypotonia is a term applied to initially floppy but otherwise healthy infants who eventually regain normal tone and motor development. The recognition of subtle histological variants in muscle cell structure is gradually replacing this nonspecific category.

Acquired muscle disease

Dermatomyositis, an inflammatory disorder of muscle, is rare in childhood. It is characterised by generalised proximal asymmetrical muscle weakness and a violaceous discoloration of the skin, especially over the butterfly area of the face, eyelids, elbows, knees and knuckles. The child is usually febrile and miserable. The ESR may be very high and an inflammatory cell infiltrate is seen in muscle obtained at biopsy. Treatment with corticosteroids often produces a permanent remission.

NEURAL TUBE ANOMALIES

The neural tube should be completely formed and closed throughout its entire length by the end of the third week of intrauterine life. The process starts at the 14th day with thickening of the dorsal ectoderm to form the neural plate. The neural plate starts folding into a groove and by about 22 to 23 days complete fusion of the groove has occurred to form the neural tube. Fusion commences in the mid dorsal region and extends towards the head and tail of the embryo.

Catastrophies at this very early stage of development may cause severe neural tube anomalies and result in intra-uterine death. Despite this fetal loss, two to three per 1000 liveborn infants have a neural tube defect of some sort, about half are due to anencephaly.

The normal development of the spinal cord

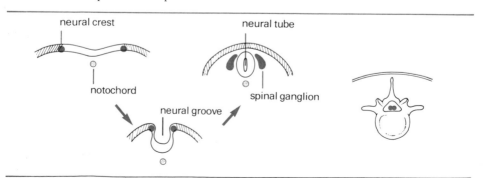

Classification of neural tube anomalies

Anencephaly		
Cranium bifidum	meningocele encephalocele	
Spina bifida	occulta cystica	meningocele myelomeningocele

Anencephaly
Anencephaly is a tragic deformity in which most of the infants are stillborn, but if liveborn survive only a few hours.

Cranium bifidum defects
Cranium bifidum defects are relatively uncommon. The minor lesions are eminently treatable; all that is required is a good skin cover, and the prognosis is excellent, for there is no associated spinal neurological lesion, and the incidence of hydrocephalus is low. An occipital meningocele, even when very large, is also treatable, although hydrocephalus is more likely. The overall prognosis is still good. On the other hand, a large encephalocele is not open to treatment, for surgery usually means either excision of a mass of brain tissue or a closure which results in raised intracranial pressure.

Cranium bifidum

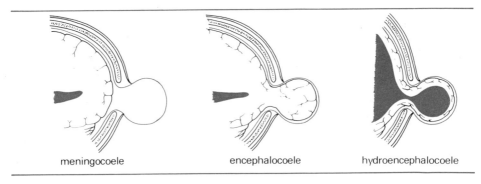

meningocoele   encephalocoele   hydroencephalocoele

Spina bifida
Spina bifida defects are common. The number of infants born with major 'open' defects has fallen considerably in the last few years due to the widespread introduction of screening procedures.

Spina bifida cystica defects vary from a meningeal sac full of cerebrospinal fluid with a normal placement of the spinal cord (a meningocele), to the exposure and complete unfolding of the spinal cord on the surface of the child's back (a myelomeningocele).

Meningocele is less common and has a good prognosis. Neurological problems with the lower limbs and hydrocephalus are rare, but partial neurological deficit affecting the bladder is not uncommon. Virtually all babies with a meningocele

Spina bifida cystica

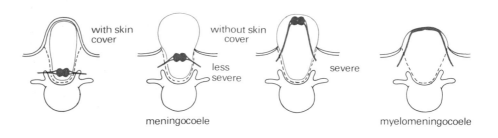

with skin cover | without skin cover
meningocoele (less severe) | myelomeningocoele (severe)

will be treated surgically in the first days of life. During infancy they may develop minor foot problems and bladder dysfunction but they usually can cope well. Children with meningoceles should be followed up throughout the whole of their growing period since neurological problems may develop with growth of the spine.

Myelomeningocele is both more common and more serious. It is usually located in the lumbo-sacral region. The range of severity varies considerably. A child with a small lumbo-sacral myelomeningocele, which is closed on the first day of life, may with careful attention have good mobility, normal bladder function and intellect. On the other hand, a baby with an extensive thoraco-lumbar myelomeningocele is likely to have no functioning motor or sensory nerves distal to his nipple line. His skin will be completely anaesthetic and therefore at risk of trauma; his trunk and limbs will be paralysed and either completely flaccid or deformed as a result of reflex activity. Involuntary movements may be seen. The bladder and bowel will be paralysed and insensitive. Hydrocephalus is present in 80 per cent of infants with myelomeningocele.

Early management. Every baby with spina bifida cystica should have full and expert assessment as soon as possible after birth to determine the extent of neurological deficit; the presence or otherwise of hydrocephalus, the extent of bony deformity of the spine; and the coexistence of any other congenital abnormality. This will permit an estimate to be made of his potential. The

Spina bifida occulta and the split notochord syndrome

spina bifida occulta

split notochord syndrome (diastematomyelia) with meningocoele

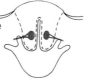

decision to operate can only be taken after a full and open discussion between surgeon and parents. Many babies with extensive defects will die within a short time whether their lesions are covered with skin or not. In these instances, early surgery would not seem to be justified. On the other hand, a baby with a lesser lesion is still at risk of infection and the complications of hydrocephalus even after surgery. It is a mistake to think that all babies will survive if operated upon and that those with uncorrected lesions will always die. One can only say that the majority of babies with minor lesions and a good prognosis will survive with treatment to adult life, and that most babies with very major lesions will die without treatment.

Survival in children with myelomeningocele showing the effect of surgical intervention (after Lorber)

Age at death	No surgery	Surgery
0–1 month	37.5%	20%
1–12 months	37.5%	20%
1–5 years	10%	10%
Survival over 5 years	15%	50%

Long term management. Once active treatment is commenced the child's management should be directed by a team consisting of an orthopaedic surgeon, a paediatric surgeon, and a physiotherapist. The facilities of an assessment unit are useful, and close contact with local schools for the physically handicapped is essential. Orthopaedic problems are particularly common in those children with unbalanced lower limb function. Urinary tract infections, urinary obstruction. ureteric reflux and urinary incontinence are common. The latter in girls may necessitate ileal loop diversion. A ventriculoperitoneal or atrial shunt is usually required to control hydrocephalus. The complications of these shunts are blockage and infection, and they may be very troublesome. The anaesthetic skin is also a problem especially in the more mobile child; pressure sores and accidental burns are likely to occur. Learning and psychological problems may add to the child's troubles in the school years but their unhappiness may be most profound when they begin to realise the full meaning of their handicap, with regard to job prospects, sex and marriage.

The quality of survival in children alive more than five years after surgical treatment of myelomeningocele (after Lorber)

18%	mild/moderate physical handicap and normal IQ
49%	severe physical handicap and normal IQ
33%	severe physical handicap and borderline or subnormal IQ

Spina bifida occulta is a common anomaly, said to occur in up to 20 per cent of normal individuals. Most people with an occult deficit are asymptomatic. Occasionally the bony defect is associated with a hairy patch or a birth mark on the back. A few children with spina bifida occulta develop a mild spastic gait, or bladder problems with spinal growth due to tethering of the cord, a split notochord syndrome, or an associated intraspinal dermoid or lipoma. Myelography may be necessary.

Hydrocephalus without spina bifida

This may result from a congenital abnormality of the brain, for example aqueduct stenosis, or it may follow an intracranial bleed, or early neonatal infection. It depends to some extent on the aetiology, but on the whole the prognosis is good and all babies should be treated. They should all have a CAT scan before surgery is performed. Later abilities are likely to be very reasonable, unless shunt complications occur.

The treatment of hydrocephalus

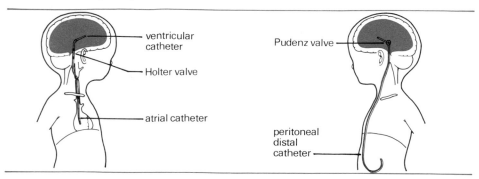

TUMOURS OF THE NERVOUS SYSTEM

Intracranial tumours are second only to leukaemia in the list of childhood neoplasia (three to five per 100 000 per year below 15 years of age). Infratentorial neoplasms predominate in this age group.

Computorised axial tomography has revolutionised the investigation of suspected brain tumour. Ideally, neurosurgical management is aimed at total resection of the tumour although this is not always possible because of infiltration or critical location. Radiotherapy has a valuable role and chemotherapy is now being introduced. Other aspects of management include ventriculo-atrial shunt insertion to control obstructive hydrocephalus, anticonvulsant therapy and dexamethasone for short term control of related cerebral oedema. In general terms the older the child and the less malignant the tumour the better the prognosis.

Intracranial tumours: clinical features

Focal neurological signs	Raised intracranial pressure	Endocrine effects
Cerebellar	headache	short stature
ataxia	vomiting	hypogonadism
nystagmus	mood change	precocious puberty
diplopia	papilloedema	diabetes insipidus
Brainstem	VI nerve palsy	
facial weakness	head tilt	
swallowing problems		
ocular palsies		
spasticity		
Cerebral		
seizures		
spasticity		

Infratentorial tumours

Cerebellar astrocytoma is a slow growing cystic tumour of the cerebellum. It presents with slowly increasing intracranial pressure and ataxia. Operative resection is very successful.

Medulloblastoma is a rapidly growing and highly malignant tumour with a more acute presentation. Complete resection is rarely possible but radiotherapy and chemotherapy are having some impact on the dismal prognosis.

Brain stem gliomata occupy a critical position in the brain stem and produce signs and symptoms of cranial nerve and long tract involvement. They are not amenable to surgery but may show long term remission after radiotherapy.

Supratentorial tumours

Gliomata of the cerebral hemispheres show a spectrum of malignancy from the more benign slow growing astrocytoma to the rapidly growing glioblastoma. They may present with focal convulsions refractory to therapy, hemiparesis and mental disturbances.

Tumours of the spinal cord. These are rare but important to recognise as the majority are benign and prompt recognition may avoid irreversible cord damage. Cord compression should be suspected in any child with gait disturbance, impaired sphincter function or back pain.

Leukaemic infiltration must also be considered in the differential diagnosis of suspected intracranial or spinal tumours.

Location of brain tumours

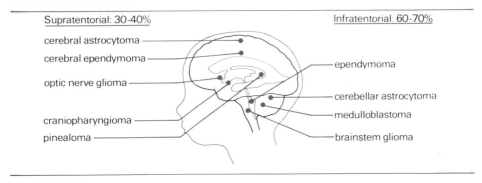

Supratentorial: 30-40%	Infratentorial: 60-70%
cerebral astrocytoma	ependymoma
cerebral ependymoma	cerebellar astrocytoma
optic nerve glioma	medulloblastoma
craniopharyngioma	brainstem glioma
pinealoma	

HEADACHE

Headache is a relatively common complaint among older children. Mild, self-limiting headaches are frequent in febrile illnesses but a severe headache of acute onset raises the possibility of intra-cranial inflammation, subarachnoid haemorrhage, leukaemic infiltration or an intracranial tumour.

Intermittent headaches may originate from a variety of problems; sinusitis, dental caries, intracranial tumours and hypertension. The majority have no obvious organic explanation and may fall into the category of periodic syndrome or tension headaches.

Migraine

Migraine is common in childhood. A family history and the characteristic symptoms of throbbing headache, visual disturbance, photophobia and nausea make the diagnosis relatively straight forward in the older child. There may be problems in the recognition of migraine in the pre-school child and it may be manifest by acute periods of distress, pallor and nausea. Attacks resulting in ophthalmoplegia or hemiparesis may occur. An underlying vascular malformation is a rare association. Treatment is initially with simple analgesics such as aspirin or paracetamol. More severe cases may benefit from non-ergotamine antimigraine preparations.

Ocular headaches

Ocular headaches result from constant muscular activity attempting to correct a latent squint or refractive error, usually long sightedness or astigmatism.

Benign intracranial hypertension

This is due to neither inflammatory nor space-occupying lesions. It usually develops in association with vomiting over a day or so, and papilloedema is present. It may be a complication of otitis media or occur after a nonspecific viral illness; rarely, it develops during corticosteroid therapy. When the diagnosis has been confirmed, currently by CAT scan, treatment is directed towards reducing the intracranial pressure in order to avoid secondary optic atrophy. A short course of high dosage corticosteroid is usually successful but may have to be complemented by repeated lumbar puncture.

ATAXIA

Ataxia refers to a disorder of movement manifest by incoordination, clumsiness and poor balance. In the young child, hypotonia and delayed motor development may be the only obvious signs.

Ataxic cerebral palsy

This is caused by malformation or damage of the cerebellum or its connections. Dandy-Walker syndrome refers to congenital absence of the foramina of Majendie and Luschka with resulting cystic dilation of the IV ventricle. Affected children have a characteristic prominence of the occipital region.

Acute ataxia

In older children this may be due to intoxication with drugs, for example phenytoin or alcohol. If the history does not reveal a cause, the rapid recovery certainly suggests it. Cerebellar ataxia may also be a manifestation of viral encephalitis, especially that caused by varicella. The differential diagnosis includes an acute presentation of a cerebellar tumour such as medulloblastoma, but the subsequent progression determines the need for neurosurgical investigation.

Friedreich's ataxia

This is the most common of the hereditary ataxias, and is an autosomal recessive condition initially characterised by pes cavus and a relatively clumsy gait. Examination reveals ataxia, loss of postural and vibratory sensation, and impaired leg tendon reflexes. There may, in addition, be optic atrophy and cardiomyopathy. The patients become increasingly handicapped and may be wheelchair-bound by early adult life.

Ataxia telangiectasis

Ataxia telangiectasis is inherited as an autosomal recessive. In addition to slowly increasing cerebellar ataxia, there are characteristic telangiectasia obvious over the bulbar conjunctiva and face. There is an associated impairment of cellular immunity which increases susceptibility to infection and may also be related to the predisposition to neoplasia.

There are rare metabolic disorders which result in cerebellar disturbances; Hartnup disease in which there is a derangement of tryptophane metabolism, and Refsum's disease in which phytanic acid accumulates.

CEREBRAL PALSY

Cerebral palsy is the leading cause of crippling handicap in children (2 per 1000). In using the label cerebral palsy, it is necessary to appreciate that the underlying lesion is permanent and non-progressive. In a developing child, however, the resulting clinical picture will not be static. The lesion is localised in the brain and, as it arises in early life, it interferes with normal development. The main handicap is one of disordered movement and posture, but it is often complicated by other neurological and mental problems.

Aetiology

The brain is usually damaged in fetal life or in the early postnatal period. In the majority of cases the precise cause may be obscure or multiple, for example birth trauma and hypoxia complicated by hypoglycaemia. Congenital malformations of the brain include congenital cysts, fusion defects, failure of normal migration of grey matter, and aplasias.

Causes of cerebral palsy

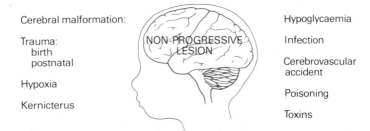

Cerebral malformation:		Hypoglycaemia

Trauma:
  birth
  postnatal
	NON-PROGRESSIVE LESION	Infection

Hypoxia		Cerebrovascular accident
Kernicterus		Poisoning
		Toxins

Classification

Spastic cerebral palsy, which accounts for 70 per cent of cerebral palsy cases, involves damage to the cerebral motor cortex or its connections, producing clasp-knife hypertonia, abnormally brisk tendon jerks, ankle clonus and extensor plantar responses.

Spastic cerebral palsy

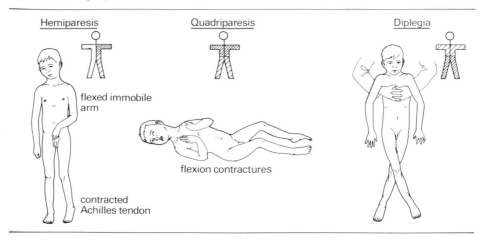

Hemiparesis   Quadriparesis   Diplegia

flexed immobile arm

flexion contractures

contracted Achilles tendon

Dyskinetic cerebral palsy or choreoathetosis (10 per cent of cases) characterised by irregular and involuntary movements of some or all muscle groups. These may be continuous or occur only on voluntary active movement. Athetosis is the commonest form with slow purposeless distal muscle movement. Choreic movements are quick, jerky and more proximal.

Ataxic cerebral palsy is associated with hypotonia, weakness, uncoordinated movements and tremor and accounts for 10 per cent of cerebral palsy.

Mixed cerebral palsy form the remaining 10 per cent of cases.

Clinical features

Infants who show poor sucking ability, increased or decreased muscle tone, abnormal reflexes, irritability, convulsions or drowsiness in the newborn period are at risk of developing cerebral palsy. However, many such infants do develop normally and great care must be exercised in anticipating future development. Usually cerebral palsy is not diagnosed until several months have passed, and when it becomes obvious that motor development is abnormal or delayed. For example, the infant may be brought to the doctor because at three months of age he is not showing real head control or at 10 months of age he is not yet sitting alone. His mother may say that he seems stiff on handling. An infant with spastic hemiplegia is sometimes noted to have developed arm and hand preference before one year. The persistence of primitive reflexes, such as the assymetric tonic neck reflex, beyond the time they usually disappear is suspicious. The characteristic involuntary movements of choreoathetosis are not usually obvious until near the end of the first year of life. Affected children are usually very floppy and show delayed motor development in infancy. Children with ataxic cerebral palsy are also hypotonic and delayed in motor development but subsequently show an intention tremor.

Management

The child with cerebral palsy requires a multi-disciplinary assessment initially to define the problem, and then to develop a structured treatment programme. Physiotherapy aims to encourage normal motor development, to inhibit abnormal motor development and to prevent contractures. The parents are taught to perform the exercises at home.

Some degree of mental handicap is seen in about 60 per cent of children with cerebral palsy. However, it should not be forgotten that children with severe cerebral palsy may have normal intelligence; this applies particularly to the dyskinetic group. Epilepsy occurs in approximately 30 per cent and is symptomatic rather than idiopathic. Visual impairment due to errors of refraction, diffuse ambliopia or optic atrophy occurs in 20 per cent. Squint due to external ocular muscle imbalance or paralysis is present in 30 per cent. 20 per cent have a degree of hearing loss which is often of the sensorineural type. Children with choreoathetosis are particularly liable to have associated deafness. Speech disorders are common and are due to a variety of causes including hearing loss, perceptual defects, mental handicap and incoordination of tongue, palate, and lip muscles.

Children with cerebral palsy often do less well in school than would be expected by their estimated abilities. One reason for this is the high frequency of perceptual defects. Behaviour disorders may be due to the frustrations of being handicapped, to strained family life brought about by the presence of a handicapped child, and to the hyperactivity which may be associated with brain damage.

Even with adequate physiotherapy, long-standing muscle weakness or spasticity is likely to produce orthopaedic deformities. These are more common in spastic cerebral palsy where the involved muscles develop fibrotic contractures. Spasticity in the adductors of the thigh may lead to dislocation of the hips and operation may be necessary to correct this. Spasticity and contracture in the calf muscles produce a fixed equinus deformity of the ankle which requires a tendoachilles lengthening operation to allow the heel to be used for walking and weight bearing. Neglect of these deformities may lead to painful osteoarthritis.

Drugs have a limited role in the management of cerebral palsy, apart from the treatment of epilepsy. Schools for the physically handicapped provide physiotherapy and speech therapy, and they have specially trained staff and equipment. There is, however, a deficiency of opportunity for the handicapped school leaver. The overlap between the pathology of cerebral palsy and mental handicap is such that many children in schools for the severely educational subnormal also have cerebral palsy.

BIBLIOGRAPHY

General
Gamstorp I 1970 Pediatric neurology. Appleton-Century-Crofts, New York
Gordon N 1976 Paediatric neurology for the clinician. Heinemann, London

Intracranial infection
Davies P A 1977 Neonatal bacterial meningitis. British Journal of Hospital Medicine 18: 425–434
Hambleton G, Davies P A 1975 Bacterial meningitis: some aspects of diagnosis and treatment.
   Archives of Diseases Childhood 50: 674–684
Illis L S 1977 Encephalitis. British Journal of Hospital Medicine 18: 412–422

Epilepsy
Bower B 1978 The treatment of epilepsy in children. British Journal of Hospital Medicine 19:
   8–19

Neuromuscular disorders
Dubowitz V 1978 Muscle disorders in childhood. Saunders, Philadelphia
Gardner-Medwin D 1977 Children with genetic muscular disorders. British Journal of Hospital
   Medicine 17: 314–340

Neural tube anomalies
Lorber J. 1975. Ethical problems in the management of myelomeningocele and hydrocephalus.
   Journal of the Royal College of Physicians 10: 47–60
Stark G D 1977 Spina bifida. Problems and management. Blackwell, Oxford

Tumours of the nervous system
Till K 1975 Paediatric neurosurgery. Blackwell, Oxford.

Celebral palsy
Blencowe S M 1969 Cerebral palsy and the young child. Livingstone, Edinburgh
Bobath K 1966 The motor deficit in patients with cerebral palsy. Clinics in developmental
   medicine No. 23. Spastics Society, London
Christensen E, Melchior J C 1967 Cerebral palsy. A clinical and neuropathological study. Clinics
   in developmental medicine No. 25. Spastics Society, London

19
Vision, Hearing, Speech

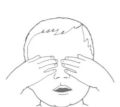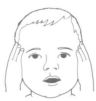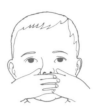

VISION

Vision is the most highly evolved of man's special senses. Binocular stereoscopic perception and interpretation requires not only an exact optic mechanism but also complex neural interconnections. The retina and eye are relatively mature at birth, and 75 per cent of postnatal ocular growth occurs in the first three years of life. Myelination of the optic pathways is, however, still incomplete at term, and experimental work has recently confirmed the clinical impression that normal development of the optic radiation and visual cortex is dependent on undistorted light reception. It is therefore essential to act promptly when, for example, a severe ptosis or a cataract threatens the visual development of a newborn infant.

Assessment of vision
Before the age of six months, vision may be assessed by the response to a moving face, a slowly moving ball and by attention to finger play. After the age of six months, the Stycar series of tests (screening tests for young children and retardates) are widely used. Vision must be considered in the context of general development.

The development of vision

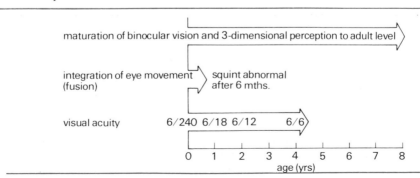

The assessment of vision

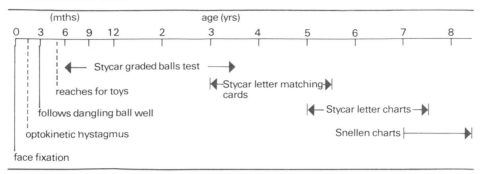

Squints

Squints are common in early childhood. All fixed squints and any squint which persists to age five or six months requires careful evaluation. Having detected a squint, expert assessment involves full examination of the eyes to exclude, for example corneal opacities, cataracts, and refractive errors. The usual cause of infantile strabismus is an ill-understood failure to develop binocular fusion at the normal time. Other important causes include refractive errors, particularly hypermetropia and astigmatism, neurological disorders which interfere with the normal function of the extraocular muscles, and eye diseases such as cataracts or retinoblastoma. Whatever the cause, the image of the squinting eye is suppressed, thereby avoiding diplopia and, if neglected, this may lead to an irreversible failure of development of the visual pathways from the squinting eye (amblyopia).

Testing for a squint

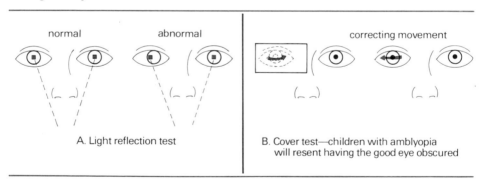

The blind child

For educational purposes a child is defined as blind if he requires education by methods which do not involve sight, for example Braille, and as partially sighted if he requires special educational consideration but can use methods which depend on sight. In practice, most blind children have some vision even it it is only recognition of light and dark, or perception of shapes.

About 500 children each year are newly registered blind or partially sighted, an incidence of approximately 1 in 2500 children. As many as 50 per cent of blind children have additional handicap; physical disability, low intelligence, hearing

Causes of childhood blindness (after Schappert-Kimmijser *et al.*, 1975)

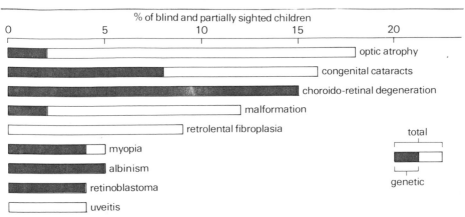

and language difficulties. In their survey of visual handicap, Fraser and Friedmann (1967) reported that the main causes of visual handicap in childhood were choroidoretinal degenerations (16 per cent), congenital cataracts (16 per cent), optic atrophy (14 per cent) and retrolental fibroplasia (23 per cent). Overall, the conditions causing blindness were genetically determined in 50 per cent of children and due to some perinatal disturbance in 33 per cent. Since this study the incidence of retrolental fibroplasia has dramatically decreased due to the greater care with which oxygen therapy is now used in the newborn period.

Blindness must be suspected where there is a pendular nystagmus or roving, purposeless eye movements. Normal children cease to show random, un-coordinated eye movements after six weeks of age. Blind babies also tend to poke their eyes in a characteristic fashion, probably to produce pleasurable visual hallucinations of retinal origin.

With the exception of cataracts, most causes of blindness in children are not amenable to medical treatment. Recent advances in cataract surgery allow their early removal in congenitally acquired cases and the infant is immediately provided with constant-wear, thin, soft contact lenses to reconstitute the optic mechanism and thereby avoid stimulus deprivation amblyopia. The results are still frequently unsatisfactory.

Parents of a blind child need expert, sympathetic advice from a very early stage. Peripatetic pre-school teachers from the Royal National Institute for the Blind often fulfil this role in the U.K. The parents must be taught to stimulate their infant using non-visual means, touch and speech. The home should be adapted so that the child can explore his environment safely. Residential school is often necessary for the blind child who needs to learn Braille. The child with partial sight may cope in an ordinary school with the help of special equipment.

HEARING

Hearing refers to the reception of noise and its transmission to the relevant areas of the cerebral cortex. A higher appreciation of sound and its interpretation, listening, is integral to language development. The fetus is sensitive to noise and from the moment of birth there is an important sound interplay between mother and infant. Hearing provides for emotional contact, language development, identity with the environment and assists in the awareness of posture and body orientation. All children should be screened for deafness by tests which are appropriate to their stage of development and it is usual for these tests to be performed at six to nine months of age, and again at the pre-school examination.

Assessment of hearing

In performing the test at age six to nine months it is essential to have a contented child in a quiet room. The examiner stands one to three feet to the side of the child and just outside his range of vision. The sound stimulus should be given at ear level. Soundmakers employed are a high pitched rattle, spoon in cup, tissue paper, hand bell and selected speech sounds, for example 'oo' and 'ss'. The final proof of adequate hearing is the comprehension and imitation of normal speech. Although pure tone audiometry has a place in defining the hearing of children, it cannot replace clinical speech tests. Whereas hearing loss of less that 20 dB normally has no effect on the child's development, a loss of over 40 dB creates problems in the development of ordinary speech. Testing over a range of frequencies may show a widespread loss or a loss purely in the high frequency zone. Deafness is classified into two categories, perceptive and conductive. In perceptive deafness there is damage to the cochlea or auditory nerve whereas in the conductive type the middle ear is damaged. Most severe deafness in children is perceptive in type and is present from birth. The two types of deafness can be distinguished in older children by pure tone audiometry. In the perceptive type, there is equal impairment of bone and air conduction of sound; in the conductive type, there is an air bone gap with bone conduction greater than air conduction.

Forty per 1000 school children have mild deafness, usually a conductive middle-ear deafness due to glue ear. Two per 1000 children have moderate

Audiograms: three patterns of hearing loss

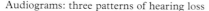

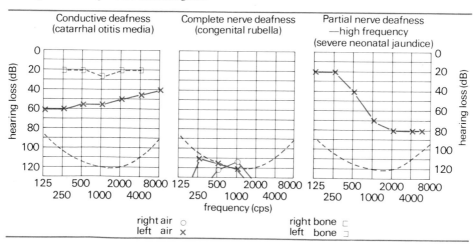

Causes of childhood deafness

Conductive deafness	Perceptive deafness

Glue ear, following otitis media (almost all cases)	1. Prenatal:
	    genetic — various types
	    congenital infection, e.g. rubella
	    maternal drugs, e.g. streptomycin
	2. Perinatal:
	    birth asphyxia
	    severe hyperbilirubinaemia
	3. Postnatal:
	    meningitis
	    encephalitis
	    head injury

deafness sufficient to require them to use a hearing aid, and one per 1000 children is severely deaf and requires special education.

More careful management and follow-up of children susceptible to otitis media will reduce the incidence of glue ear. In established cases of glue ear the deafness is usually reversed by aeration of the middle-ear by means of a grommet inserted in the tympanic membrane, or by removal of the hypertrophied adenoids which often block the Eustachian tubes.

There is no specific therapy for perceptive deafness but if there is some residual hearing, a hearing aid is useful. This is simply a device for amplifying sounds within the frequency range of the spoken voice. There are problems in that the receiver is not selective and is liable to cause distressing exaggeration of environmental and background noises, for example rustling clothes. Careful instruction in its use is required as well as attention to such items as the ear piece. It must be emphasised that the provision of an aid is only part of a more general process of rehabilitation and education. Parents of the young deaf child need expert guidance on how to encourage him to talk and develop language. Such help is given by the peripatetic teacher of the deaf. Many moderately deaf children can attend a normal school, but the more severely affected require specialist education, either at a school for the deaf or in a partially hearing unit attached to a normal school.

SPEECH AND LANGUAGE

Language is essential to our culture as it provides the symbolic code for communication and for our thought process. The early development of vocalisation (exploratory sounds) and verbalisation (meaningful sounds) is closely linked to the mechanisms of hearing and listening.

There is a wide age range among normal children for the development of vocabulary. Some may be excellent at non-verbal communication and clearly have a well developed inner language. In others, the physiological basis of speech development is intact but is hindered by detrimental family relationships, social factors or psychiatric disturbances. It is also recognised that children in institutional care have delayed speech development and this is probably due to a less intense interpersonal relationship.

Assessment of speech

Speech development must be considered in the context of the wide range of normal development. The parents of the two-year-old boy with obviously normal development but a vocabulary of only 10 to 20 words may be comparing him with the little girl of similar age down the road with a vocabulary of 200 words. Both are within the normal range. Assessment must consider general development as well as environmental factors. Comprehension and free conversation during play are useful guides before embarking on more specific diagnostic exercises. An experienced speech therapist plays a valuable role in assessing and treating these children, and will be able to make a distinction between comprehension and expressive language delay.

The developmental speech disorder syndrome

This term embraces those children who are of normal intelligence and have no obvious anatomical or physiological problem with speech production. It is more common in boys and there is often a family history. In mild cases there is no delay in language development, the difficulty lies with articulation particularly of consonants. This mild form has a good prognosis and the family must be encouraged to promote speech by games and other reward activities. More severe degrees reflect actual language delay and require more formal therapy. It is always essential to ensure that hearing is normal.

Causes of speech delay (after Ingram)

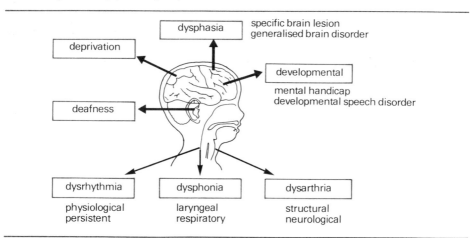

Dysrhythmia

It is common for children between three and four years of age to have a so-called physiological stammer. This corrects itself spontaneously and must not be made a focus of attention. A more persistent stammering or stuttering has a familial predisposition. In younger children, therapy is largely directed towards diverting attention away from the speech difficulty with the expectation of spontaneous improvement in many cases. In older children, more formal exercises such as syllable timed speech may be necessary for the most disruptive cases.

CLEFT LIP AND PALATE

The middle third of the face develops as the result of migration and fusion of mesodermal folds covered by ectoderm. The earlier or primary palate creates the olfactory pits, and failure of fusion results in unilateral, bilateral or, rarely, median cleft lip. The secondary palate originates from folds on either side of the tongue. These rise above the tongue and fuse in the mid-line to form the true palate. Cleft palates occur when tissue migration is disorganised or obstructed by the tongue. It is sometimes the result of a small mandible.

Cleft lip and palate are common, 1 in 600 births. The majority are isolated abnormalities but they may be part of a chromosomal or other malformation syndrome. The family history is often positive, and most clefts are determined by polygenic inheritance which influences the threshold to ill-defined environmental factors. Occasional cases have been linked to maternal corticosteroid therapy. One-third of clefts are limited to the lip, one-quarter to the palate and the remainder involve both.

Management. The alarming facial appearance calls for prompt counselling of the parents, preferably with 'before and after' photographs to emphasise the successful outcome of corrective surgery. Feeding problems can usually be overcome by using a soft teat with an enlarged hole and by nursing the baby erect. Those with a cleft lip may cope with breast feeding.

The aims of surgery are to provide a good cosmetic result and an adequate speech mechanism. The usual practice is to repair the cleft lip at three months of age and the palate at six months or later. Too early a repair may interfere with mid-facial growth. An orthodontist may be able to provide a plate to reduce the cleft size during the waiting period.

In later years additional specialist help is required to overcome Eustachian tube obstruction, speech delay and dental problems.

Pierre-Robin Syndrome refers to severe micrognathia with a secondary cleft palate. The affected infants are susceptible to feeding and respiratory problems, and require expert nursing until the mandible grows.

Treacher-Collins Syndrome encompasses a spectrum of ear and facial malformations caused by first and second pharyngeal arch developmental failure.

BIBLIOGRAPHY

Critchley M 1973 The dyslexic child. Heinemann, London.
Drillien C M, Drummond M B 1977 Neurodevelopmental problems in early childhood. Blackwell, Oxford.
Fraser G R, Friedman A I 1967 The causes of blindness in childhood. Johns Hopkins, Baltimore
Holt K S, Reynell J K 1967 Assessment of cerebral palsy ii. Vision, hearing, speech, language, communication, and psychological function. Lloyd-Luke, London.
Ingram T T S 1961 A description and classification of common speech disorders associated with cerebral palsy. Cerebral Palsy Bulletin 3: 57.
Morley M E 1972 The development and disorders of speech in childhood. 3rd edn. Churchill Livingstone, Edinburgh.
Schappert-Kimmijser J, Hansen E, Haustrate-Gosset M M, Lindstedt E, Skydsgaard H, Warburg M 1975 Documenta Ophthalmologica 39: 213.

20
Mental Handicap

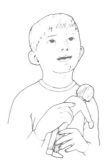

The level of medical care provided within a community may be assessed by the prevalence, identification and care of those who are severely mentally handicapped. Better services result in fewer people being affected, and the early recognition of those that are. The care offered must also be as supportive and humane as the community can afford.

The words used to describe the mentally handicapped have changed with the years for they quickly become terms of derision (e.g. moron, idiot, cretin, mongol); and currently 'mentally retarded' is being abandoned. As a group, however, these children may be defined as having a low mental ability and learning problems. The severely handicapped have difficulty in learning to walk, dress and communicate. The more mildly affected have difficulty acquiring skills to look after themselves, and earn a living.

Aspects of mental ability or intelligence can be measured by a variety of tests. They measure what an individual has achieved at the time of the assessment and,

The population distribution of intelligence and current classifications of mental handicap

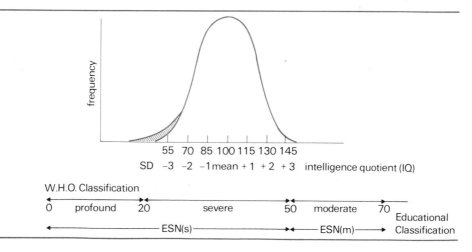

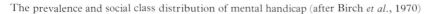
The prevalence and social class distribution of mental handicap (after Birch et al., 1970)

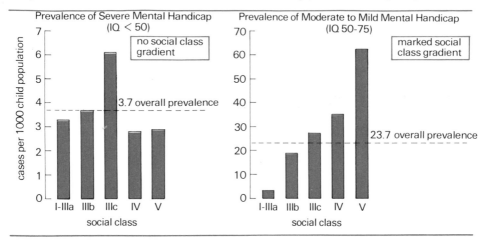

although they may be a guide to what he might achieve, they do not necessarily measure his potential. The results of the tests are expressed as a quotient, the child's 'mental' age over chronological age. The distribution of intelligence follows a Gaussian or normal distribution with a distortion in the lower range due to the effects of deleterious environmental and social factors. Fetal and early infant death counteracts some of this excess.

It is helpful to divide those with low intelligence and who require special education into two groups, mild and severe. The mildly handicapped are composed largely of those in the lower range of the normal distribution, with IQs in the 50 to 70 range. They often come from families of low intelligence and poor social background. The severely handicapped with IQs below 50 usually have some organic disorder; a recognised inherited disorder, a brain deformity or have suffered a severe injury which has permanently damaged the brain. Obviously there is some overlap between the two groups.

Causes of mental handicap (after studies of Rutter et al., 1970; and Birch et al., 1970)

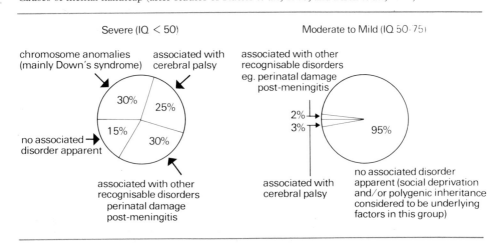

The classification in the table below emphasises the extensive list of disorders which may contribute to mental handicap; each Chapter in this book contains problems which may produce this end result. The diseases discussed in the remainder of this chapter warrant a separate section, not because of their frequency, but because they do not fit conveniently into other categories.

A classification of the recognised causes of mental handicap

Causes of mental handicap	Examples
A *Genetic*	
1. Chromosomal disorder	Trisomy e.g. Down's syndrome
2. Metabolic disorder	Aminoacid e.g. phenylketonuria
	Carbohydrate e.g. galactosaemia
	Organic acid e.g. isovaleric acidaemia
3. Storage disorder	Gangliosidoses
	Lipidoses
	Complex carbohydrates
	Mucopolysaccharidoses
4. Cerebral degenerative disorder	Leucodystrophies
5. Structural disorders	Tuberose sclerosis
	Familial hydrocephalus
B *Intrauterine*	
1. Congenital infection	Cytomegalovirus
	Rubella
	Toxoplasmosis
2. Drugs	Phenytoin, alcohol
3. Cerebral malformations	Hydranencephaly, porencephaly
C *Perinatal*	
1. Problems during pregnancy	Pre-eclamptic toxaemia
	Hypertension
	Antepartum haemorrhage
	Premature onset of labour
2. Problems during labour and delivery	Prolonged labour
	Fetal distress
	Trauma
	Asphyxia
3. Neonatal problems	Intraventricular haemorrhage
	Hypoglycaemia
	Infection e.g. meningitis
	Jaundice
D *Postnatal*	
1. Trauma	Accidental or non-accidental injury
2. Infection	Encephalitis, meningitis
3. Anoxia	Asphyxia, status epilepticus
4. Metabolic and endocrine	Hypoglycaemia, hypernatraemia,
	Hypothyroidism
5. Malnutrition	
6. Poisoning	Lead
7. Psychological	Infantile psychosis/autism

→ neuronal dysfunc⁼, atrophy, mental deterior⁵
motor, fits, visual → coma + †.
20 known storage diseases affect N.S.

STORAGE AND OTHER CEREBRAL DEGENERATIVE DISORDERS

Neuronal storage disease - defic. lysosomal enzymes

Gangliosidoses *accum ⁼ metab's → ballooning + death.*

Tay-Sach's disease is the most frequent of these rare disorders. It is due to *(lack enz HEXOSAMIN-ASE –A)* the abnormal accumulation of ganglioside GM_2 in the grey matter. The developmental regression is usually obvious by six to nine months of age with increasing motor weakness. An exaggerated startle response to sound, hyperacusis, is an early sign. Visual inattention and social unresponsiveness are part of the deteriorating course which includes convulsions and difficulties in swallowing, and ends in death by three to five years. A cherry red spot at the macula is characteristic of this degenerative disorder. The diagnosis may be confirmed by measuring serum hexosaminidase activity. Prenatal detection is possible, but as 80 per cent of cases mark the first appearance of the condition in families, it is far more valuable to identify at risk couples before they reproduce. The high frequency of the heterozygote in Ashkenazi Jewish populations has been a stimulus to successful voluntary detection programmes.

Other gangliosidoses include a generalised form with hepatosplenomegaly and skeletal deformities, GM_1 type 1, and a variety with later onset neural presentation, GM_1 type 3. The measurement of specific enzyme activity enables precise identification.

other lysosomal disorders inv N.S :–

Neural lipidoses

Gaucher's disease may be classified into neuronopathic and nonneuronopathic or visceral varieties. The former presents in infancy with feeding problems, stridor, and spasticity. There is prominent hepatosplenomegaly and Gaucher cells can be identified in marrow or liver biopsy. Death occurs within months. The non-neuronopathic form presents later in childhood or early adult life with hepatosplenomegaly, pancytopenia and bone involvement. It is compatible with a reasonable life span.

Niemann-Pick disease also causes abnormal storage in the reticuloendothelial system and two of the four recognised varieties are neuronopathic. It may

The biochemical basis of Tay-Sach's, Gaucher's and Niemann-Pick disease

Disorder	Storage material	Deficient enzyme
Tay-Sachs	Ganglioside, GM_2 — ceramide – glucose – galactose – N-acetylgalactosamine / N-acetylneuraminic acid	hexosaminidase
Gaucher's	Cerebroside — ceramide – glucose	glucocerebrosidase
Niemann-Pick	Sphingomyelin — ceramide – phosphoryl choline	sphingomyelinase

resemble Tay-Sach's disease and have a cherry red macular spot. It can also present in the differential diagnosis of neonatal hepatitis. Typical foam cells can be found in marrow and liver biopsy.

Mucopolysaccharidoses

These complex carbohydrate storage disorders typically cause abnormal accumulation in fibroblasts and chondrocytes resulting in coarsened skin, corneal clouding, skeletal dysplasia and hepatosplenomegaly. The manifestations vary and not all have neural involvement. There are currently seven or eight varieties which can be distinguished by the enzyme defect and the major storage substance, dermatan, heparin or keratan sulphate and its excretion in the urine.

Hurler's syndrome is the best recognised form and results from the deficiency of α-L-iduronidase.

Hurler's syndrome

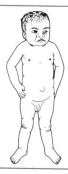

grossly retarded development

coarse facies
hazy corneas
enlarged tongue

cardiac abnormalities

hepatosplenomegaly
umbilical hernia
claw hand
joint deformities

urine:
    dermatan sulphate
    heparan sulphate

The mucolipidoses resemble the mucopolysaccharidoses but lack the urine products. Sophisticated biochemical studies are required for their precise identification.

White matter degenerative disorders

These present with progressive motor deterioration and spasticity. There is associated intellectual loss, progressive blindness due to optic atrophy, and convulsions.

Metachromatic leucodystrophy is the most commonly recognised variety and usually becomes obvious in the second year. Sulphatides accumulate in nervous and other tissues due to deficiency of the enzyme, aryl sulphatase. The diagnosis is made by demonstrating metachromatic material in urinary sediment or tissue biopsy, and establishing deficient aryl sulphatase activity in white cells or cultured fibroblasts.

MALFORMATIONS ASSOCIATED WITH MENTAL HANDICAP

A number of conspicuous malformation syndromes are associated with handicap. It is also important to document minor anomalies for these may also provide clues

De Lange and infantile hypercalcaemia syndromes

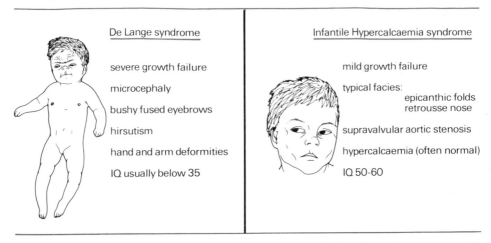

De Lange syndrome

severe growth failure

microcephaly

bushy fused eyebrows

hirsutism

hand and arm deformities

IQ usually below 35

Infantile Hypercalcaemia syndrome

mild growth failure

typical facies:
　　　　　　epicanthic folds
　　　　　　retrousse nose

supravalvular aortic stenosis

hypercalcaemia (often normal)

IQ 50-60

to underlying major disorders. A single minor anomaly is relatively common, 14 per cent of newborn infants, but the presence of three or more anomalies carries a 90 per cent risk of an associated major defect. Particular attention should be paid to eyes, ears, palate, hair pattern, hands and feet. There are invaluable reference atlases which link malformations with defined syndromes.

Microcephaly

Microcephaly refers to a head size below the normal range. It has a common but not invariable association with mental handicap. A neonate with a small head whose rate of head growth parallels the normal percentile lines probably has a prenatal cause. A neonate who has a normal sized head but whose rate of head growth deviates until it falls below the normal range probably has suffered brain damage in the perinatal period.

Prader-Willi and Seckel syndromes

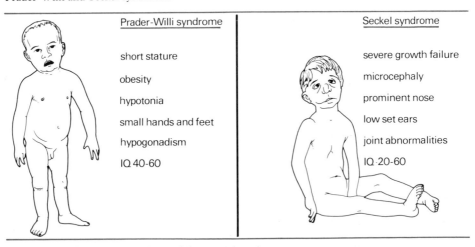

Prader-Willi syndrome

short stature

obesity

hypotonia

small hands and feet

hypogonadism

IQ 40-60

Seckel syndrome

severe growth failure

microcephaly

prominent nose

low set ears

joint abnormalities

IQ 20-60

The identification and treatment of mental handicap

Developmental assessment should be available for all infants, and for those where suspicion arises there must be ready access to the skills of a multi-disciplinary assessment team. It is important that prompt, confident reassurance is given to the parents of children who demonstrate innocent variation of development, and that sensitive explanation is provided where abnormality is likely. Many local authorities keep 'at risk' registers of children with complicated birth histories, but at least 30 to 40 per cent of eventually handicapped children are not included.

It is seldom that specific treatment is possible for mentally handicapped children but those involved must be alert to such a possibility. Lead intoxication is a primary aetiological factor in very few, but many of these children show pica and are at risk of ingesting paint flakes or contaminated soil. Hypothyroidism and aminoacid disorders, particularly phenylketonuria, are readily excluded by appropriate biochemical tests. Progressive deterioration in performance emphasises the need to look for metabolic, storage or neurodegenerative disorders. Further clues may be provided by an unusual smell of the skin or urine, by hepatosplenomegaly or by retinal abnormality. Modern techniques and the identification of specific enzyme deficiencies have improved the yield of such investigations. There is almost no place for brain biopsy.

Investigations which may identify the cause of mental handicap

Total blood count	Cerebrospinal fluid examination
Lymphocyte inclusions	Skull X-ray
Thyroid function tests	Electroencephalography
Serum aminoacids	Computerised axial tomography
Plasma lead level	White blood cell enzymes
Fasting glucose and calcium level	Lymphocyte electron microscopy
Blood acid-base balance	Fibroblast culture studies
Urine aminoacids	Liver biopsy
Urine mucopolysaccharide screen	Marrow biopsy

Specific treatment. Dietary manipulation assists a small but important group

Inborn errors of metabolism: possible therapy

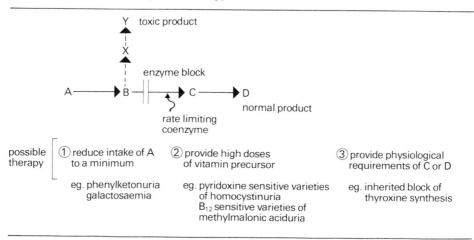

of children with inherited disorders of carbohydrate, aminoacid or organic acid metabolism. We have not yet devised a satisfactory means of replacing deficient enzymes within the tissues, and the blood-brain barrier may prove to be an impenetrable obstacle. Prevention through accurate diagnosis of index cases and genetic counselling provides the only successful method of control in the majority of these disorders.

General management. Handicapped children and their families require the resources of a multi-disciplinary approach. In addition to general assessment, the child's social, motor, language, hearing and visual abilities must all be considered. A therapeutic programme must begin as early as possible with parents playing an active role together with physiotherapists, speech therapists, and play counsellors. Health visitors and social workers assist the parents in coming to terms with their problems and advise on financial and equipment help. Seizure disorders and behavioural problems may require specific drug therapy.

The Education Act of 1970 legislated for special schools to be available for all handicapped children. Recently, the Warnock Report (1978) recommended more integration of handicapped and non-handicapped children for educational purposes. Although schools are classified as dealing with the E.S.N. (M) or E.S.N. (S) categories the system has to be flexible to accomodate co-existing physical problems. Children in the IQ range 50 to 70 often achieve some independence and benefit from the high staff pupil ratio available in E.S.N. (M) schools. 80 per cent are capable of an open occupation and the remainder are provided with employment in sheltered workshops, adult occupation centres. Children with IQ below 50 are rarely independent and often need to be dressed and fed. They may not be able to speak and require constant attention. Education at E.S.N. (S) schools is essentially aimed at training the children to do simple social tasks. As these children become older the parents find it increasingly difficult to look after them. Up to the age of 14, only about 25 per cent are in residential care but after this age the proportion increases rapidly. Residential facilities vary considerably but there is a tendency towards smaller units which attempt to retain the family structure and links with the surrounding community. Those remaining at home when they leave school usually attend an occupational centre run by the local social work department.

BIBLIOGRAPHY

Birch H G, Richardson S A, Baird D, Horobin G, Illsley R 1970 Mental subnormality in the community. A clinical and epidemiological study. Williams & Wilkins, Baltimore.
Griffiths M 1973 The young retarded child. Churchill Livingstone, Edinburgh.
Hewett S 1970 The family and the handicapped child. Allen & Unwin, London.
Kershaw J D 1973 Handicapped children. Heinemann, London.
Kirman B H 1972 The mentally handicapped child. Nelson, London.
Mackay R I 1976 Mental handicap in child health practice. Butterworth, London.
Rutter M, Graham P, Yule W 1970 A neuropsychiatric study in childhood. Spastics International Medical Publications. Heinemann, London.

21
Behaviour

Until recent years, doctors treating children tended to ignore unusual or deviant behaviour, believing its correction to be the responsibility of the parents or, if the problem was particularly troublesome, the psychiatrist, social worker, teacher, or the welfare services. However it is a mistake for a family or hospital doctor caring for children not to have studied the behavioural disturbances, for on the one hand many childhood illness are associated with some disturbance in behaviour, indeed some organic disease may present with a behaviour problem, and on the other hand children at conflict with themselves or their family or their surroundings, may present with symptoms which mimic organic diseases.

In the first part of this Chapter, behavioural problems which are thought to be due to brain damage, brain dysfunction or a delay in brain maturation are discussed. In the second part the interactions between the child, his family and his surroundings which might produce conflicts are outlined and illustrated. In the third part some of the effects on the child of deviant behaviour by the parent are considered. Overlap between the sections is inevitable.

PHYSICAL ILLNESS

Diseases affecting the brain

General. It is obvious that any illness which affects the brain might alter a child's personality and affect his behaviour. One parent, a bird-watching enthusiast, recognised unusual behaviour in his own youngster some weeks before his child was admitted semiconscious with diabetes. The list of diseases, metabolic, traumatic, infective, neoplastic which may affect the brain and its function is endless, all may have associated behaviour problems, some of which are easily recognised and understood, but others, for example the odd behaviour of a child with a cerebral tumour, may be overlooked for some time. Their precise relationship to the physical illness is not always clear. There are, for example, many reasons why a child after severe head injury might be unfriendly and withdrawn. Children with perceptive problems, deafness and blindness, may

Classification of causes of psychiatric syndromes in childhood

- Diseases which interfere with vital supplies to the brain:

- Perceptive disorders

- Brain pathologies:
  epilepsy
  mental retardation

- Developmental delays:

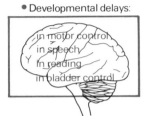

in motor control
in speech
in reading
in bladder control

- Psychiatric syndromes:

tics
hyperkinetic syndrome
'minimal brain damage'
autism

develop their own patterns of behaviour which to others appear odd and sometimes unacceptable. However the main subjects of this section are not the variations in behaviour which occur in children with organic disease or of children with perceptive problems, important though these are, but brain conditions which present and are recognised by the peculiar behaviour patterns they produce.

Epilepsy is due to an involuntary, uncontrollable impulse from the brain which produces an episode of abnormal behaviour. The usual forms of that behaviour, grand mal, focal epilepsy, petit mal have been discussed elsewhere. Psychic equivalents, with clouding of awareness, confusion states, automatic motor behaviour patterns, angry outbursts are thought to be rare in children. Epilepsy of whatever form is associated with increased incidence of behavioural disturbance. This might be related to the brain dysfunction or to the drugs used to control the fits, or to the handicap epilepsy brings to the child in his relationships.

Mental handicap whether due to obvious brain injury or to an uncertain mix of genetic and early environmental factors may present primarily with behaviour difficulties. These disturbances may be more of a burden to the child, his parents and his teachers, than his basic learning problem. Whether, for example, aggressiveness, negativism, self-destruction or repetitive behaviour in retarded children is due to their abnormal brain function or a consequence of how they are handled in early life is an important question to be considered if appropriate management programmes are to be devised.

Maturational delay

Children with mental handicap have a generalised delay in development and usually end up with reduced abilities in all areas, so-called global retardation. However the delay may be in one area only and with time, the child may learn to overcome the difficulty or to bypass it. Thus the child may have a functional delay in motor control, hearing, speech, bladder control etc. As we all develop in different ways and at different rates, and end up with different levels of ability, each identified group contains children in the extremes of the normal range, children held back for a variety of reasons, as well as specific functional disorders.

Clumsiness, or motor dyspraxia, in its severe form may result in a child being so uncoordinated that he has problems at home, at school and at play. His school work is untidy as a result of poor eye-hand coordination, and he performs badly at sports, particularly ball games. Such children are delayed in learning to dress themselves and have difficulty in keeping themselves tidy. They continually knock things over and frequently fall over themselves. The academic and social difficulties which follow can cause the child considerable unhappiness and lead to behavioural problems if they are not recognised and dealt with sympathetically. Specific physiotherapy programmes may help.

Specific reading retardation. Reading is a complex activity which requires a great number of skills, and therefore reading difficulties might be due to a variety of factors. For example children with a general learning problem are slow to read, children who are understimulated or badly taught are slow to read, and children who have a perceptive problem are slow to read. But apart from those in which a reading delay might be anticipated, there are many otherwise normal children, who have specific reading retardation. Some experts consider that 4 to 8 per cent of school children have such a problem. Boys are more often affected than girls and there is often a family history. Usually the children are a little slow to develop speech and characteristically they have even more difficulty with spelling than with reading so that, for them, dictation is a nightmare. They may also have difficulty with handedness. There is an argument for screening all children for specific reading retardation not only so that their reading exercises can be approached with insight and sympathy but also to ensure that their general education is not hampered by their limited reading ability. Dyslexia and 'word blindness' have been names given to the most overt form of this problem.

Specific speech and language delay. Hearing, intellectual, or psychosocial impairment are more common factors leading to speech delay than a specific developmental disorder. Nevertheless there are a small group of children, around 2 per cent, of those with speech delay, who have normal intelligence and hearing and come from a happy, stimulating environment but who are unable to speak clearly. They require a personal educational programme.

Nocturnal enuresis. Involuntary emptying of the bladder during sleep is a common and troublesome problem. In round terms the majority of children are dry at night by 3 years of age, some 10 per cent plus regularly wet the bed at 5 years of age, and somewhat less than 5 per cent still do so at 10 years of age. One or two in every hundred will have an organic problem, either a congenital abnormality of the urinary tract, a urinary infection, polyuria or neurogenic bladder. A careful history, thorough examination and urine examination for glucose, infection and specific gravity should exclude these possibilities. Only rarely on the history of nocturnal enuresis alone is radiological investigation of the renal system justified. In another small percentage nocturnal enuresis will be the presenting symptom of a child emotionally upset. Gentle probing enquiry should bring this to light and point the interview into the appropriate direction.

In the majority, clinical enquiry gives no indication of the aetiology. Often there is a family history and there will be relatively more children from poor and unhappy homes than might be expected. It might be hard to refute the parents suggestion that their child's bladder capacity is too small or that they pass excess amounts of urine during the night. Some physicians recommend exercises to enlarge the bladder capacity. Physiologists have postulated immature circadian rhythms, psychiatrists on the other hand have suggested that when children, in the mystery of sleep, wet themselves and their bed, they are saying that they want to be comforted like a baby, they are frightened or that they are making a hostile gesture in the security of their bed about something that has happened to them during the day.

Many children improve, some surprisingly quickly with whatever method of management is used, whether it be habit training with star charts, lifting at night, drugs or a pad and bell. Suggestion and encouragement are perhaps the most helpful. Tricyclic drugs for example imipramine 25 mg for the child under 30 kg body weight and 50 mg for those over, work at least temporarily in about a third. The greatest claim has been made for the bell alarm which is placed in the child's bed so that the alarm rings when the child wets. It is said to help over two thirds of those who can be brought to use them.

Faecal soiling. Although it may seem appropriate to discuss faecal soiling after nocturnal enuresis, as a problem it has more in common with those disorders precipitated by conflict. There is far less reason to believe that, in the majority, it is due to a delay or abnormality in the development of brain function. Faecal soiling usually occurs during the day. Most children are clean by $2\frac{1}{2}$ years of age and soiling may be viewed as abnormal after 4 years of age and certainly by the time the child goes to school.

It may take three fairly distinct forms. In one, sometimes called encopresis, the child has bowel control but passes the formed stool in unacceptable places, for example behind the curtains in the lounge, on the wallflowers in the garden, indeed everywhere except in the toilet. Sometimes the act is performed in a secretive manner and sometimes it is meant to be provocative. Usually the child has problems which cannot be resolved easily and expert advice is required. Children inappropriately or inadequately trained, or who are mentally or socially slow form a second group. In these children a formed stool is passed, sometimes in the toilet but usually in the pants. A firm, consistent training programme should help these patients. Set-backs during bowel upsets whether from inappropriate food or infections are to be expected. Children who are chronically constipated

Susan

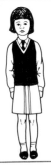

Current problem:	Other problems:	Background:
faecal soiling	intermittent constipation nocturnal enuresis low intelligence	mother: epileptic six children, not coping. father: unemployed aggressive and intolerant. school: poor progress and unpopular

Susan—aged 11 yrs | family needs support |

often present with soiling. The insensitive distended rectum cannot stop soft faeces passing round the hard impacted masses and oozing out. These children continuously soil themselves and always smell. The soiling disappears after the constipation has been corrected.

Tics

Tics are sudden repetitive coordinated movements of no apparent purpose. They can affect any muscle groups but commonly take the form of blinking, facial grimacing, twisting the head, or shrugging the shoulders. The average age of onset is two years and it has been reported that as many as 4 per cent of children develop them at some time. Tourette described a bizarre syndrome where vocal tics, often rude words, accompany gestures which might be equally embarrassing. In 25 per cent of children with tics there is a family history. In some there is evidence of brain damage or other features of delayed maturation. The majority are precipitated by stress. Usually the tics disappear, sometimes in weeks or months, often in late adolescence, and rarely do they persist into adult life.

Hyperkinetic syndrome

In children with the hyperkinetic syndrome there may be a family history, evidence of a developmental delay or a history which suggests that the child might have had 'minimal brain dysfunction' or 'minimal brain damage'. In some there is little evidence to suggest any of these alternatives.

The children are not so much clumsy as apparently overactive. They never sit still, they are distractable, they never settle down, they are destructive, impulsive and excitable. It is when they first go to school that they appear to be at their most difficult and it may be then that their problem first comes to light.

In adolescence, though the hyperactivity is less, their learning difficulties with socially disruptive behaviour may lead to further problems. As adults they are more likely to have trouble with the law, or need psychiatric help.

Management starts with a careful evaluation of the child's problems and continues by full discussions with parents, teachers and anyone else concerned. Each programme is individual. Once the child is under regular sympathetic observation the effects of drugs can be assessed. Brain stimulants, methylphenidate and dextroamphetamine, benefit over half the affected children; the tricyclic antidepressants may also help.

Autism and childhood psychosis

Schizophrenia can begin in late childhood, the symptoms are similar to those found in adults. Adults who develop schizophrenia have often shown unusual behaviour when they were youngsters, but the pattern is not characteristic so prediction and maybe prevention is not yet possible. Bizarre or psychotic behaviour is also seen in encephalopathies and in the severely retarded. About half the children with psychosis have a cluster of clinical features which suggest a specific disorder, infantile autism.

Characteristically, autistic children fail to develop social relationships, they are slow to speak and have little non-verbal communication. They also follow ritualistic behaviour patterns and endlessly perform repetitive movements.

Parents seek advice because they wonder if the child is deaf and again later because of delay or absence of speech development. Often the infant's behaviour has been unusual from birth and only occasionally is the child's development for the first year or so apparently normal. Over half the children are mentally retarded as well and these have the worst prognosis. Even those with average intelligence have great difficulty coping when they grow up. Only a few manage to be gainfully employed and they rarely marry.

Autism is rare: in a population of one million some 20 to 40 children might be identified. They need to be under the care of experts in special schools but because of its rarity it is difficult to provide this for all children whilst maintaining strong home links. Drugs currently play only a small part in management, they may help if there is an associated sleep problem.

THE INTERACTION BETWEEN THE CHILD AND HIS WORLD

A child may develop symptoms of physical disorder or behaviour problems or educational difficulties due to conflicts and confusion within himself, or with his family, with his peers, with school or with society at large. If a school girl gets stomach-ache because she hates her ballet lessons or dislikes her new step-father, then eliciting that information may be just as important for that child as testing the urine in another suspected of having urinary infection. This section merely points to some of the more obvious factors which might lead to problems.

The child

Acute organic disease frightens children possibly more than adults, and they show it in different ways according to their maturity. It can be difficult to distinguish the symptoms and signs due to this reaction from those due to the underlying pathology. A terrified two-year-old with croup may improve dramatically in the arms of a friendly confident capable nurse or become even worse if placed on a strange bed surrounded by flashing lights and stainless steel.

Chronic organic disease makes extra demands on the child. Some children cope marvellously well but in others the continuing difficulties are just too much and secondary symptoms or behaviour problems add to their difficulties. The burden of the disease for some children can be very heavy; what, for example, can be said to an adolescent with muscular dystrophy or cystic fibrosis when he learns by one means or another of the prognosis of his condition? Sometimes it is the parents who cannot accept or have difficulty managing the child's condition. It is always sad when a child with asthma exaggerates his bronchospasm or a child with diabetes deliberately breaks diet to precipitate hyperglycaemia in order to gain admission to hospital where they feel more secure, and where the pressures of coping either with the family or the outside world are avoided.

Deformity and disability present at birth may lead to problems if one or both parents have difficulty accepting their own abnormal child; they feel ashamed about him when they should be showing him off. Later as the child grows up he may have trouble at school, for children go through a period of wanting to be the same and of mocking those who are different. Just being different can lead to problems.

Claire

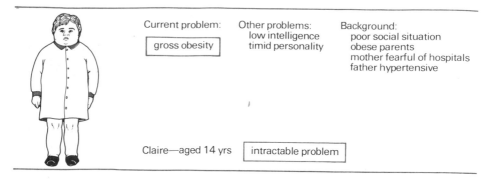

Current problem:

| gross obesity |

Other problems:
low intelligence
timid personality

Background:
poor social situation
obese parents
mother fearful of hospitals
father hypertensive

Claire—aged 14 yrs | intractable problem |

Intelligence is determined by a mixture of genetic and environmental factors. Happily, in the main, parents get children of similar abilities but misfits occasionally occur, a slow child in an academic family, an awkward child in an athletic family, a gifted child in an average family, a swan amongst ducks, all may lead to conflict and result in bodily symptoms, behaviour disturbances and underachieving.

Temperament likewise appears to be genetically and environmentally determined. A child's temperament is not only a factor in the risk of disorders developing but may also determine the mode of expression. An outgoing, extrovert child is more likely to develop behaviour problems, while a sensitive, timid child is more likely to internalise conflicts and have disorders of bodily function. The success of any management programme depends on those concerned knowing the child for whom they are making plans.

The family

A great deal has been written recently about the qualities required of parents. A child needs not only food, warmth and physical protection but also to be loved, to feel important, to be stimulated and encouraged to make the most of his abilities, and to be controlled and guided in the ways of his society. It is the privilege and responsibility of parents to meet these needs and most parents delight in the task. Many factors, some beyond anyone's control, can interfere with the relationship between parents and child.

Maternal deprivation. The bond between mother and child is fashioned at birth and secured over the first weeks of life. If others care for her sick child the mother may not develop that blind love and devotion which is so essential for his early well being. Separation from parents, particularly the young child from his mother, even for brief periods may not only have immediate effects on the infant, for example uncontrollable screaming or quiet withdrawal, but have more lasting effects as well. For most families brief periods of separation are not as harmful in the long term as was originally thought but in the context of certain family relationships they can be. Most children tolerate such events without lasting effect, but clearly they should be avoided if possible, particularly in the early years. If either the mother or her dependent infant needs hospital care, they should be admitted together if it is at all possible. One is often important in the other's recovery.

Family breakdown. Unhappily for children in western societies divorce rates are increasing, couples seeking divorce are tending to be younger and the duration of their marriages are shorter. Illegitimacy rates are also increasing, so are the numbers of mothers with young children who go out to work. Such situations add to the child's problems and may limit the care he receives.

Parental abilities and attitudes. If a parent is sick, what of the child? If a child has stomach ache it is well to ask about the family symptoms. Children are quick to note how adults gain sympathy and avoid the unpleasant, and they assume that there is no reason why they should not use the same tactics. A parent with a chronic illness may add to the child's anxieties and responsibilities and push the child beyond his limit. A parent with a psychiatric disorder, for example, depression, may have a devastating effect on the child. Sometimes it is the child's illness which draws attention to the mother's need. The effect that the death of a parent has on a child varies with his maturity. A disturbed child may be considerably helped by having the opportunity to talk frankly about it with a sympathetic but uninvolved adult.

Even when both parents are well and able to provide a comfortable home, their attitudes and expectations of their children can still lead to difficulties. In the extremes they may over-protect them or over-discipline them or ignore and reject them or they may wish to dominate them, even when they are capable of being independent. On the other hand, they may have unrealistic expectations of their abilities; for example, a mother who expected a six-month-old infant to use a pot, a father who expected his children to move at the blow of a whistle, a professional woman who thought her seven-year-old should realise when she wished to be left alone.

Adoption. The situation of a couple longing for children that they cannot have and adopting into their family an unwanted child has its own peculiar problems. Inevitably the child has those characteristics, appearance, abilities and personality determined by his genetic makeup from his parents but also he is influenced by the environment provided by his new home. As neither parents nor child are perfect, it is not surprising to find that the adopted child is more likely to

John

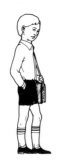

Current problem:	Other problems:	Background:
stole money from school and home to buy sweets	high IQ reading retardation	unmarried mother who despised and did not mention his father. Catholic school taught the sanctity of marriage

John—aged 8 yrs | he wanted to be told about his father

develop behaviour problems (which may be due in part to inherited characteristics) and the parents must be aware of this. Nevertheless the future of the adopted child is undoubtedly better than if he had not been adopted at all.

Children in care. It has been said that bad parents are better than no parents. This is not true. However, in the absence of a larger family to embrace a child who loses both parents, the best efforts of the social services often fall well short of the child's needs. It is easy to be pessimistic about the long-term prognosis of such children. Professor Michael Rutter, at the conclusion of his book on maternal deprivation, points out that many children build happy and successful lives out of appalling childhoods and recommends that we seek the secrets of their success so that we might more effectively help others to avoid an unhappy outcome.

Environment
Deprivation. Ineffectual parents tend to be poor and to live in bad housing in deprived sections of the town or country. It is difficult to be sure of the extent that a child's problems are due to his make-up, the care and attitudes of his parents or to his physical surroundings. But there is no doubt that poverty, overcrowding and poor housing, are associated not only with increased rates of illness and death in infancy and childhood but also behaviour problems and school failure. It is so difficult for children from such backgrounds to become good parents themselves. The poor are at a threefold disadvantage; they are more likely to fall ill, they have less family reserves to meet new problems and they are less able to make use of the support the state provides. Even in the U.K. with a National Health Service, the deprived are still at a disadvantage in comparison with the middle classes.

Neighbourhood. Wealth is relative, and poverty as defined in western societies need not bring misery. It has been shown that the prevalence of health and social problems vary considerably from one community to another with apparently similar levels of wealth, housing, and services. In some communities there is stability and mutual responsibility, in others there is aggression, cruelty and conflict. Race, culture, religion, industrial troubles can all lead to a family being rejected by the neighbourhood. Families continually on the move may create problems of identity for their children.

School. School is where children go to work, where they make friends and

Peter

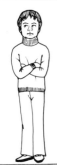

Current problem:	Other problems:	Background:
unprovoked outbursts of aggressive behaviour	severe epilepsy low intelligence nocturnal enuresis	low birth weight abandoned by teenage mother. fostered— then adopted

Peter—aged 14yrs   requires protective environment in special school

enemies, where they test out their temperament against others, where they find out how other families think and behave. So problems at school may be far more than difficulties with learning. A child who has difficulty with his school such that special education is considered necessary should have a thorough and expert medical assessment so that the restraint due to a medical condition is reduced to a minimum.

BEHAVIOURAL PROBLEMS

From what has been said so far it can be appreciated that many factors may contribute to the genesis of any particular problem which brings a child to the doctor's attention. The physician is particularly concerned with symptoms which suggest physical disease but have their origins in a psychological disturbance, and with behavioural problems which are a consequence of a physical disorder either as a direct effect of brain disturbance or indirectly due to the difficulty the child has coping with his illness or handicap.

The pre-school child

Feeding problems. Interaction between an uncertain or insecure mother with a healthy baby or a happy mother with a determined or difficult baby may lead to the baby vomiting, refusing food or failing to gain weight satisfactorily. Sometimes the problem is resolved by patience and counselling either from the health visitor, relative or friendly neighbour but it is not uncommon for a child to have to be admitted to hospital to exclude an organic cause and to reassure both mother and her baby.

Sleep problems. Adults used to a regular biological rhythm differ in their tolerance of the baby's desire for a feed in the middle of the night. Occasionally infants appear to scream and cry through most of the night and this may be tolerated when the baby is young and weak but a playful demanding toddler in the middle of the night can stretch the patience of most parents. The temptation for the parents is to take the child in their bed or for one or other parent to sleep with the child to comfort him but this is really no solution and can lead to further problems. Adults without sleep perform poorly in their work and this adds to the strain. In this situation there is an argument for giving the infant a sedative in a

Jason

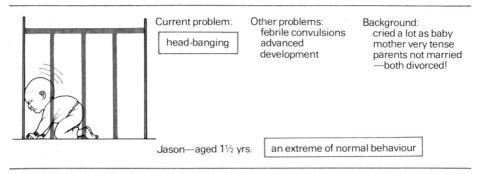

Current problem:
head-banging

Other problems:
febrile convulsions
advanced
development

Background:
cried a lot as baby
mother very tense
parents not married
—both divorced!

Jason—aged 1½ yrs.   an extreme of normal behaviour

dose which ensures that he sleeps well for at least six hours each night. This helps him to establish a normal sleep habit and gives his parents a chance to regain their equilibrium. The sedative should be given in increasing dosage until it is effective and then maintained for some weeks. It is important to explain to the parents the purpose of the exercise.

Breath-holding attacks. Infants and toddlers quickly find that they can control their parents by refusing to do what they are asked. For example, they may refuse to eat or to go to the toilet, but perhaps their most dramatic card is to refuse to breathe. Breath holding attacks to the point of going unconscious, when they may or may not provoke a fit, are not uncommon. They certainly terrify the parents and may reduce them to quivering.slaves. From the medical point of view it is important to distinguish the episodes from convulsions due to other causes and to reassure parents about the nature of the attacks. In the vast majority of cases the children come to no harm. These determined, often stubborn youngsters need to be handled firmly and consistently.

Rhythmic behaviour. Head rocking, head banging, thumb sucking, self stimulation, baby behaviour, and many other variants may all occur during normal development. They are more likely to appear when the child is uncertain, anxious or tired. In the very disturbed, autistic or retarded child they can become bad habits and strategies need to be devised to avoid or suppress them.

Delayed development and regression. Understimulation with or without undernutrition may limit a child's development and growth. It is not surprising perhaps that a child left alone for hours with no toys in a high rise flat is quite withdrawn, apathetic, and has little muscle tone or strength, and delayed motor, social and mental development.

Bowel and bladder control. Again inappropriate training or anxiety and conflict will interfere with the development of bodily control and appropriate social habits. Noctural enuresis which in the main is probably due to a disorder in maturation and encopresis have been discussed in the first part of this Chapter.

School children

Recurrent abdominal pain. One of the common symptoms which bring children to clinic are recurrent pains usually in the abdomen or head, occasionally in the limbs. A few will have organic disease so all require a careful clinical evaluation. In others it may be a cry for help, the child having a psychiatric disorder or a terrible domestic situation. But for the majority, the clinical investigations will be negative and there will be no major psychosocial problems. There may have been mild or moderate disturbances in the child's life, or they may not be being as successful as they would like or fear they cannot maintain the standards expected of them. Often they are children of good ability with greater self-control and sense of responsibility than the average.

A thorough examination and reassurance with explanations will help many. However in those referred to hospital, a good percentage continue to have recurrent pains into adolescence and adult life. Headaches rather than abdominal pains tend to persist.

Jane

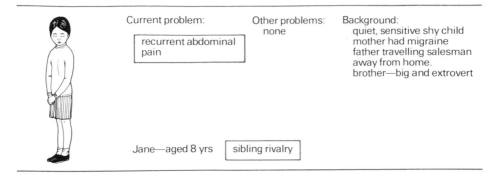

Current problem:

recurrent abdominal pain

Other problems:
none

Background:
quiet, sensitive shy child
mother had migraine
father travelling salesman
away from home.
brother—big and extrovert

Jane—aged 8 yrs   sibling rivalry

Periodic syndrome describes a condition when attacks of abdominal pain are associated with severe vomiting. The vomiting can sometimes result in dehydration to a degree that requires correction by intravenous therapy. In this situation it is difficult to believe that the child has not got an organic disease but so far no pathology has been identified. However in its milder form it merges with the clinical entity of 'recurrent abdominal pain'.

School refusal and truancy. Illness is the commonest reason for school absence. Sometimes children are kept away from school to help in the home. It is important to distinguish these two categories from those children who refuse to go to school because they are anxious, frightened or depressed, or those children who play truant from school because they dislike the atmosphere in which they appear to fail and are subject to ridicule and as they see it, to unfair discipline.

Conduct disorders. Often parents are concerned because their young children are unacceptably aggressive, destructive, cruel or antisocial. Again individual tolerance will depend on the family and the community. In some lively teenagers, outbursts of aggressive, destructive, foolish or antisocial behaviour may be dismissed as high spirits but in others living in inner city areas with mixed cultures and limited outlets it results in delinquency.

Emotional disorders. Children, like adults can get unduly anxious; they may suffer from unreasonable fears and they can have outbursts of hysterical behaviour. By nature, children are optimistic and confident about the future, but occasionally even without obvious cause they can become severely depressed and seriously attempt suicide. These children should have the counsel of a child psychiatrist.

Anorexia nervosa. In this odd condition, young people either just before or during puberty, deliberately avoid food so that they lose weight, and they often go on losing weight till they become tragically thin. It is thought that they have an irrational fear of growing up, of becoming sexually and physically mature. Usually they are able youngsters if somewhat obsessional and precise. Rarely are there major psychological problems which need attention.

As they can starve themselves to death, some management must be attempted but as no pathology or avoidable environmental factors are usually identified, it

Alison

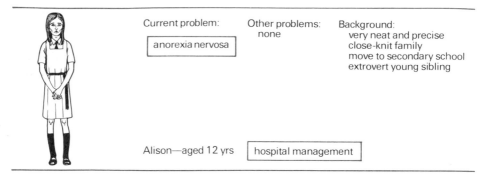

Current problem:

anorexia nervosa

Other problems:
none

Background:
very neat and precise
close-knit family
move to secondary school
extrovert young sibling

Alison—aged 12 yrs   hospital management

has to be symptomatic. It sounds somewhat crude, but the most effective approach appears to be to remove all the child's privileges and return them one by one as she begins to eat more and more. Antidepressive drugs may help.

Management

The above paragraphs merely list some of the symptoms and problems which children under medical care may have. Management includes recognising them for what they are, identifying the contributing factors and conferring with the other people concerned. The latter may include the family doctor and other members of the primary care team, the health visitor, the school teacher, school health services and school welfare officers, the educational psychologist and social service workers. When, after review, a programme of care has been agreed, it is essential that a person is identified to be responsible for counselling the child and parents and ensuring that all concerned are properly informed. Being thorough at the outset can avoid many problems later. With the more intractable emotional and conduct disorders a child psychiatrist will be the key person, but the majority will fall within the responsibility of the health visitor or the family doctor or the paediatrician.

THE MALTREATMENT OF CHILDREN

Deviant behaviour by adults may take the form of injuring their children. Child murder, child cruelty, child neglect, child abuse, child molesting and the use of children for pornography all fall into this category. The obvious examples are easily recognised, but defining the limits of child abuse or child neglect is difficult. It might be considered that it is the right of every child to be allowed to develop to his full potential. Child abuse could then be defined as any action or omission by an adult responsible for that child which either temporarily or permanently interferes with that development. In a real world we must settle for something less. What we are able to achieve is a good measure of our success as a society. In this section we will not be concerned with mental or social abuse or educational ineptitude, not because these are unimportant, but because they are not primarily medical problems. Similarly child cruelty and murder will not be considered further.

Child abuse

Clinical features. Non-accidental injuries and other forms of child abuse occur when parents, at their wits end, strike out at their helpless but demanding infant. It also happens when ignorant, inept, cruel, selfish, irresponsible or mentally sick parents do not exert reasonable self-control. Gripping and shaking the baby may produce finger tip bruising on his chest and arms. Forcing his

Gripping injuries

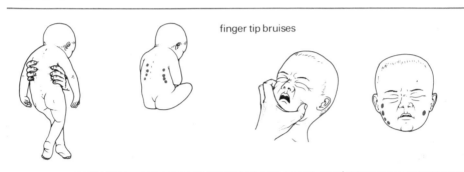

finger tip bruises

mouth open to give food may cause similar bruises on the cheeks. The frenulum may be torn or the palate scratched by objects pushed in the mouth. Slapping and hitting the infant may cause black eyes or characteristic strap marks. The skin of attacked infants may also show scratches, bite marks, cigarette burns or scalds. Rough handling may fracture long bones, ribs or skull. Swinging the baby by the legs or arms can cause epiphyseal separation at the end of the long bones. Squeezing the limbs with rotation can separate the periosteum and cause periosteal haematomas. Repeated injuries of the same bone leads to large callus formation. Banging the head not only produces fractures of the skull but haemorrhages in the eyes and occasionally blindness.

Shaking the head can tear superficial veins over the brain and cause subdural haematomas. The child may weather the initial injury, but the blood clot may then draw in fluid; the infant then develops the clinical features of a space-occupying lesion of slow onset. He may present with vomiting or fits or changes in the level of responsiveness and activity. The fontanelle is full and there may be papilloedema

Some non-accidental injuries

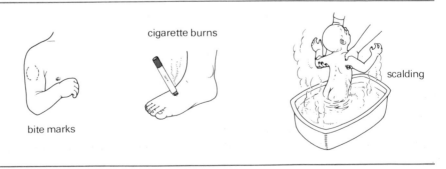

cigarette burns

scalding

bite marks

Bony injuries

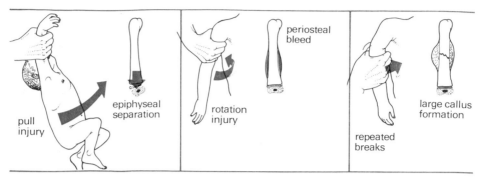

and retinal bleeds. This injury may kill the child; if it does not, if often leaves him mentally retarded, hemiplegic or blind.

All the baby's injuries must be noted in detail and photographed if possible.

A careful enquiry is essential. The parents often delay in bringing the child for medical attention. Their story does not accord with the injuries. Their explanation for the injuries may change if they are pressed. Their concern for the child may be inappropriate, they may show too much concern or anger or they may be off-hand and indifferent. Often they are relieved when hospital admission is advised. Sometimes they will talk at length about their own anxieties and problems and say how difficult and demanding the baby has been. It is very important to record precisely the history as it is given, with an evaluation of the parents' attitudes.

The injury which can kill or leave the child with severe brain damage

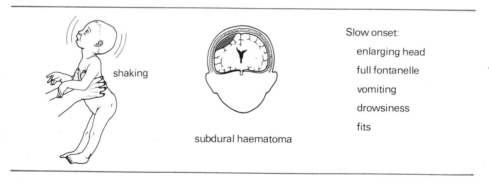

Child abuse occurs in families from all walks of life but it is more common in the under privileged and in families where actions speak louder than words. As Professor Kempe has suggested, the setting in which child abuse might occur includes a number of elements:

1. The parents have usually had troubled childhoods themselves; they may be from broken homes or have suffered deprivation or abuse themselves when children.

2. There are problems with the marriage; for example the marriage may be between two young people from disturbed homes who married for the wrong reasons, perhaps because they wanted to leave home or were in need of affection. Some people mistakenly believe that a pregnancy will help to reverse a breaking relationship.
3. The child may be difficult to rear, he may have been premature or have a blemish or handicap. More often than not the child's problems are imaginary, the baby's first cry is seen as rejection, he fails to respond as his mother feels he should to her and this is felt to be his fault. An unloved child may be difficult, a difficult child may be unloved.
4. Against this background there may be added stresses, for example the father in trouble with the law or there may be financial or housing problems.
5. Finally, there are no life lines available, no close friends to whom the parents can turn for advice, support and relief.

Management. If a health visitor, social worker or casualty doctor suspects non-accidental injury the child must be admitted to a place of safety until a fuller enquiry has been made. This might be a police station, a social service institution or a hospital. If his parents are deliberately injuring him, society has a responsibility to protect him. If the parents are unwilling to release their child then he may have to be taken from them on the grounds laid down to obtain the necessary care order.

Whilst providing temporary protection, the primary medical responsibility is to identify and treat the injuries, attend to the child's general well being, and to exclude possible contributing factors and alternative diagnoses. It is equally important for others to evaluate the parents and the family situation and provide support and guidance if this is appropriate.

The distribution of the bruises is usually diagnostic. Babies when they begin to walk frequently fall and bruise their foreheads and shins, but do not bruise their upper arms and chests. Nevertheless bleeding diseases should be excluded. Brittle-bone disease is a rare condition where bruising as well as bone fractures occur with the slightest injury, but the fractures are in the shaft and not at the end of the long bones. Although some bony injuries are obvious, others are not, so a full skeletal survey by radiography is essential.

The social work team will usually take the lead in planning the strategy for management, but they depend on the full cooperation of medical and nursing personnel involved and the police. Initial policy is usually worked out at a case conference held as soon as possible after the diagnosis is firm. Subsequent management will depend on the background and on the attitudes of the parents. When investigations have been completed a full case conference with representatives from all agencies concerned in attendance is held to decide what legal action is required, what social work activity is to be attempted and what medical surveillance is desirable.

Many children may be allowed home, initially under supervision, and although they may not live happily ever after they do appear to thrive and to be content. Occasionally it is necessary to take the child away from his parents and put him into care of others. The decisions are very difficult and even those with most knowledge and experience can get it wrong. Unhappy experiences in this area can harden the hearts of the wisest and kindest of men and produce vicious reaction in others.

Child neglect
A child may also be harmed by omission. This might be due to unavoidable circumstances, or ignorance or ineptness on the part of his guardians as well as deliberate attempts to hurt or punish him. The children are generally under-nourished and undersized, the skin and hair are often in poor condition and they may be dirty and infested. Nasty rashes may be present in those places where the most dirt collects, the skin creases and nappy area.

Deprivation
A child in a repressive atmosphere may appear to be well nourished and clean, but still fail to thrive, his hands and feet may be cold and small, and his growth suppressed. These more subtle forms of negligence or abuse are more difficult to recognise and define. The management as with most of the problems in this Chapter includes a thorough clinical evaluation, a detailed enquiry about him, his family life and his neighbourhood, and a programme of care which is realistic and accepted by all concerned.

BIBLIOGRAPHY

Helfer R E, Kempe C H 1968 The battered child. The University of Chicago Press, Chicago
Pinkerton P Childhood disorders. Crosby Lockwood Staples, St Albans, U.K.
Rutter M 1972 Maternal deprivation reassessed. Penguin, London
Rutter M, Herson L 1977 Child psychiatry. Modern approaches. Blackwell, Oxford
Smith S M (ed) 1978 The maltreatment of children. M.T.P. Press, Lancaster

Index